WO 196
£66.99
03

Chronic Wound Management

THE EVIDENCE FOR CHANGE

Chronic Wound Management

THE EVIDENCE FOR CHANGE

Edited by

RAJ MANI

University of Southampton Hospitals Trust NHS
Southampton, UK

The Parthenon Publishing Group

International Publishers in Medicine, Science & Technology

A CRC PRESS COMPANY

BOCA RATON   LONDON   NEW YORK   WASHINGTON, D.C.

Published in the USA by
The Parthenon Publishing Group
345 Park Avenue South, 10th Floor
New York, NY 10010, USA

Published in the UK and Europe by
The Parthenon Publishing Group
23–25 Blades Court, Deodar Road
London, SW15 2NU, UK

Library of Congress Cataloging-in-Publication Data

Chronic wound management : the evidence for change / edited by Raj Mani.
     p.   cm.
Includes bibliographical references and index.
ISBN 1-84214-084-1 (alk. paper)
1. Wound healing. 2. Wounds and injuries–Treatment. 3. Evidence-based
medicine. I. Mani, Raj.

RD94.C476 2002
617.1'4–dc21   2002033320

British Library Cataloguing in Publication Data

Chronic wound management : the evidence for change
    1. Wound healing   2. Wounds and injuries – Treatment –
    Evaluation
    I. Mani, Raj
    617.1'4'06
    ISBN 1-84214-084-1

Typeset by Martin Lister Publishing Services, Carnforth, UK
Printed and bound by Butler & Tanner Ltd., Frome and London, UK

Contents

List of principal contributors   vii

Foreword   ix
V. F. Falanga

Preface   xiii

1   Introduction   1
Chronic wound management: a global perspective
T. J. Ryan

2   What is evidence?   11
M. J. Campbell

3   Medical therapy for leg ulcers   23
J. Kantor and D. J. Margolis

4   Compression for venous leg ulcer management   35
P. Vowden and K. R. Vowden

5   The lessons learnt from wound healing in HIV-infected patients and the need   57
for change of management
K. Jönsson and S. Mzezewa

6   Changes in chronic wound management: perspectives from Tamil Nadu,   73
India
C. V. Krishnaswami, N. S. Raji, K. M. Ramakrishnan and M. Babu

7   Burn wound management: how to prevent a burn becoming a chronic   81
wound
L. Téot and S. Otman

8   Changes in diabetic foot ulcer management   95
M. Edmonds and A. Foster

9   Pressure ulcer studies: reasons to change   113
M. Romanelli, D. Mastronicola, A. Magliaro and S. Siani

10   Mucosal inflammation of the gastrointestinal tract and healing   129
V. Mani

11   From the wound healing laboratory: any evidence for change?   135
R. Mani

12   Models for healing   145
      F. Gottrup

13   The role of surgical intervention in chronic wounds   159
      C. P. Shearman

14   Conclusion   167
      C. P. Shearman and R. Mani

      Chronic wound management illustrated   169

      Index   203

List of principal contributors

M. J. Campbell
Professor of Medical Statistics
Institute of Primary Care
Northern General Hospital
Sheffield, UK

M. Edmonds
Consultant Physician
Diabetic Foot Clinic
King's College Hospital
London, UK

F. Gottrup
Professor of Surgery
Copenhagen Wound Healing Center
Bispebjerg University Hospital
Copenhagen, Denmark

K. Jönsson
Professor of Surgery
Department of Surgery
University of Zimbabwe
Harare, Zimbabwe

C. V. Krishnaswami
Consultant Physician
The Diabetes Department
Voluntary Health Services Hospital
Chennai, India

R. Mani
Consultant in Clinical Science and
   Honorary Senior Lecturer Vascular Group
Southampton University Hospitals Trust
Southampton, UK

V. Mani
Consultant Gastroenterologist and
   Honorary Senior Lecturer
Beaumont Hospital
Bolton, UK

D. J. Margolis
Consultant Physician
Department of Dermatology
Center for Clinical Epidemiology and
   Biostatistics
Philadelphia, Pennsylvania
USA

M. Romanelli
Consultant Dermatologist
Department of Dermatology
University of Pisa
Pisa, Italy

T. J. Ryan
Emeritus Professor of Dermatology
Slade Hospital
Oxford University
Oxford, UK

C. P. Shearman
Professor of Vascular Surgery
Department of Vascular Surgery
Southampton University Hospitals Trust
Southampton, UK

L. Téot
Consultant in Plastic and Reconstructive
   Surgery
Service des Brûlés
Hôpital Lapeyroine
Montpellier, France

P. Vowden
Consultant in Vascular Surgery
Department of Vascular Surgery
Bradford Royal Infirmary
Bradford, UK

Foreword

In all fields concerned with the acquisition of knowledge, as well as the integration and interpretation of empirical or experimental findings, one often sees an evolutionary process of thinking at work. Medicine is no exception. Certain ways of addressing clinical and experimental questions, identification of the needs to improve the knowledge base, even the formulation of hypotheses, they all seem to fall naturally into place. I have always been impressed by how clinicians and scientists working independently around the world will often choose to investigate the same problem and frequently come up with similar hypotheses. The exact elements underlying this collective evolution in our thinking are hard to trace. It could be that published writing and personal interactions at scientific meetings play a large role in defining what is important and what needs to be done next. However, I believe there is more to it than that, for there seems to be an overall dominant force, cutting across different fields.

Anyhow, I am reminded of such matters as I read this fine work edited by Dr Raj Mani on *Chronic Wound Management: the Evidence for Change*, for it fills an important need and seems to be right in step with the way the field of chronic wounds is moving. This textbook is a very timely and useful compendium of what constitutes the present evidence in the treatment of chronic wounds, as well as containing some tantalizing suggestions of yet-to-be proven therapies but which are readily available. For many years now, the field of wound healing, that of chronic wounds in particular, has been inundated by demands for evidence. As I was stating in the previous paragraph, this is part of the overall evolution of our times: the emphasis on going beyond personal experience. We face this emphasis at our meetings, in our journals and, if we are in a teaching environment, in the way students and trainees view and judge our way of practicing medicine. It used to be, not too long ago, that one would treat a few patients with a given therapy and suggest positive conclusions that many clinicians would readily accept. No more. It used to be that one would combine certain treatments, each one of them not actually proven to work, and strongly suggest the power of the combination. No more. It used to be that one would take rather limited personal experience or data of uncertain relevance to conclude that a therapy did not work or was detrimental to the healing process. No more. Now, I do not mean to say that such things were done maliciously and knowing that the conclusions were wrong. On the contrary, it was a way of being helpful. However, in the last several years, the entire context has changed, and an evolutionary process in our thinking has taken place. It is now a different world, one where we are much more accountable for the way we interpret published information and treat patients.

This textbook, while providing ample discussion of evidence-based treatments for chronic wounds, holds yet another important solid link that ties the different chapters together. This is an angle I had not previously seen emphasized, or at least not as comprehensively stated. I am referring to the discussion of how chronic wounds are treated globally, and of the challenges facing us in improving the outcome and alleviating the suffering of all patients with wounds, not just those in the Western world. Clinicians who are used to sophisticated dressings and bandages, growth factors, bioengineered skin, and a host of other advanced therapies need a constant reminder that such treatments are not available in poorer countries. The problems there are different, immense. As we are reminded in this textbook, complications from infection, acquired immunodeficiency, inadequate facilities and care, these are the cards that those patients are dealt. Within that context, an interesting statement made in this textbook caught my attention. It was said that, in some countries with such limited budgets, it may not even be ethical to spend an inordinate amount of money to prove the effectiveness of a given therapy; that money could have been put to better use to take care of the more basic needs of patients. Not ethical to test for evidence – interesting. I found it interesting because, in a perverse way, we in the Western world are facing a similar problem but in reverse. Let me explain. Let us hypothesize that a pharmaceutical company will spend hundreds of millions of dollars to pursue ambitious and cogent research objectives, develop a new treatment, and test it in clinical trials. When regulatory approval finally comes, it would seem that the process is over and that the goal has been achieved. However, enter reimbursement. Now, the task will be to convince government and private insurers that the treatment should be reimbursed. That is not easy, considering that these agencies have their own fixed budgets, just like the poorer countries we were discussing, and that there are so many other unmet medical needs. After all, there is cancer, and cardiovascular disease, and AIDS. Even in wound care, there are many treatments that are reimbursed already. Some may argue that some therapies should not be reimbursed at all because there is no evidence they are effective. However, the fact is that they are being reimbursed, even as they

prevent reimbursement of new and more effective treatments. The bottom line is that our hypothetical truly effective treatment that has just been approved for use is now less available than it would seem. When it comes to practicing evidence-based medicine in wound healing, another example of the strange similarities between our more advanced medical system and poorer nations can be seen in our clinics. In many countries, including the United States for example, the evaluation of patients will need to include whether they can afford the treatment we prescribe. Reimbursement issues will have to be dealt with, and not just the evidence for that treatment. A compromise is often made at the bedside, but I am afraid that in some cases it would not stand the scrutiny of evidence-based medicine.

These days, as one discusses evidence-based treatments, I also hear some frustration about how the emphasis on evidence has become a tool for insurers to deny reimbursement for a given therapy. This is partly true, especially when by necessity there is only anecdotal or incomplete experimental evidence for that treatment. Elsewhere, I have referred to this problem as the 'dark side' of evidence-based medicine. However, when we place everything in perspective, we will realize that, by emphasizing evidence, we have gained much more than we have lost. True, we may have difficulty in obtaining some expensive or more complex treatments for patients with unusual and difficult-to-heal wounds. However, by emphasizing evidence, the effectiveness bar has been raised for the majority of our patients. Ignorance or unfamiliarity with wounds is no longer a valid excuse for clinicians. With the focus on evidence-based treatment, there has been a concomitant emphasis on the more basic aspects of wound care with which all clinicians should comply: compression for venous ulcers, off-loading for pressure-induced wounds, the need for thorough debridement, wound bed preparation. Indeed, the emphasis on evidence and the numerous clinical trials performed in the last few years have made basic wound care better.

There are two important issues about evidence-based chronic wound management that we will need to address in the next few years. One challenge is how to eliminate the reimbursement of treatments that are probably ineffective or which, at the very least, require new clinical trials to make their case. As stated, such treatments are 'grandfathered in' and are difficult to remove from the list of reimbursed items. Their reimbursement interferes with the acceptance of new and more effective products. Working with government and other insurers, we need to develop a process that will allow us to analyze our options. The second issue is that, in my view, even when evidence is available and properly presented, adherence is not made to that evidence. This is an interesting phenomenon, and is not necessarily linked to reimbursement issues or how expensive a certain product or clinical approach is. There is a lag period before clinicians adopt new knowledge and alter their way of practicing. Repeated exposure to the evidence is often needed and, in some cases, it would seem that an actual mandate is required for change to take place.

As elegantly detailed in this textbook, there is much of which to be proud in the management of chronic wounds. While many unanswered questions remain, and while the evidence for certain approaches is still sketchy, rather remarkable progress has been made. The basic aspects of wound care are much more robust than they were even a few years ago, and the introduction of new and exciting products has also improved basic wound care. Not adhering to certain therapeutic principles for which there is reasonable evidence will eventually become untenable. The old maxim of 'Do no harm' remains a sound principle. However, it will become increasingly clear that one can do much harm by not providing what are established, evidence-based treatments.

Vincent Falanga, MD
Professor of Dermatology and Biochemistry
Boston University
and *Chairman of Training Program*
Roger Williams Medical Center

Preface

Several times in the last few years, a tale from south Indian folklore relevant to chronic wound healing has crossed my mind. It runs as follows: there was a young man who spent most of his days rolling a boulder all the way up a hill, only to release it and watch it tumble down. That this man was frivolously wasting his time became village gossip to an extent where the elders became concerned and decided that there was a need to visit the site. The date was set for this visit and a meeting with the young man. The delegation included a retired physician. On the occasion, when asked to account for the reason for his behavior, the young man replied that he had a bad knee. One of the elders informed the young man that this condition would be treated back in the village, to which the young man answered 'My father had bad knees and spent his days in bed, as your medicines wouldn't work. At least I am active, this keeps me happy.' His actions were based on pure personal experience and observation – he did not await the outcome of a randomized controlled study to determine the best course of action for him. There are a number of morals in this story; these are left to readers to decipher.

This book project has been an enjoyable experience because my colleague contributors delivered their chapters in good time while being available for discussion and debate as needed. I shall remain eternally grateful to all of them. I would like to express a special debt of gratitude to Luc Téot and Finn Gottrup for their encouraging perspectives during the formative stages of this book. I thank my friends Geoff Fairris and Paul Weaver for giving me their time and the benefit of their valuable clinical experience in commenting on specific chapters. The course of this project development has been almost 'laminar flow' because of the calm stewardship of Grant Weston who has been very easy to work with over the tenure of this development.

Now a few essential acknowledgements. I shall always be indebted to Carol Collins for her ability to attend to details; for reasons unknown, these seem to fly past me with ease.

To my wife and children, when I am apparently absent-minded or inactive, they should remember the story of the young man on the hill.

Finally to my mother, whose contribution to my work and existence increases as I age. Is it merely anatomical and physiologic details that are replicated in DNA? There is much more to learn for us all.

Raj Mani
October 2002

Introduction
Chronic wound management: a global perspective

1

T. J. Ryan

In this book, several experts give updates on aspects of wound healing. Consequently, the introduction will focus on areas of ignorance. These will be examined, pointing out gaps in our knowledge of the pathogenesis of chronic wounds and the gold standards required for their management.

The scenario must be set by first defining chronic wounds and reiterating briefly how wounds heal.

CHRONICITY

A chronic wound, by definition, is not an acute wound and therefore it is not following timely healing or the sequence of healing that characterizes the ideal. The ideal includes rapid control of hemorrhage with an only transient subsequent inflammatory response to injury and, before a few days have passed, the complete clearance of damaged tissue. Ischemia, even to a slight degree, would necessitate a better blood supply to be grown in the form of granulation tissue, to support a wound bed fit for subsequent epithelialization. Finally, there is a remoulding of the wound bed with a variable degree of scar formation (Figure 1.1). All of this is interrupted or delayed in a chronic wound.

The causes of chronicity have been described in a table of local, general and health service organization defects (Table 1). Locally important is the failure of apposition of a healthy wound edge due to space occupancy by blood exudate and fibrin. There may be infective and necrotic tissue or foreign bodies, and a surgical failure to bring the wound edges together. A failure of blood supply is a common cause of non-healing, underlying nearly all chronicity and sometimes due to too much tension or swelling in the wound edge.

Chronic wounds often show a lack of uniformity or of homogeneity of blood supply. This is seen in the pattern of blood flow or it is observed as a variation in the proximity of the blood vessel to the tissue supplied (Figure 1.2). There may not only be ischemia but also damage from reperfusion.

Much of the failure inherent in chronic wounds in the developing world[1] especially, but also in the elderly and chronic sick of the developed world, is due to factors such as poor nutrition, which may be systemic, local in the tissue or both, or to failure of the immune system. Overriding all of these causes of delay is the poverty of the person affected. Limitation of access to best practice is a common cause of poor healing. It characterizes the 'developing

Table 1 Factors delaying wound healing

Global	General	Local
Building inadequate	Age	Inadequate blood supply
No access to transport	Malnutrition	Hematoma formation
Health care worker	Cancer	Foreign body implantation
knowledge	Anemia	Necrotic tissue
availability	Systemic infection	Wound infection
Patient compliance	Steroid treatment	Radiation therapy
Management support	Vitamin and trace metal deficiency	Recurrent trauma
	Cancer chemotherapy	Duration of surgery
	Diabetes	Experience of surgeon
	Jaundice	Suture material
	Uremia	Wound tension
	Obesity	Absence of nature's secret remedy
	Hypothermia	
	Anti-inflammatory drugs	
	Gender	
	Genetic defects – skeletal or adhesion proteins	

world', and it is usually due to inequalities in the provision of the necessary financial support of the health service. It can be found even in the developed world.

Major advances in our knowledge have occurred quite rapidly during the last decades of the 20th century, but their dissemination has been limited to a few who have cultivated a special interest in the field. All the data on cytokines and growth factors that dominate research into healing seem to have displaced earlier knowledge and, although Hippocrates, Galen and Ambroise Paré are still mentioned, some of the research that dominated the literature in the first 60 years of the 20th century is now forgotten or unread. Until antibiotics became widely available in the mid-20th century, the main concern was infection. Fifty years later, it has been forgotten that Eusol and Dakin's solution were life-savers, invented in the worst conditions of trench warfare, and all the hand-washing that was a beneficial habit of the first half of the century, bequeathed by Lister and Florence Nightingale, was slipping out of fashion by the end of the 20th century. It is argued that, in a modern wound healing unit, trench warfare conditions should not be simulated. We can do better! However, the world's most numerous wounds are still dirty and arrive late for the most expert attention.

When Howard Florey (1953) published the lectures that had been given over the previous few years in Oxford's General Pathology and Bacteriology course, he encouraged the reader to know about the direct observation of skin wounds into which a window had been inserted[2]. The experiments of Clark and Clark on the rabbit's ear and observations of the hamster cheek pouch (Figure 1.3) or bat wing were visual and therefore very informative[3]. Every stage of wounding and repair could be observed *in vivo* through a microscope. These series of daily observations of wound healing were the most detailed ever made. They were clearly described and covered the topic of *in vivo* wound observation in a manner that has never been surpassed.

Later advances in the histopathology and histochemistry of excised wounds gave rise to several landmarks, as observers produced serial observation of all stages of wound healing and began to take an interest in the techniques of skin grafting[4–7]. Gillman, writing in the same period, was interested in fibrin as a barrier or as a scaffold and the influence of the dermis on the epidermis. The control of epithelial mitosis gave rise to the Chalone theory (Bullough) and observations on the effects of vitamin C and vitamin A in wound healing were admired by both Florey[2] and Gillman[6].

The one person whose work of the mid-20th century has attracted the greatest contemporary interest is Winter[8]. By demonstrating that moist wound healing is preferable to drying out, he and Scales made obsolete the fan at the end of the bed, which cooled and dried chronic wounds, and they provided a rationale for a new industry producing proactive moisturizing dressings.

Gillman made the point that both granulation tissue and scars are new organs of repair as distinct to regeneration[6]. The latter, with its scarless healing and absence of inflammation and granulation tissue, has progressed to the contemporary studies of healing in the embryo. Gillman also suggested that healing was transiently identical to neoplasia. Exact clarification of what this means is possibly the most complete advance made in biological studies of the past 50 years. What initiates and stops healing is clearly a story that has parallels in the field of cancer. Interestingly, Gillman pointed out that, for the first 2 or 3 days after injury, acute inflammation is devoid of mitotic activity. It is exudative non-proliferative inflammation. The older wound is proliferative, and it also eliminates damaged tissues by apoptosis, necrosis and extrusion. The surgeon's role is to assist the healing process by reducing hemorrhage and exudate by providing good drainage in the first phase and assisting in the debridement of the wound in its later phases. The harm done by suturing and the effect of tension-induced ischemia and of stitch abscesses led to important refinements of surgical skills, and numerous studies followed in the mid-20th century. Calnan quoted Trevor Roper, who in a history of World War II was always conscious of what might have happened[9]. It is a question that can stimulate research: 'what if this step is not taken?'

In every case, one point is certain – no step can be omitted that will result in acceleration of normal acute wound healing. Conversion of a chronic wound to an acute wound by excision and apposition of the wound edges brings the rate of healing up to that of an acute wound, but the rate is no faster than that.

ACCIDENT PREVENTION

Can one prevent wounds? Well up to a point of course one can. 'Accident prone' means 'prone to carelessness'. Not to care about wearing crash helmets or seat belts or being careless with fireworks have little to do with intelligence or knowledge, but much to do with judgment and priorities. There are some who are inherently optimistic and believe accidents will not happen to them, and they will always take a chance that the dead branch against which they place their ladder will not break. Judgment is impaired by alcohol and by fatigue, but also by optimism.

Governance too must play its part in making correct judgments. The prevalence of burns has been much reduced in the developed world by legislation against inflammable materials. Such legislation has mostly not reached the developing world, where clothing and bedding may be highly inflammable and the household fire an open one. On the other hand, in the developing world, there is education about environmental dangers. Most children will know that the buffalo is a dangerous beast and more complex dangers are often covered in initiation ceremonies. The Aboriginal child may be safer than a Western child in the Australian bush. Respect for weapons may make those who use them learn how to use them safely.

The practice of first aid and expedition medicine are taught in the expectation of saving lives, but also to prevent acute wounds from becoming chronic[10]. The protection of a burnt limb by rapid cooling and then covering to prevent infection is one example. It has also been found that persons who learn first aid are less likely to have accidents. First aid teaches priorities and provides order in the management of casualties. The most at-risk are treated first. Avoiding danger becomes an exhortation taking precedence over diagnosis. Careful assessment of the casualty precedes management. Help is sought by making sure that the correct information about location and number or types of casualty is given.

WHAT IS ESSENTIAL WHEN LITTLE ELSE CAN BE AFFORDED?

In every trial of a new dressing, it is compared to gauze and the latter inevitably can be shown to delay healing. It is, however, all that is available in the developing world. The Western world has found Eusol and Gentian Violet to be either toxic or carcinogenic, but this is all that is available from the West in the developing world.

The African in Tanzania, for example, is told that traditional medicine is unscientific and its prescription package, which is an oral custom, may take into account spirits, evil influences and environmental effects. It is all they can afford, and it is locally available and sustainable[11].

The West exports agents with an out-of-date expiry date, often without a data sheet or any other instructions. Consequently, strong steroid creams may be used as emollients. There is, of course, the *WHO Model of Essential Drugs* (www.who.int-medicines) prepared as a result of international advice. It takes into account appropriateness, sustainability and cost. The evidence base for many of the most commonly used agents, especially in

the case of topical agents used in wound healing, is admittedly inadequate[12]. A review of the Essential Drugs list is under way, but the criteria for inclusion will need to be flexible and it will be difficult to meet gold standards.

In every nation there should be at least some basic therapy available to all, preferably at low cost. In at least one training school or tertiary (regional) referral unit, gold standards should be aimed for. The world needs elite units to export gold standards and there should be at least one in every country. As an example, in Tanzania the management of lymphedema requires that affected communities are taught low-cost, self-help measures for morbidity control of their enlarged limbs; washing the skin, elevation and movement costs nothing and everyone can do it[13]. On the other hand, few can afford manual lymphatic drainage containment bandaging or hosiery, which are the centerpieces of management in the developed world. In a country such as Tanzania, where AIDS is an epidemic, the differential diagnosis of early lymphedema due to Kaposi's sarcoma must be thought of and other causes of lymphedema well managed. The associated lymphedema of the scrotum and the accompanying hydrocele is also part of the picture. Next to blindness, lymphedema has been assessed as the commonest cause of disability and, for some, the full picture of elephantiasis (Figure 1.4) results in destitution. The difficult case will not respond to self-help measures and there is no economic justification for the gold standard management of such a problem to be made available everywhere. By contrast, it would be unjust not to have at least one center in every country where the management skills for difficult cases can be taught and other important themes such as team development can be practiced.

Another example is the person affected by leprosy who walks around with a foot ulcer. The straps of his shoe are nailed to the sole and the nail is projecting into the wearer's foot

(Figure 1.5). It should be possible to prevent this at any health center, replacing the nail with adhesive. At the same time, there should be a few centers where the management of the ulcer itself and the preparation of footwear can be of a gold standard. Special units are also required for the management of burns; many hospitals in the developing world have the same degree of lack of control of bacterial surveillance as in the developed world, cross-infection with antibiotic-resistant bacteria being rife. Some leading hospitals are apparently unable to afford masks and gloves and a clean environment is not maintained. Hand-washing should be practiced everywhere but may be difficult where there is a shortage of water. Nevertheless, in each leading hospital there should be at least one area fully equipped and correctly supervised where gold standards can be observed and from which their practice can be disseminated. It may be too costly to distribute gold standards far afield but at least there should be one unit where the teaching of gold standards can be observed.

TRADITIONAL MEDICINE VERSUS BIOMEDICINE: THE NEED FOR INTEGRATION

The history of management of wounds by herbal medicine, honey or maggots is a long one[14]. These agents are locally available, sustainable and at low cost. Of course, in elite units of the West, there are more efficacious remedies, but it can be argued that the needs of the developing world are so great that the elite units should be providing evidence that traditional medicine is safe and effective. The Wound Healing Unit in Oxford has collaborated with African, Chinese and Vietnamese traditional healing systems to provide proof of safety and efficacy of wound healing agents[15]. In collaboration with the Global Initiative for Traditional Systems (GIFTS) of Health, it has adopted the policy that, if an agent is little used, then no more need be done than note its existence, but, if it is widely used, then its availability and sustainability should be supplemented by attention to its safety. A safe and frequently used agent that is cheap can be promoted, especially if it gives satisfaction and enhances well-being. Studies of efficacy should follow, if they can be done without expense and there is likely to be a clear outcome. Expensive studies, which are ultimately not taken into account, are immoral because money can be better spent in the developing world[12].

Biomedicine has always favored a chemical explanation for the disease and its treatments. Contemporary wound healing explanations are dominated by cytokines and growth factors. Treatments that are single chemical agents are preferred by the scientist and by evidence-based medicine. Traditional medicine is often poly-pharmacy with multiple herbal agents, the exact content of which is unpredictable. However, if the tradition is followed with respect to identification of the time of harvesting, cultivation in the correct soils and the procedures for producing the medicine are standardized, up to a point, then as in Chinese medicine no harm can be expected due to variation in content of the active principle.

Asian medicine is more tolerant of physical theories of causation and management; energy or 'chi' is perceived as essential and balance is far less a chemical phenomenon than Western medicine's *milieu intérieur* subscribed to for more than a century.

Acupuncture is widely used to promote healing (Figure 1.6) and its role has perhaps done more to support the view that 'there is something there which we don't understand' rather than 'it is wishful thinking'. Western medicine uses mechanical or physical forces within wound healing in the form of tissue expansion, tissue compression, anti-gravitational therapy, the application of vacuum or warming devices, cryotherapy and manual lymphatic drainage (a form of massage) and laser therapy. These are examples of accepted systems of applying physical forces. The vascular system is perhaps best suited to concepts of balance[16] – there is cardiac output versus peripheral resistance, there is Starling's law of forces in and outside a blood vessel wall, and there is vasomotion, which is a control of flow properties of blood – all of which entertain a concept of balance. Whether it is Chinese medicine or biomedicine, in the field of vascular medicine there is a common language leading to mutual understanding[16].

Western medicine tends to think of the benefits of exercise and mobilization (Figure 1.7). Other systems think of control of posture and movement, often also including attention to correct breathing.

THE TRANSDUCTION OF BIOCHEMICAL SIGNALS BY MECHANICAL FORCES

Except perhaps in the field of orthopedics, the relationship of structure to the distribution of chemical effects and the influence of mechanical forces on both have so far been neglected. The orientation of fibers is important for the skin; it is tangential in the upper dermis, whereas in the mid-dermis the fibers have a horizontal disposition. These are determinants of mechanical forces and the direction of their effects. The role of the water content of ground substance has been emphasized as a factor producing tension in a series of papers by Gniadecka[17] and others by Ryan (Figure 1.8). The importance of the fibrin clot and platelets initiating the effect of contractile forces on a wound has been emphasized. They are dissolved by fibrinolysis and the effect that this has on the grip and stick of contact adhesion between cells and the connective tissue has also been discussed[18]. Due to the cholesterol content of cell membranes and the effect

of mechanical distortion of cell membranes on the flip–flap pattern of kinases attached to the membrane, they have a fluidity that allows them to either maintain a position within the cell membrane or to extend into the cytosol or externally outside the cell membrane[19]. At a very basic level, this fluidity means that processes like phosphorylation, which are necessary for contact and adhesion, may be impaired by mechanical forces, just as they may be impaired by stereochemical interference by added chemical structures. As cells are attached to fibers and the forces experienced are dependent on their length and flexibility, distortions may be felt further afield than simply by the cell membrane. It becomes important to recognize the significance of the orientation of these fibers and thus the tangential orientation of fibers in the upper dermis, and the horizontal disposition of fibers below that level can have a profound effect on skin behavior. Even studies of the importance of depth of skin burns have so far ignored the significance of the orientation of fibers in the upper dermis to the integrity of epidermal function. Most recently, the expansion of the water content of the upper dermis (Figure 1.9) leading to an effect on the permeability component of vascular endothelial growth factor (VEGF), due to tensions felt in the upper dermis, has been put forward as an explanation of its angiogenic effect[20].

THE CONCEPT OF VULNERABILITY

The vulnerable are more likely to develop wounds from stimuli that, in the less vulnerable, are instantly assuaged or repaired. The triggers, such as trauma and infection, that cause subclinical responses that are not overt produce exaggerated responses in some persons who are vulnerable[21]. These are clearly clinically manifest. A typical example is dermatographism, which are scratches with an exaggerated triple response, affecting between 5 and 10% of the population. Another example is the Koebner phenomenon, typically seen in psoriasis close to a lesion during an active phase, where the slightest trauma, which in the normal person would produce no response, results in the development of psoriasis at the site of injury (Figure 1.10). It is known as the isomorph response and there are other diseases such as lichen planus or viral warts which can do the same. Vulnerability of certain regions of the body is also well known: the eyelids tend to be particularly sensitive to topical cosmetic agents which produce irritation only at that site. The legs are more vulnerable because of the chronic effects of venous hypertension. The diabetic is also more vulnerable, due to a failure in the normal response to injury, having a high resting blood flow, but unable to increase blood supply to a level required for repair. Loss of pain awareness, as in diabetes mellitus, or pressure injury, in persons who are unconscious or paraplegic, are more likely to produce ischemic necrosis at that site. Some genetic diseases, such as the absence of Type VII anchoring filaments of collagen in epidermolysis bullosa, or C_1 esterase inhibitor deficiency, are all clear examples of vulnerability.

Acquired vulnerability may be specific, as for example, a contact sensitivity to a particular topical agent such as the primula or the antibiotic neomycin. At the other end of the immune spectrum, protection from infection and repair responses may be impaired in patients affected by AIDS.

Damage to tissues insufficient to produce a wound can be stored as a memory that summates with a subsequent injury. This is observed in the Schwartzman phenomenon or in the heightened reactions of the tissues in Behçet's syndrome or in pyoderma gangrenosum (Figure 1.11). The tendency to form keloids is another pattern of vulnerability.

PAIN RELIEF

Pain relief is an end-point of management that is sometimes more appropriate even than the aim of complete healing[22]. The quality of pain has recently received more attention. Thus its periodicity, its focus to a particular site and depth and its response to awareness or interference of sleep are all factors which may require different degrees of management of pain. Thus whether it is stabbing, continuous, diffuse or localized, burning, stinging or aching, pain may correspond to different patterns of neural conduction. It may be a response to different mediators of inflammation.

The language describing the various syndromes in which pain is exaggerated after wounding has undergone a change from time to time. Causalgia and *oedeme bleu* are terms that have been replaced first of all by reflex sympathetic dystrophy and, most recently, complex regional pain syndrome. As described, in a recent commentary in *The Lancet*, the cause of this problem is uncertain, but 'At the heart of this controversy is the difficulty of understanding how such a devastating syndrome can develop after an injury that sometimes is trivial and that in many cases seems to heal quickly'. The devastating syndrome is described as follows:

'Patients typically describe a burning sensation in the affected limb that is aggravated by movement, handling, temperature changes and psychologic distress. Patients often guard their limb protectively; normal movements are limited and muscles show sign of wasting. The limb also often swells, sweats excessively and is warmer or cooler than the contralateral limb.'

There is some evidence of reduced sympathetic vasoconstrictor activity which is followed by a secondary change in which adrenergic supersensitivity over-compensates for the loss of sympathetic vasomotor control.

The peripheral and spinal disturbances that might provoke or maintain such a condition are discussed by Drummond[23], who concludes that there is a possibility that the syndrome can be explained by failure of inhibitory spinal or supra-spinal influences on nociceptive transmission, and refers to the transformation of normal arousal and attentional processes into the neuronal pathways that mediate or suppress information. Some neurologic syndromes associated with severe non-healing remain to be explained. Extreme examples include those which have a cultural basis, such as the stigmatization which is seen predominantly in women of the Catholic faith and which produces non-healing, painful, repetitive wounds simulating those of the wounds of Jesus Christ. By contrast, the painless non-inflammatory, deeply pierced skin wounds of some Asian ceremonies are equally unexplained (Figure 1.12).

MULTI-CULTURAL ASPECTS OF CARING

Those who manage wounds and especially chronic wounds should understand that religious beliefs may intensify under stress and that beliefs may influence wound healing. Caring for persons with chronic wounds, so that dignity is not lost and personal values are not demeaned and independence is encouraged, is the basis of good management in a multi-cultural scenario. As described above, pain relief is one end-point and, as Bowsher has described[24], for most of us who lie on a bed of nails, the experience, though not acutely painful, is most uncomfortable and soon becomes intolerable. But some people, by process of something akin to auto-hypnosis, can become tolerant to such pain and, as Bowsher showed, this is not naloxone reversible. The management of wounds is complicated by belief and especially by religion. Most Africans first go to traditional healers from whom they benefit. Colonialization by missionaries who looked for the 'true faith' or by settlers who wanted labor resulted in traditional healers being labeled as 'witch doctors' and their suppression was attempted. At the same time, the Western colonial influence established hospitals which have never succeeded in managing the majority of their populations. The traditional healer is so often the leader, the ceremonial chief, or equivalent to a priest and may share with his/her patients beliefs in a completely different causation of disease, including wounds. Happenings which produce wounds or processes which lead to non-healing may be interpreted as an offence to ancestors or to being bewitched. Processes such as being undressed by Western doctors or being subjected to digital and rectal examinations are deterrents. Self-esteem, which is often necessary for complete healing, or the death of a patient in a community, requires attention to the details of naming and correctly identifying, as well as the appropriateness of manner in handling both the living and the dead. For those who believe in reincarnation, amputation is highly undesirable. Some of this is important even for wound healing. Fortunately in the developed world, and led by the nursing profession, questions such as 'What is the meaning of living with your venous ulcer' are now seen as important to the management of these patients[25].

References

1. Ryan TJ. Wound healing in the developing world. In: Nemeth AJ, ed. *Wound Healing in* *Dermatology Clinics*, Vol 11. Philadelphia: W.B. Saunders, 1993:791–800

2. Florey H. *Lectures in General Pathology*. London: Lloyd Luke Medical Books, 1954, 1–733

3. Clark ER, Clark EL. *Am J Anat* 1939;64:251

4. Arey LB. Wound healing. *Physiol Rev* 1936;16:327–406

5. Billingham RE, Russell PS. Studies in wound healing. *Ann Surg* 1956;144:961–81

6. Gillman T. Possible importance of dermal–epidermal interactions in the pathogenesis of human and experimental wound healing and skin cancer. In: Rook A, Champion RH, eds. *Progress in the Biological Sciences in Relation to Dermatology*, Vol 2. Cambridge: Cambridge University Press, 1964:113–33

7. Gillman T, Penn J. The healing of cutaneous wounds. *Med Proc South Afr* 1956;2:121

8. Winter GD, Scales JT. Effect of air drying and dressings on the surface of a wound. *Nature (London)* 1963;197:91–2

9. Calnan JS. *Epithelium in Wound Healing Symposium*. Oxford: Medicine Publishing Foundation, 1982:2

10. Anderson SR, Johnson CJ. Expedition health and safety: a risk assessment. *J Roy Soc Med* 2000;93:577–62

11. Bodeker GC, Ryan TJ, Ong C-K. Traditional approaches to wound healing. *Clin Dermatol* 1999;17:93–8

12. Ryan TJ. Health for all (Editorial). *J Altern Complement Med* 2001;7:303–6

13. Ryan TJ. Lymphatic filariasis: management of lymphoedema. *Africa Health* 2001;23:9–11

14. Bernstein RM. *Honey, Mud and Maggots and Other Medical Marvels*. New York: Macmillan, 1999:1–279

15. Ryan TJ. Integrated treatment of chronic wounds. In: *Health in the Commonwealth 1998/99*. London: Kensington Publications, 1998:298–9

16. Ryan TJ. Studies of the microcirculation in China. *Tropical Doctor* 1997;27:48–51

17. Gniadecka M. Studies on cutaneous water distribution and structure. *Forum Nordic Dermatovenerol* 2000;5(Suppl 1):1–24

18. Ryan TJ. Pathophysiology of non-healing chronic wounds: biochemical control of grip and stick. In: Janssen H, Rooman R, Robertson JIS, eds. *Wound Healing* – Janssen Biomedical Science Series. Petersfield, UK: Wrightson Biomedical Publishing, 1991

19. Ryan TJ. Biochemical consequences of mechanical forces generated by distension and distortion. *J Am Acad Dermatol* 1989;21:115–30

20. Ryan TJ, Thoolen M, Yang YH. The effect of mechanical forces (vibration or external compression) on the dermal water content of the upper dermis and epidermis assessed by high frequency ultrasound. *J Tiss Viab* 2001;11:97–101

21. Ryan TJ (ed.). Microvascular injury. In: *Major Problems in Dermatology*, Vol 7. London: Lloyd Luke Medical, 1976:416.

22. Hofman D. Practical pain management associated with wounds. *Oxford European Wound Healing Course Handbook*. Oxford: Positif Press, 2002:110–15

23. Drummond PD. Mechanism of complex regional pain syndrome: no longer excessive sympathetic outflow? *Lancet* 2001;358:168–9

24. Bowsher D. Ability to lie on bed of nails not due to endogenous opioids. *Lancet* 1980;i:1132

25. Ebbeskog B, Ekman SL. Elderly people's experiences, the meaning of living with venous leg ulcers. *J Eur Wound Manag Assoc* 2001;1:21–3

What is evidence?

2

M. J. Campbell

INTRODUCTION

We are now in the era of 'evidence-based health care' (EBHC). There are different types of evidence and this chapter will consider the strengths and weaknesses of different approaches. EBHC requires that we should consider critically all evidence that a treatment works or an agent causes a disease. This requires a systematic assembly of available evidence followed by a critical appraisal of this evidence. Before this paradigm of review and appraisal, it had been considered sufficient to understand the pathophysiologic process of a disorder and to prescribe drugs or other treatments that had been shown to interrupt this process. Historically, the practice of medicine has been based on history-taking, clinical examination and treatment of symptoms based on the accepted pathophysiology of the condition. Two examples serve to illustrate how this can mislead. Sackett and co-workers[1] give an example of a finding that patients who displayed ventricular ectopic beats following a myocardial infarction were at high risk of sudden death. Drugs were then widely prescribed to suppress these ectopic beats, on the assumption that removing the cause would reduce the effect. However, subsequent randomized controlled trials, which examined clinical outcomes and not physiologic process, showed that use of these drugs actually *increased* death rates rather than decreased them and their use is now strongly discouraged. The second example concerns neonatologists who always kept premature babies lying on their fronts. One tacit assumption was that, should the baby vomit, the baby would be less likely to inhale it. This practice was extended to all babies. However, subsequent epidemiologic studies showed that babies who were habitually put on their fronts were at higher risk of sudden infant death. A 'back to sleep' campaign was initiated and the sudden infant deaths in England and Wales dropped from some 2000 per year to less than 600. The argument for putting babies on their fronts was not *evidence-based*.

We are now encouraged to only use therapies for which there is good evidence of effectiveness. The UK Government has set up NICE, the National Institute for Clinical Excellence, to consider which treatments are effective and also cost-effective for use in the National Health Service and thus effectively compel clinicians to use evidence-based medicine. Last year, they were asked to produce guidance on the use of debridement for difficult-to-heal surgical wounds[2]. This chapter will consider how the NICE review used the available evidence, both from studies and from expert opinion, to give guidance in this area.

The structure of this chapter will be in two parts: the first part will consider the general problem of assessing evidence and the second part will look at a specific example, namely the NICE appraisal of difficult-to-heal surgical wounds.

EVIDENCE AND PROOF

Discussion of EBHC begs the question: what is evidence? Let us start with the problem of *proof*. Philosophers have long argued over this problem. In mathematics, the Greeks demonstrated rigorous proofs of *theorems* (literally God-like things) and they thought of these as general laws. Thus, we know for certain that the Pythagoras Theorem is true. The question arises as to whether one can have similar certainty in other areas of human enquiry. In natural science, Francis Bacon (1561–1626) described the work of scientists as collecting information and adducing natural laws. However, the Scottish philosopher, David Hume (1711–1776), concluded that no number of singular observations, however large, could logically entail an unrestricted general statement. Just because event A follows event B on one occasion, it does not follow that event B will be observed the next time we see event A. It does not logically follow, in the manner that a mathematic theorem is true, that A will always follow B if we observe A following B on 2, 20 or 2000 occasions. The point here is that simply *observing* an association is not proof that an association exists. There may, however, be real reasons why two events are associated and, in general, one would hope to discover these. Thus, if we observed that 20 consecutive bedridden patients developed pressure sores, it does not logically imply that the 21st patient will. However, it does suggest an association, which it would be foolish to ignore.

'Hume's problem' troubled philosophers from his day to the present. It seemed to discourage trying to make sense of nature. It was not until the 20th century that Popper came up with the idea of falsifiability. Laws cannot be shown to be either true or false. They are held *provisionally* true. Observations cannot be used to prove the laws, but can falsify them. Hume's famous example is that the universal law 'all swans are white' cannot be proven, no matter how many swans one sees, but it would take but a single black swan to refute the law. This has direct bearing on statistical inference, where one sets up a null hypothesis and then tries to refute it. Failure to reject the null hypothesis does *not* mean that one should accept it, simply that we do not have enough evidence to reject it. Clinical trials are set up with the null hypothesis that there is no effect of treatment on outcome and then we try to disprove it. However, we can never prove a null effect. As a topical example, this has considerable implications when trying to show that the combined measles, mumps and rubella vaccine does not cause autism. All we can do is demonstate that, if there is a risk, then the risk is very low. It is up to those taking the risk to decide whether it is lower than the competing risks associated with measles.

The light that this may shed on EBCH is that *guidance is only provisional*. It is based on the best evidence available at the time. We can collect more evidence and, if this concurs with the existing evidence, it may give us greater confidence in our guidelines, but cannot prove them. Later evidence may contradict the existing theories.

This approach may seem rather negative, but in fact it is liberating. What Popper's philosophy gives scientists is the freedom to try their best, without claiming God-like omnipotence, such that any statements are assumed true for all time. It gives scientists a model whereby criticism of existing models is actively encouraged and is a legitimate occupation for a scientist. It enables us to differentiate good scientific theories from bad ones; in good ones one can devise experiments to attempt to falsify the theory. However, we should not fall into the trap of relativism – all theories are equally valid. Falsifiable theories that withstand attempts to disprove them are to be preferred over ones that have no such evidence. It is worth pointing out, however, that often the choice of *which* experiments to do is a social or

Table 1 Strength of evidence (weakest to strongest)

Case series
Case–control study
Quasi-experimental study (non-randomized prospective study)
Open randomized controlled trial
Single-blind randomized controlled trial
Double-blind randomized controlled trial

political decision. Thus, lack of evidence may not be the fault of the theory, but rather the lack of political will to test the theory.

However, outside of physics and mathematics and in the more fallible fields of medical science, the nature of human variability has meant that universal laws are rare. There are obvious laws, such as if you deprive a person of oxygen they soon die, but they are the exception. Give a person a large dose of arsenic and they do not inevitably die. Rather than universal laws, medical science is concerned with a number of basic questions such as: does exposure to substance A increase the risk of disease B? Does treatment C cure more people with disease D than other therapies? In the 19th century, Koch devised a number of questions that could be used to try to decide whether a specific bacterium caused a disease. These were modified by Bradford Hill[2] to a general examination of whether exposure to an event, be it an environmental exposure or a medical treatment, would increase the risk of disease, or a cure, respectively. The Bradford Hill criteria are: temporality, consistency, coherence, strength of association, biological gradient, specificity, plausibility, freedom from or control of confounding and bias and analogous results found elsewhere. Temporality means that the effect follows the cause and not vice-versa. Thus a fall in lung cancer deaths in UK men succeeded a drop in the numbers of smokers by some 30 years, lending weight to a causality link between smoking and lung can-

cer. Consistency means that the same fall in lung cancer deaths has been observed in other countries where smoking prevalence has fallen. Coherence means that different studies, such as case–control studies and cohort studies, show similar effects. Strength of the association suggests that the stronger the effect the more plausible the causality. For example, smokers have 10 times the risk of lung cancer compared with non-smokers. The idea concerning the biological gradient is that if heavy smokers are at greater risk than light smokers, then the case for causality is strengthened. Specificity suggests that, if the link were causal, the smokers would be mainly at risk from respiratory disease and not from other unrelated diseases such as road accidents. A confounding variable is one that is related to the exposure and the outcome, but not in a causal pathway. For smoking, genetics has been argued as a confounder. The impulse to smoke may be genetic – certainly if parents smoke then children are more likely to smoke. Also the risk of lung cancer may be controlled by genes. If the genes for smoking and lung cancer were linked, then it would appear that smoking and lung cancer were causally related. However, if the genetic theory were true, it would have a hard time to explain away the other causal evidence such as temporality.

Just as in philosophy we cannot prove a universal law, so in medicine we cannot prove absolutely a causal effect. Hill's criteria increase the likelihood of a causal effect, but cannot give an absolute proof. Hill himself admitted 'none of my nine viewpoints can bring indisputable evidence for or against the cause-and-effect hypothesis and none can be regarded as a *sine qua non*'[4]. Hill's criteria should not be regarded as a checklist, but rather as an *aide-mémoire*.

This leads to the use of statistical ideas[5]. We devise a model, based on a hypothesis about the data. This is usually a null hypothesis, i.e. there is *no* effect. We then observe an experiment, or a survey, and obtain some results. We can deduce the probability of getting the observed data (or data more extreme from the null model), when the null hypothesis is true. If this probability is small, then we reject the null hypothesis. We say the result is statistically significant. Note that failure to reject does not mean we accept the null hypothesis, although, provisionally we are willing to entertain it. Failure to reject may mean that the study is too small – it lacks power. We should calculate a confidence interval about the observed effect, and believe that the truth is likely to lie within this interval. An underpowered study will have a wide confidence interval. This means that, with a small study, the results will be compatible with a large range of possible hypotheses.

To properly understand power, we need to consider an alternative hypothesis. This specifies that the treatment will have a particular effect. For example, in a trial to compare three- and four-layer compression bandages, the null hypothesis might be that the cure rate at 3 months is 50% for both treatments. The alternative hypothesis is that the three-layer bandage has a cure rate of 50% and the four-layer a cure rate of 60%. The difference, 10%, is the effect size. The power for a study of a given size is the probability of getting a statistically significant result, given that the alternative hypothesis is true.

Despite the impossibility of proving equivalence, one can design trials to demonstrate it. To do this we need to specify a difference, within which we are prepared to say groups are equivalent. For example, we might concede that, if a difference in cure rates of 5% between the three- and four-layer bandages was observed, we would take them to be equivalent. Usually equivalence trials need larger numbers than conventional trials[6]. Above all, simply because a difference is not significant does *not* mean that treatments are equivalent.

HIERARCHY OF DESIGNS

Suppose we now wanted to evaluate a particular therapy – compression bandages for leg ulcers, for example. There is a well-known 'hierarchy' of designs that gives an increasing weight of evidence from different types of study[5,6]. These are described in Table 1. It is noteworthy that this evidence is for testing prior hypotheses relating to therapies. There is a whole branch of research methodology – qualitative research – that has equal validity, but it is largely involved in exploring and developing hypotheses.

The weakest level is the so-called *case-series*. An eminent nurse writes a note to say that he or she has tried a particular compression bandage in patients with venous leg ulcers and has achieved excellent results. There are many criticisms of this design. Firstly, we do not know how the patients have been selected; the nurse may have an unerring eye for selecting those who are likely to recover anyway. Secondly, without further evidence of the natural history of the disease, we do not know whether the patients may have recovered naturally, without intervention. Thirdly, we do not know whether this type of compression bandage is better or worse than any other.

This leads to the second level of evidence, which is the *case–control study*. This can be used for looking at the effectiveness of established therapies. We examine a group of patients, some of whom have improved and some of whom got worse. We then look to see what proportion of cases and controls were treated with the particular compression bandage in question. If there is a statistical difference with, for example, a greater proportion of people treated with the bandage in the cases, we might conclude that the bandage is effective. The main problems of this design are that we have no idea *why* patients would be given one therapy rather than another; for all we know, it might be directly related to outcome. For example, those with the worst ulcers are given four-layer bandages.

For new therapies, we might try a 'before-and-after' design. For example, if we have always treated patients with a three-layer bandage and we then introduce a four-layer bandage, we can compare the outcomes before and after the introduction of the new therapy. This is a very plausible scenario. After all, Fleming did not need a clinical trial to demonstrate the efficacy of penicillin. Prior to the discovery and use of penicillin, most people with certain bacterial infections died, but afterwards they survived. The main disadvantage of 'before-and-after' designs is that we have no idea whether the patients in the two groups are comparable. Whilst it is hard to imagine the natural history or incidence of a disease would change when a new therapy is introduced, it is plausible that the way the disease is diagnosed and patients recruited for treatment have changed. As an example, Christie[7] looked at survival after stroke before and after the introduction of a CT scanner. Patients who had a scan were matched by age, sex and level of consciousness with patients who had a stroke before the introduction of the machine. Survival was better after the scan than before. However, Christie then chose a control group consisting of patients who had *not* had a scan *after* the introduction of the machine and matched them to another group of stroke patients who were admitted before the CT machine. Again, survival was better after the introduction of the machine. Two possibilities are that other types of stroke therapy had improved over the period that the machine was introduced or that patients with milder disease were being admitted to hospital after the machine was introduced.

A rather stronger design is a prospective one called a *quasi-experimental design*. Sometimes, this is described as a cohort design, although, usually in epidemiology, cohort designs are purely observational, i.e. there is no direct intervention. In this instance, patients from one clinic, for example, are given the four-layer bandage and patients in another clinic act as a control group and get standard therapy. The difficulty here is that again patients in the different clinics may not be comparable.

A design that is often used in Health Services Research is a community intervention design. This is an extension of a quasi-experimental design. For example, the cure rates for chronic ulcers are observed in two clinics. A new intervention is introduced in one clinic, and after a period of time the cure rates are again measured. An important point is that the subjects at each time point are *different*. Also the allocation of the intervention to the clinic/community is done for pragmatic reasons, such as convenience.

The type of design which provides the strongest type of evidence is the *randomized controlled trial*. In this, patients are allocated treatment by some form of random mechanism. In this way we can ensure that *in the long run* patients before treatment will be comparable in the intervention and control groups. Clearly, if one knew which were the important prognostic factors, one could match the patients in the intervention and control groups. The advantage of randomization is that known and unknown factors will tend to balance out in the long term.

A further refinement is to blind (or mask) the patients as to which treatment they are receiving, which yields the single-blind trial, and to blind both the patients and the person doing the evaluations, which yields the *double-blind randomized controlled trial*. There are clearly extensions to this, since one could also blind the care givers and data analysts. Often with wound trials, which involve large pieces of equipment, it is impossible to blind the patient. However, there are feasible ways of blinding assessors by use of videos of patients or photographs of wounds. Where these are completely impossible, it is important to use objective measures such as wound diameter. The reason for the intellectual attraction of the double-blind randomized controlled trial is that it is the *only* design that can give us an absolute certainty that there is no bias in favor of one group compared to another at the start of the study.

ADVANTAGES AND DISADVANTAGES OF RANDOMIZED CONTROLLED TRIALS

There is some controversy over how much emphasis should be placed on the pre-eminence of randomized controlled trials over other forms of evidence. On the one hand, for example, it has been argued that scientific committees should turn down any non-randomized study because of its 'inherent bias'[8]. On the other hand, it has been argued that randomization is unnecessary when the effect of an intervention is so dramatic that the contribution of unknown confounding factors can plausibly be ignored, for example, defibrillation for ventricular fibrillation[9].

Randomization may be inappropriate where a trial would have to be of disproportionate size and duration, and thus expense, if it were to detect very rare long-term adverse effects or the impact of policies designed to prevent rare events. For example, no adverse events were detected in trials of the anti-inflammatory drug benoxaprofen, involving some 3000 patients. However it was subsequently found, from post-marketing surveillance, to have been associated with 61 deaths[10].

The main problem of randomized controlled trials relates to the issue of the generalizability. The process through which patients become involved in trials, including differential participation by centers, practitioners or patients may limit the confidence with which the results can be applied in routine practice. It may be argued that non-randomized studies, which often have more inclusive entry criteria and procedures, may include subjects that are more representative of the population to whom the results may be applied. Even the process of recruitment, in which only individuals willing to be randomized will be recruited, may introduce hidden biases that make subjects unrepresentative of the reference population. Randomized controlled trials have been criticized because they often exclude patients about whom clinicians may seek advice on treatment. They may exclude women, the elderly, those with strong preferences and those with multiple pathology or severe disease.

A further concern is the setting, which may not be typical of those in which most people are treated; the trial may take place in a center of excellence, which is not where most people experience therapy. Thus the results from a trial might show larger benefits than would be experienced in general practice.

Randomization may be misleading where the process of random allocation may affect the effectiveness of the intervention. This can arise when subjects cannot be blinded to the intervention because the intervention requires their active participation, which in turn will be affected by their underlying beliefs and preferences. Consider a trial of effectiveness of clinical audit in improving the quality of wound care. This would be difficult because effectiveness depends on the attitudes of the participating clinicians. In some circumstances, experiments may be impossible in practice as clinicians may not accept that there is uncertainty about the relative merit of different interventions and thus deem a trial unethical. It is possible that a preference for a treatment will enhance its therapeutic effect (or perhaps preference for another treatment will reduce the effect of the offered treatment)[11]. An example of such a trial might be a trial of psychotherapy compared to pharmacologic treatment for depression. Randomized controlled trials, by necessity and design, ignore people's preferences and so may underestimate the main effects. Unfortunately, when people have strong preferences, randomization is difficult; one cannot randomize between enthusiasts for a treatment and those who strongly reject it.

A major criticism of non-randomized trials is the possibility that groups being compared differ in prognostically important characteristics. The key question is whether the potential for allocation bias can be identified and, if present, whether it can be overcome in the analysis. This may be possible if the outcome measure can itself be measured prior to and after therapy. For example, if the outcome is wound diameter, it would be helpful to have a baseline measurement as well. The main problem is that, in the absence of a truly random allocation method, there is no way of knowing that the allocation method is not biased. This is also true when the method is random but is not concealed so that the treatment allocation can be predicted in advance. Thus, for example, allocating treatments in order A,B,A,B is not random and can be predicted. Although one can argue that the order that the patients arrive in the trial is random, it has been found from bitter experience that knowledge of the eventual treatment can affect recruitment to a trial and thus bias the comparison groups. Investigators, knowing which treatment a patient will get if they enter the trial, may be influenced as to whether that patient is actually entered. Similarly, if patients knew what therapy they were likely to get, they may also be influenced. It does not take a great deal of imagination to imagine one is suffering from an incurable disease, when a possible new cure is announced. How many of us would volunteer for the placebo?

The problems for and against randomized controlled trials have lead Peto and co-workers[12] to argue, at every available opportunity, that we should be conducting large, simple randomized controlled trials. These mega-trials should have as unrestricted an entry as possible and recruit tens of thousands of patients, or possibly every incident case of a disease in the country. Their very size and nature means that the treatment groups would be comparable and the trials generalizable.

The arguments for and against randomized controlled trials are summarized in Table 2.

COMPARISON OF RANDOMIZED AND NON-RANDOMIZED STUDIES OF THE SAME THERAPY

A recent review compared randomized and non-randomized trials[13]. It found no obvious patterns; neither randomized controlled trials nor non-randomized studies gave consistently larger or smaller estimates of treatment effect. A greater effect might occur if patients receive higher quality care or are selected in a way that gives greater capacity to benefit. A lower estimate of treatment effect may occur if the way the patients are selected to the randomized controlled trials produces a study population with less capacity to benefit than would be the case for a non-randomized study. Also, for unblinded randomized controlled trials, a lower estimate may be obtained if there exists a strong patient preference in favor of one treatment.

The authors found that large clinical databases that contain detailed information on patient severity and prognosis have been used instead of randomized controlled trials[13]. Where the database subjects are selected according to the same inclusion criteria, the

Table 2 Arguments for and against randomized controlled trials

Argument	Comment
For	
Balances known and unknown prognostic factors – only method which guarantees bias free comparison	Guarantee is only true with infinite sample size. Requires a large sample to balance a moderate number of covariates
Use of a control group	Allows for the fact that patients can recovery naturally
Blindness means that psychologic effects should be minimized	Many therapies struggle to retain blindness for a long period of time, especially if the treatment works
Against	
Highly selected group of patients – not generalizable	Design trials which allow wide selection criteria, including elderly people
Patient preference may alter outcome	This is a problem with unblinded studies
Does not reflect the way therapies are used in practice	The solution is to use more naturalistic trials

treatment effects of the two methods are of similar size.

IMPROVING THE QUALITY OF REPORTING OF RANDOMIZED CONTROLLED TRIALS

There is a wide variety in the quality of the conduct and reporting of randomized controlled trials. A recent document describes items that should be reported, to indicate that the trial has been conducted to a high standard[14]. These include:

(1) The method of randomization should be reported. The allocated treatment group should be unknown to the investigator until after the patient has been recruited to the trial;

(2) Where possible, the treatment should be blind to the patient and the investigator. Where it is impossible to blind treatment to the patient, it is sometimes possible to blind the evaluator. For example, if the patients are to be interviewed about their experiences of a particular therapy, the interviewer could be kept in ignorance of the therapy the patient has had;

(3) As many patients as possible should be followed up. Drop-outs should be reported by treatment group;

(4) Where the trial is set up to investigate differences in therapies, analysis should be by intention to treat (ITT). This means that subjects should be analyzed by the treatment they were randomized to and not the treatment they received. Thus subjects who do not comply with therapy will be analyzed as if they received therapy. Subjects who drop out of the trial, but for whom outcome measures are available, should be included in the group to which they were randomized for analysis. This tends to lead to conservative estimates of treatment effects, but reflects more closely what happens in real life, where subjects are not compelled to take treatments. ITT is important for validity, since people often drop out of trials for reasons related to outcome, such as they fail to make progress or they are cured. Use of ITT maintains the integrity of the groups as

they were randomized, since we know that we make unbiased comparisons between these groups. However, ITT should *not* be used in trials designed to demonstrate that two treatments are equivalent, since this will bias the study toward demonstrating equivalence.

The alternative to ITT, which specifies in the protocol that analyses of subjects should be by the treatment they actually receive, is called a per protocol analysis.

NICE REPORT – WOUND CARE TECHNOLOGIES: DEBRIDING AGENTS

Most surgically sutured wounds heal without complication. However, in some cases wound healing can be delayed due to the presence of infection or wound breakdown. This can result in wounds becoming cavity wounds that necessitate healing by secondary intention. Other surgical wounds that are not sutured but left to heal by secondary intention include abscess cavities such as peri-anal abscesses or breast abscesses.

Debridement involves the removal of devitalized, necrotic tissue or fibrin from a wound. The effectiveness of debridement has not been confirmed by clinical research, although it is generally agreed that wounds that contain devitalized and necrotic tissue require debriding[15,16]. There are many different methods that can be used to debride a wound. These are broadly classified as surgical/sharp, biosurgical (maggots), mechanical, chemical, enzymatic and autolytic (see Table 3).

The review[3] looked at eight databases, including MEDLINE, EMBASE and the Cochrane Controlled Trials register. Only randomized controlled trials or quasi-experimental studies were considered. Only studies that reported an objective measurement of wound healing were included in the review, although patient outcomes, such as ease of use or pain, were reported in some of the included studies

as well. Only studies reported in English, German, Dutch or French were included.

A total of 137 studies identified by the main searches were excluded, as they did not meet the inclusion criteria. The main reason for exclusion for the majority of the remaining studies was that they did not investigate surgical wound healing by secondary intention. Most looked at either sutured wounds or chronic wounds, such as venous leg ulcers, pressure sores and diabetic foot ulcers. Twenty-nine studies were excluded because they had no objective measure of healing, 20 because they had no control group and eight because they were case studies. Some of the studies were excluded on a number of these criteria. Twenty-three were reported in a language not covered by the review (15 in Russian).

Seventeen studies met the inclusion criteria, all of which used autolytic methods of debridement. Fifteen of the studies were randomized controlled trials and two were quasi-experimental studies. Four different types of debriding agent were used in the included studies. These were dressings using: foam, alginate, hydrocolloid and dextranomer polysaccharide beads. Gauze or gauze-based dressings were used as a comparator in 14 trials.

Fourteen trials were for surgical wounds. Of these, five of the studies related to healing by secondary intention after pilonidal abscess excision. Four of the surgical studies investigated the treatment of postoperative wounds from toenail avulsions.

QUALITY OF INCLUDED STUDIES

In general, the quality of the reported trials was poor. Only three of the 14 surgical wound trials reported the method used to randomize participants to different intervention groups. In one trial, patients were allocated numbers and those with even numbers were treated with the intervention dressing, whereas those with odd numbers received the standard

Table 3 Types of debridement methods

Classification	Technique	Comments
Surgical	Sharp instrument (scalpel or scissors)	Quick but imprecise
Biosurgical	Larvae therapy	Maggots destroy dead tissue by liquefying it with enzymes and ingesting it. There is no available guidance with which to select patients for this technique. There is a degree of unacceptability and a degree of uncertainty about adverse effects from damage to live tissues by maggots.
Mechanical	Wet-to-dry dressings, wound irrigation, adherent dressings	May remove viable tissue at the same time
Chemical	Hypochlorite solution	It has been argued that free radical generation may cause damage
Autolytic	The body's natural process of debridement	Can be enhanced by promoting a moist wound environment, using dressings such as hydrocolloids, alginate and foam dressings and polysaccharide beads or paste
Enzymatic	Topical enzymes	Target specific necrotic tissue

dressing. Treatment allocation is thus unlikely to have been concealed from those conducting the procedure and so the study was considered quasi-randomized. Detailed information regarding blinding was not reported in most trials.

Follow-up was relatively complete (greater than 80%) in 10 out of 13 surgical trials. None of the seven trials of surgical wounds that were deemed to have no drop-outs reported using an ITT analysis or a per protocol analysis, so it was impossible to ascertain if non-compliers had been included in the analysis correctly.

Only one of the trials of surgical wounds reported the blinding of the outcome assessors to treatment allocation.

Nine of the 14 surgical trials reported information on baseline characteristics, which included the initial wound size. Seven of the trials were judged to have used an appropriate test to analyze the data. Three trials did not report what statistical test had been used. Three trials did not use any statistical analysis to compare treatment groups.

Trials were relatively small (median sample size 43). As was discussed earlier, small trials that are not significant are very difficult to interpret.

In summary, the majority of trials reported in the systematic review suffered methodologic flaws.

FINDINGS OF THE REVIEW

One of the surprising findings of the review is that the clinical effectiveness of debridement itself had never been formally evaluated, despite having been in use for some 200 years and being common practice in wound management.

The review found four studies that compared silicone elastomer foam versus traditional moist gauze. No significant difference in healing time was found. One small poor-quality trial showed a slight difference between polyurethane foam and gauze dressings. One trial failed to show a difference in mean healing time comparing polyurethane foam and silicone foam. Three trials compared alginate dressing to traditional gauze and in two of them a statistically significant difference in mean healing time was found. No other significant comparisons were found.

One critical fact in supporting the review is that *all* the relevant evidence has been assembled. This means that the review should publish a careful summary of its searching techniques and that the reviewers searched the 'gray' (unpublished reports and company documents), as well as peer-reviewed publications. Interested parties are given a chance to produce evidence of studies that the reviewers may have missed.

NICE APPRAISAL: COMMITTEE'S DECISION

What was the committee to make of the evidence? The evidence put before them included not only the review, but also manufacturers' submissions, patient evidence and expert opinions. Manufacturers' submissions may consist of case studies – patients who have received a benefit from a particular therapy, which, it is claimed, would not have been achieved in the absence of the therapy. If good-quality trials were available, then these would have precedence in helping to form opinions. In their absence, the committee have to weigh trial and observational evidence, together with expert and patient opinion. For example, patients attested to the painful nature of having impregnated gauze removed from wounds and the possible revulsion from the use of larval therapy. In addition, the committee had to decide whether evidence from the field of chronic wound healing could be carried over to the healing of surgical wounds. On this point, the opinion was that it would be unsafe to assume that therapies that worked for chronic wounds could be assumed to work for surgical wounds.

The committee's conclusions can be found in the Final Appraisal document[17]. The document states:

> 'There is a suggestion that modern dressings have a beneficial effect on healing, compared to traditional gauze dressings, especially for toenail avulsions. Due to methodologic flaws, these results should be interpreted with caution. For outcomes other than healing, modern dressings suggested benefit for surgical wounds but not toenail avulsions; however, these outcomes are hard to assess and particularly subject to bias, especially in unblinded studies. ... Any evidence taken from single case studies should be treated with caution. There is no evidence to support the superiority of one type of modern dressing over another.'

These documents are usually only given a 3-year period of validity. Accruing evidence may change the advice in later years.

The conclusions are based on a number of different sources: trials, quasi-experimental studies and expert and patient opinion. Note that 'absence of evidence is not evidence of absence'. The guidance is not saying that there is *no* difference in the outcomes from different types of modern dressings, simply that in some cases the evidence was poor and in others absent. Trials may subsequently be conducted in these areas and then the guidance may be altered.

An important outcome from the review is a clarification of where evidence is lacking and where further research should be aimed.

CONCLUSION

Advisory bodies have to make decisions about medical treatments based on evidence. It is their duty to ensure that all available evidence is made known to them. The best evidence is from double-blind randomized controlled trials. However, it is often the case that these are of poor quality or not available. When trial evidence is available, it does not necessarily give consistent results. Decisions have to be made by making the best of available evidence and it is most important that any guidance is clear when based on 'mere' clinical opinion.

A further decision that advisory bodies have to make is not only to decide whether a therapy is effective, but also *cost*-effective. A therapy may have a small but significant effect, but be extremely expensive and so its use would mean that other patients would be deprived of other treatment.

CONFLICT OF INTEREST

The author was technical lead for the NICE appraisal team for the guidance on debridement for difficult-to-heal surgical wounds.

ACKNOWLEDGEMENTS

The author is grateful to Nicky Cullum, Jon Nicholl, Raj Mani and Alicia O'Cathain for their helpful comments on this chapter.

References

1. Sackett DL, Richardson WS, Rosenberg W, Haynes RB. *Evidence-based Medicine: How to Practice and Teach EBM*. New York: Churchill Livingstone, 1997

2. Gilman EA, Cheng KK, Winter HR, Scragg R. Trends in rates and seasonal distribution of sudden infant deaths in England and Wales, 1988–92. *Br Med J* 1995;310:631–2

3. Lewis R, Whiting P, ter Reit G, O'Meara S, Glanville J, for the National Institute for Clinical Excellence. A rapid sytematic review of the clinical effectiveness and cost effectiveness of debriding agents in treating surgical wounds healing by secondary intention. NHS HTA Programme, 2000: www.nice.org.uk/pdf/Woundcare HTA report.pdf

4. Bradford Hill A. The environment and disease: association or causation. *Proc R Soc Med* 1965; 58:295–300

5. Campbell MJ, Machin D. *Medical Statistics: A Commonsense Approach*, 3rd edn. Chichester: John Wiley, 1999: chapter 2

6. Campbell MJ. Design and analysis of research studies in wound healing. In Mani R, Falanga V, Shearman CP, Sandeman D, eds. *Chronic Wound Healing: Clinical Measurement and Basic Science*. London: WB Saunders, 1999:170–8

7. Christie D. Before and after comparisons: a cautionary tale. *Br Med J* 1979;279:1629–30

8. Ellenberg JH. Selection bias in observational and experimental studies. *Stat Med* 1994;13:557–67

9. Black N. Why we need observational studies to evaluate the effect of health care. *Br Med J* 1996;312:1215–18

10. Opren scandal [Editorial]. *Lancet* 1983;1:219–20

11. McPherson K. The best and the enemy of the good: randomised controlled trials, uncertainty, and assessing the role of patient preference in medical decision making. The Cochrane Lecture. *J Epidemiol Community Health* 1994;48:6–15

12. Peto R, Collins R, Gray R. Large-scale randomized evidence: large, simple trials and overviews of trials. *J Clin Epidemiol* 1995;48:23–40

13. Britton A, McKee M, Black N, McPherson K, Sanderson C, Bain C. Choosing between randomised and non-randomised studies: a systematic review. *Health Technol Assess* 1998;2:13

14. Moher D, Schultz KF, Altman DG. The CONSORT statement: revised recommendations for improving the quality of reports of parallel-group randomized trials. *Lancet* 2001; 357:1191–4

15. Bradley M, Cullum N, Sheldon T. The debridement of chronic wounds: a systematic review. *Health Technol Assess* 1999;3:iii–iv, 1–78

16. Rodeheaver G, Baharestani MM, Brabec ME, *et al*. Wound healing and wound management: focus on debridement. *Adv Wound Care* 1994;7: 22–36

17. National Institute for Clinical Excellence. Guidance on the use of debriding agents and specialist wound care clinics for difficult to heal surgical wounds. London: National Institute for Clinical Excellence, 2001

Medical therapy for leg ulcers

3

J. Kantor and D. J. Margolis

INTRODUCTION

Chronic wound care has changed little over the past century; compression, debridement, dressing changes and other features of wound care familiar to many practitioners are practiced in much the same way as they were over 100 years ago. The use of medical therapies – both systemic and topical – in treating these wounds remains an exception to this rule. Recent studies on everything from pentoxifylline[1-4] to recombinant growth factor therapy[5-7] have made the world of therapeutics a dynamic place. Given the mood of excitement surrounding growth factor therapy and tissue engineering, however, it is important to appreciate that these treatments are, in many cases, mere adjuncts to the foundations of wound care that have been practiced for a century or more. Indeed, medical therapy for chronic wounds must occur within the context of a comprehensive wound-care regimen. Even the most advanced growth-factor therapies will be ineffective if a wound is not off-loaded, debrided or dressed appropriately.

This chapter is not inclusive of all possible therapies for chronic wounds, but discusses some of the most common medical therapies for leg ulcers. Since most medically managed leg ulcers are of either venous, diabetic neuropathic or pressure in origin, these will represent the clinical focus of this chapter[8]. Both systemic and topical therapies are addressed, although details of dressing choices are not a part of this chapter.

PENTOXIFYLLINE

Pentoxifylline is a trisubstituted xanthine derivative that has been used to treat a variety of systemic disorders, most notably intermittent claudication[1]. Theorizing that its beneficial effect for vaso-occlusive disease could extend to therapy for venous ulcers, several studies have explored the potential benefits of pentoxifylline in treating patients with venous leg ulcers.

Most recently, two randomized trials were conducted to evaluate the efficacy of pentoxifylline therapy. These trials are the subject of a recent critical commentary[1]. A study by Dale and co-workers[4] evaluated pentoxifylline 400 mg three times daily with limb compression versus limb compression and placebo. The investigators utilized the probability of healing by 24 weeks of therapy as their primary end-point. Despite finding an absolute risk difference of 11% favoring pentoxifylline therapy, this result was not statistically significant. The failure to attain statistical significance may be secondary to the sample size, since this study was powered to detect a 20% benefit over standard care.

A second study evaluating the use of pentoxifylline in a higher dose did demonstrate a statistically significant benefit of pentoxifylline therapy over placebo when taken as 800 mg three times daily[2]. The median time to healing was 71 days for the pentoxifylline group versus 100 days for the placebo group ($p = 0.04$). There was no significant improvement over placebo for patients treated with 400 mg three times daily (median time to healing was 83 days). It is therefore possible that pentoxifylline has a beneficial effect on venous ulcers, but that this effect is only seen at higher doses than have traditionally been used to treat intermittent claudication.

A separate Cochrane Collaborative Review also supports the efficacy of pentoxifylline for the treatment of these wounds[3]. Given the results of these two recent clinical trials, it appears that pentoxifylline may represent a reasonable choice when deciding on adjuvant medical therapy for venous leg ulcers. Still, both clinical trials found only a modest benefit in patients treated with pentoxifylline. Given the relatively low incidence of side-effects reported in these trials, however, pentoxifylline – as either 400 mg or 800 mg three times daily – should be considered in patients with venous ulcers. Nevertheless, clinicians must ultimately decide whether a possible 10% absolute risk difference in healing by 24 weeks is worth both the practical and financial cost of pentoxifylline.

ANTIBIOTIC THERAPY

Clinicians, in a zealous attempt to maintain an aseptic wound environment, often begin the treatment of patients with chronic wounds with either oral or topical antibiotics. This practice stems from a very reasonable concern, particularly in patients with diabetes, that superficial wound colonization or perhaps infection might progress to deeper tissue infection and then to osteomyelitis. This could ultimately lead to limb amputation[9].

While this is certainly a logical approach, it is predicated on the assumption that wound infection – and the ensuing osteomyelitis and limb amputation – can be prevented by prophylactically administering antibiotic therapy. A controlled trial evaluating the use of antibiotic therapy in patients with diabetic foot ulcers, however, failed to detect a significant benefit of antibiosis[10]. The host of problems associated with the *laissez faire* use of antibiotic therapy (including everything from drug side-effects to antibiotic-resistant organisms), coupled with a dearth of evidence to support antibiotic use in this population, translates into a strong argument against the routine use of systemic antibiotic therapy among patients with uncomplicated chronic wounds. The logic for using systemic antibiotics may also be predicated on diminishing wound bio-burden (i.e. the colonization in tissue infection of the wound by bacteria). While there is ample evidence that graft take is impeded if more than 10^6 bacteria per gram of tissue can be cultured, there is no conclusive information that systemic antibiotics can be used to diminish the concentration of wound bacteria and this problem is probably best handled by debridement[11–14].

Similarly, topical antibiotic preparations have also not been shown to improve the probability of treatment success[14,15]. Furthermore, they are formulated for use on intact skin and thus their absorption and efficacy on a wound have usually not been evaluated.

When clinical evidence of wound infection exists, systemic antibiotic therapy should be initiated. The choice of individual agent, as well as the route of delivery (parenteral versus oral) must be tailored to the individual clinical situation[16]. A patient presenting with a fulminant wound and Gram-negative sepsis should clearly be started on parenteral therapy, while an individual with peri-wound erythema and warmth without obvious systemic involvement could likely be started on oral therapy.

Choice of antibiotic agent must be geared toward the suspected organism. Empiric therapy is appropriate early in the course of care[16]. While acute wound infections often occur secondary to Gram-positive bacteria, particularly epithelial flora, chronic wounds may be colonized or infected by a broader array of organisms, including Gram-negative and anaerobic bacteria. Thus, therapy must always be chosen based on the clinical circumstances of the presumed wound infection.

The value of wound cultures derived from swabbing the wound is questionable. Wounds, like intact epithelial surfaces, are colonized by numerous bacterial species and therefore microbiologic diagnoses based on swabbing the wound surface have little if any bearing on the organisms responsible for the wound infection *per se*[16]. A deeper tissue sample is therefore needed in order to appropriately ascertain the presence and nature of the infecting organism. In diabetic foot ulcers, where surgical debridement is a cornerstone of standard therapy, tissue samples may be taken after debriding the surface eschar. For patients with venous leg ulcers that often do not necessitate aggressive surgical debridement, the decision to surgically remove a deep tissue sample for microbiologic analysis must be reached after considering risks and benefits[17,18].

Oral agents for the treatment of infections in foot ulcers may include cephalexin, clindamycin and the fluoroquinolones[16]. Parenteral antibiotics should be chosen based on the susceptibility patterns of the responsible organisms. Studies have suggested that agents such as imipenem/cilastin, ampicillin/sulbactam, piperacillin/tazobactam and third-generation cephalosporins such as cefoxitin and ceftazidime may be effective in treating these infections[16,19]. Importantly, when patients have serious complications necessitating parenteral antibiotic therapy, they must also be evaluated for other systemic complications such as electrolyte abnormalities and possible surgical intervention.

Topical applications of bleach, Dakin's solution or other skin cleansers or antiseptic agents are generally ineffective at preventing or minimizing infection, since the bacterial infections representing the root cause of the problem are generally deeper than the superficial layers of the wound reached by these topical agents. More importantly, while these harsh chemicals are indeed effective at killing bacteria *in vitro*, they exert a similar destructive effect on the granulation tissue necessary for wound healing and have been demonstrated to have cytotoxic effects. Rather than improving healing rates, topical application of these chemicals is believed to result in poor healing since the granulation tissue is being repeatedly injured by their application. Normal saline or water is probably the least toxic skin-cleansing agent. However, overly aggressive irrigation, even with normal saline, may also be damaging to the wound bed and may lead to the traumatic removal of granulation tissue needed for appropriate wound healing.

VITAMINS, ELEMENTS AND MINERALS

Few practitioners dispute the importance of adequate nutrition for promoting wound healing. Despite the assumption that vitamin and mineral supplementation may aid in healing these wounds, few studies have addressed the potential benefits of this supplementation in a rigorous fashion. Supplemental vitamin C is often prescribed for patients with chronic wounds. The well-known effects of excessive ascorbic acid deprivation, as seen in scurvy, include a susceptibility to non-healing wounds. Some reports have evaluated the use of vitamin C as an adjunctive wound-healing agent with mixed results[20,21]. While supplementing vitamin C intake for patients with a known deficiency would be prudent, the role of excessive so-called mega-dosing with ascorbic acid is questionable. Given the prevalence of malnourishment in the community of adults with chronic wounds, the low cost of ascorbic acid and the low incidence of side-effects secondary to supplementation with a water-soluble vitamin, it would certainly be reasonable to provide vitamin C supplementation, especially in those with pressure ulcers, the population of chronic wound patients most likely to be malnourished.

Zinc has been used for more than a century as a topical adjunct for the care of chronic wounds[22]. Unna believed that the zinc paste in his boots had a beneficial effect on healing; it now appears more likely that the continued popularity of the Unna boot for patients with venous leg ulcers stems from its compressive effects on the lower extremity in patients with venous ulcers[23]. One study demonstrated a debriding effect of topical zinc paste in pressure ulcer patients, although it is not clear whether this effect improved the likelihood of healing[21]. Another study suggested that topical zinc oxide improves healing in both arterial and venous ulcers[22]. However, a study in porcine skin suggested that the only beneficial action of zinc on the wound bed was that it aided in inhibiting bacterial growth[24]. While oral zinc supplementation as a systemic therapy has not been formally evaluated, it would not be unreasonable to provide patients with a multivitamin on a daily basis in order to optimize their vitamin and mineral intake.

Magnesium, whether in milk of magnesia or antacid form, has also been evaluated as an adjunctive therapy for pressure ulcers[21]. A small, randomized, controlled trial in pressure ulcer patients failed to detect a benefit of antacid therapy; notably, this study may have been under-powered to demonstrate an effect of antacid[25]. Other studies have evaluated combination zinc acetate spray and aluminum hydroxide ointment and have reported a benefit of this therapy in a cohort of nursing home patients with pressure ulcers[26].

No studies have effectively evaluated the role of a daily multivitamin in patients with chronic wounds. Other unexplored therapies include iron supplementation. Adequate tissue iron levels are needed for appropriate metabolic functioning and indeed mildly decreased iron levels may be associated with hair loss[27]. Since granulation tissue represents an environment of rapid cell proliferation, it is possible that wound healing may be sensitive to mildly decreased levels of iron, although this has yet to be demonstrated. Several studies have addressed the efficacy of rutosides in decreasing the edema associated with venous insufficiency[28–33]. Results appear to be promising and these drugs may be useful in patients with venous ulcers, since these wounds generally cannot heal in the setting of persistent edema. Moreover, reducing the edema of venous insufficiency may reduce the likelihood of future wounds. Finally, case series evaluating the role of gold leaf for chronic wounds have been published, although they failed to demonstrate a beneficial effect[34].

GROWTH FACTORS

The popularity of using autologous or recombinant growth factors to mediate the healing process has ballooned in recent years. While animal models of chronic wounds have for almost 20 years shown that growth factors can be used to improve wound healing, only recently have growth factor-based therapies become available. Like other therapies discussed in this chapter, however, it is important to keep in mind that these therapies are not a panacea for healing all wounds. The principles of good wound care – maintaining a moist wound environment, off-loading if needed and compression for venous ulcers – remain the pillars of wound care.

One of the first clinically available growth factors was autologous platelet releasate (PR)[35]. Available as a proprietary product at a group of wound centers, PR is derived by drawing a patient's blood and then exposing it to a plastic that encourages platelet degranulation. This platelet soup, composed in large part by platelet-derived growth factor

(PDGF), is then injected into the patient's wound. Presumably it is the super-physiologic levels of PDGF that are responsible for the action of PR, although this has not been demonstrated. The rationale behind this approach is that the patient's own growth factors are used to stimulate increased wound-healing activity. While this technique has been in use clinically for over a decade, a recent study using propensity scores demonstrated a modest beneficial effect of this therapy[35]. An important finding of this study was that the most severe wounds were those least likely to heal with standard care alone, but most likely to benefit from PR. Although this is a proprietary product, the technology behind the manufacture of PR is publicly available and may be undertaken by individual hospital centers of clinicians. A cost-effectiveness analysis suggested that, while PR appears to increase the proportion of patients healed after 20 weeks of care, it remains a costly therapy[36].

Despite the apparent effectiveness of autologous PR for treating diabetic neuropathic foot ulcers, its efficacy has not been established in randomized clinical trials. Recently, recombinant PDGF-BB (becaplermin) has been approved by the US Food and Drug Administration (FDA) for use in diabetic neuropathic ulcers. Four studies evaluated the efficacy and safety of topically applied becaplermin and concluded that this pharmaceutical is both safe and effective[6,7,37]. Becaplermin is applied once daily and dressing changes are made every 12 h, alternating between becaplermin and saline-moistened gauze. Like all treatments for diabetic foot ulcers, the effectiveness of becaplermin is predicated on the assumption of continued good wound care, including off-loading and twice-daily dressing changes. The efficacy studies demonstrated a modest benefit of becaplermin, which increased the percentage of wounds healed at 20 weeks by an absolute margin of 10–20%. Given that approximately

30% of diabetic neuropathic ulcers heal by 20 weeks with standard care alone[38], this added benefit appears to represent a clinically significant difference. This topical medication was well-tolerated. Patients who fail to heal after 20 weeks of active treatment with becaplermin should be re-evaluated to assure that their failure to heal may not be attributed to other causes, such as a previously unnoticed arterial component. The greatest shortcoming of becaplermin therapy is its cost; as a recombinant, newly released product, many healthcare providers were initially reluctant to prescribe becaplermin. A cost–effectiveness analysis of treatment options for diabetic foot ulcers has now been published, suggesting that becaplermin therapy may represent a cost-effective adjunct to standard care for diabetic neuropathic foot ulcers of more than 8 weeks duration[36]. A potential shortcoming of becaplermin therapy is the fact that its efficacy has not been explored in patients with the most severe diabetic foot ulcers. Given that PR appears to evince a more dramatic effect for patients with the most severe wounds, it would be useful to study whether becaplermin is similarly well-suited to the treatment of these deep and recalcitrant wounds. While the original becaplermin studies focused on its efficacy in healing diabetic foot ulcers, some recent work has been done evaluating its role for the treatment of pressure ulcers as well[39]. This study concluded that becaplermin had a significant effect on healing pressure ulcers after 16 weeks of therapy, although further research is needed before this therapy can be recommended.

Another growth-factor product that has been studied recently is granulocyte colony-stimulating factor (GCSF). GCSF is produced endogenously and is known to induce terminal differentiation and release of neutrophils from the bone marrow[40]. GCSF may play a central role in the body's response to infection and this is suggested by evidence that GCSF concentrations rise during sepsis, regardless of immunologic status. Diabetic foot ulcers are often complicated both by frank infection and by the impaired ability of a patient with diabetes to respond to infectious challenges. A recombinant GCSF product (Filgrastim) has been produced and studied as a subcutaneous treatment for patients with infected diabetic foot ulcers. In a randomized, controlled trial, recombinant GCSF was administered once daily for 7 days to patients with infected diabetic foot ulcers[41]. Patients treated with recombinant GCSF appeared to fare better than those treated with placebo on several counts. Median time to bacterial eradication (median 4 days versus median 8 days) for patients treated with placebo, time to resolution of cellulitis (7 days versus 12 days), hospital stay duration (10 versus 17.5 days) and duration of required intravenous antibiotics needed (8.5 versus 14.5 days) were all significantly shorter in the group of patients treated with recombinant GCSF. From a clinical perspective, none of the patients treated with GCSF required surgery, while four out of 20 patients treated with placebo required surgical intervention. Side-effects were limited to a mild leukocytosis among patients treated with GCSF, although this was largely secondary to increases in the neutrophil count and returned to normal within 48 h after cessation of therapy. Another recent study of patients with limb-threatening diabetic foot ulcers found that the incidence of amputation was significantly lower in the group of patients treated with GCSF than in the placebo arm[42]. These findings suggest that GCSF may play a role in the treatment of patients with infected diabetic foot ulcers, although further efficacy and safety trials are still needed. Potential applications may also extend to treating uninfected diabetic foot ulcers and other chronic wounds, since reducing the risk of infection may aid in improving the outcome for these patients as well.

SKIN ALTERNATIVES

In addition to growth factors, one of the most exciting and burgeoning areas in wound research involves alternatives to traditional skin grafting. While skin grafts were occasionally used in some centers in order to aid in the closure of recalcitrant wounds, the difficulties associated with harvesting the donor graft, as well as the complexities associated with inducing closure of the grafted site (as well as the donor site) meant that this was a procedure that could not be undertaken lightly.

Graftskin (Apligraf) is a bilayered skin equivalent that includes both dermal and epidermal components[43]. Graftskin has been approved by the US FDA for the treatment of both venous and diabetic neuropathic foot ulcers. Graftskin is manufactured by harvesting neonatal foreskins and extracting both keratinocytes and fibroblasts which are then separately cultured to create the epidermal and dermal components, respectively. In a study of 208 patients with diabetic foot ulcers, Graftskin resulted in a significantly higher percentage of wounds healed by 12 weeks of care than conventional standard care alone (56% versus 39%)[43,44]. Graftskin was also noted to significantly increase the rate of wound closure in an analysis of mean time to healing. A separate randomized, controlled trial of 183 patients with diabetic foot ulcers of more than 2 months' duration found that patients treated with Graftskin were significantly more likely to heal after 12 weeks of therapy (55% healed versus 36% healed, $p = 0.008$)[43]. Finally, looking at another clinically important outcome, incidence of lower-extremity amputation at 6 months, patients treated with Graftskin had a significantly lower likelihood of amputation (6.3% versus 15.6%)[43]. This finding is particularly important, since, while a healed wound remains the outcome of choice that is evaluated in most studies, one of the most important reasons to treat diabetic foot ulcers aggressively is to avoid amputation, which itself is associated with an increased risk of (further) morbidity and mortality.

Graftskin has also been studied for the treatment of venous leg ulcers[43,45]. In a study that enrolled 240 patients, those treated with Graftskin along with standard care (compression) had a significantly greater percentage healed than those treated with compression alone (57% versus 40%) after 24 weeks[46]. Notably, secondary analyses evaluating the relative efficacy of Graftskin in older wounds of more than 1-year duration demonstrated that the benefit of Graftskin appeared most significant for patients with older wounds (47% versus 19%). Among patients with wounds of less than 1-year duration, there was no statistically significant difference in the percentage healed after 24 weeks for those treated with Graftskin or placebo (66% versus 73%).

While Graftskin is a bilayered skin substitute, another product, Dermagraft, is a tissue-engineered dermis derived from the foreskins of neonates[47,48]. Fibroblasts are isolated from these foreskins and are then grown on a polygalactin scaffold. Fibroblast proliferation leads to secretion of dermal collagen, fibronectin, glycosaminoglycans and growth factors that are then embedded within this matrix. Dermagraft thus represents a synthetic human dermis that need not be tissue-matched to individual patients and that may be applied directly over the surface of a wound bed. Several studies have evaluated the efficacy and safety of Dermagraft for use in diabetic foot ulcers. Both pilot studies and larger randomized, controlled trials enrolling more than 280 patients demonstrated a significant effect of Dermagraft on the healing of these wounds[48,49]. Like becaplermin, active treatment with Dermagraft appears to afford an approximately 15–20 absolute percent increase in the proportion of patients healed by 12–32 weeks, an apparently clinically – as

well as statistically – significant difference. Like becaplermin, however, Dermagraft is relatively costly, although the increased immediate costs must be weighed against the added effectiveness of this therapy over standard care, as well as the ostensibly decreased likelihood of serious wound infection and amputation for those treated with this dermal equivalent[50]. Dermagraft is currently approved for use in several countries, including Canada and the United Kingdom, but is not yet available in the US.

PAIN MANAGEMENT

Until recently, the subject of adequately treating the pain associated with chronic wounds has received scant attention. A flurry of recent interest in the inadequacy of prevalent pain management protocols has revived interest in this important area, although there remain no evidence-based studies of pain management for chronic wounds[51–54]. Since many chronic wounds last months to years, the chronicity of pain management needed presents an added challenge to the clinician caring for patients with these wounds. Pain management protocols vary by both geography and setting and therefore presenting a universally applicable set of protocols for pain management would be inappropriate. Ideally, patients should be treated with the minimum amount of medication that can lead to adequate analgesia. A reasonable approach is to begin with non-steroidal anti-inflammatory agents (NSAIDs), such as acetaminofen, and progress on to pharmaceuticals that include codeine or other narcotics. Patients who are expected to be on long-term pain medication should receive longer-acting narcotics, such as timed-release morphine (MS Contin). While not widely used, methadone is also effective at relieving severe pain and is particularly appropriate for patients who will be in need of long-term analgesia. If NSAIDs are used on a chronic basis, monitoring for gastrointestinal side-effects is advisable.

THERAPEUTIC OPTIONS BY WOUND ETIOLOGY

The three most common etiologies of chronic wounds are pressure ulcers, venous leg ulcers and diabetic neuropathic foot ulcers. While many of the agents discussed in this chapter have been designed to treat more than one of these wound types, it is important to stress that simply because a therapy has been shown to be effective for one type of wound does not translate into universal efficacy for treating all chronic wounds.

While several adjunctive agents have been approved for use in patients with diabetic foot ulcers and venous ulcers, few have been approved for use in patients with pressure ulcers. In part, this stems from the fact that the factor most responsible for the failure of pressure ulcers to heal is continued pressure on the wound bed. No amount of adjunctive therapy can counteract this effect. Whereas venous leg ulcers may fail to heal due to changes in the wound matrix, and diabetic foot ulcers may fail to heal due to changes in the microcirculation, most pressure ulcers are simply wounds secondary to pressure that will fail to heal until the pressure is relieved. In its clinical practice guidelines, the Agency for Health Care Policy and Research of the US Department of Health and Human Services rates the level of evidence supporting the use of various adjunctive therapies for pressure ulcers. These guidelines suggest that electric stimulation may be of benefit in patients with recalcitrant stage II pressure ulcers and for stage III and IV pressure ulcers (strength of evidence = B)[20]. The guidelines point to the results of several clinical trials that included a total of 147 patients that demonstrated modest improvement in the percentage of patients healed after a course of electric stimulation therapy. Because facilities for safely and effectively administering electrotherapy are limited and definitive studies have yet to be performed, this therapy has not been used widely. Other therapies, such as the use of hyperbaric oxygen, have only been evaluated in the context of case series. Further clinical investigation would be needed before recommending this therapy. Moreover, *in vitro* evidence suggests that the effects of topical hyperbaric oxygen therapy are limited to the superficial dermis and therefore there is, at this point, little evidence to support its use in patients with pressure ulcers. Various forms of light therapy have also been evaluated for the treatment of pressure ulcers[20]. These studies have not employed a clinical trial methodology to address the efficacy of infrared, ultraviolet or low-energy laser light forms in treating these wounds and therefore there is insufficient evidence to recommend their use in these patients. Many of the adjunctive therapies discussed in this chapter, including pentoxifylline, growth factors and skin equivalents have yet to demonstrate efficacy in the context of pressure ulcers and therefore cannot be recommended for these wounds.

The standard of care for venous leg ulcers remains limb compression. Many studies have used a modified Unna boot or multi-layered compression bandage. The precise method of obtaining compression seems to be less important than the overall goal of reaching approximately 30 mmHg of pressure[55,56]. Patients with venous stasis in the absence of ulceration should wear compression stockings in order to minimize the chances of re-ulceration. Adjunctive therapies that have demonstrated efficacy include pentoxifylline and Graftskin, although the relatively modest benefits afforded by these therapies mean that individual clinicians and patients must decide whether to proceed with these therapies.

Patients with diabetic neuropathic foot ulcers have perhaps the most varied potpourri of approved adjunctive treatment options.

Ulcers with a significant vascular component are usually studied separately, since the origin is distinct (despite its prevalence in a diabetic population) and the approach to treatment is initially surgical correction of the compromised vascular flow. Standard care for neuropathic diabetic foot ulcers includes saline-moistened gauze dressings on a twice-daily basis, surgical debridement and off-loading of the affected limb[38]. Adjunctive medical therapies for these wounds include platelet releasate, becaplermin, Graftskin and Dermagraft (outside of the US). As with venous ulcers, the benefits associated with most of these therapies are reasonably modest, although they may be clinically significant.

FUTURE DIRECTIONS

More than any individual therapy, the future of wound care will be guided by the methods used to study the efficacy of novel therapies for the treatment of chronic wounds. Certainly, gene therapy approaches to improving the prognosis of patients with chronic wounds appear to be promising and advances in other growth factor and skin substitute therapies may lead to further advances as well[57]. Still, no amount of basic scientific research can improve the lives of individuals with these wounds unless effective clinical trials are performed to assess the efficacy of potential therapies. Therefore, there is a need for appropriately powered and designed clinical studies of novel – and existing – therapies. Indeed, many of the medical treatments discussed in this chapter, including vitamin supplementation, are not so much ineffective as not-proven-effective for treating these wounds. Before global treatment recommendations can prudently be made, further research into the efficacy of these, as well as other, therapies is needed[20].

Finally, perhaps the most important message regarding the care of patients with chronic wounds is that, despite all the advances in medical therapies, the provision of standard care for wounds is the most important single step that can be taken in increasing the likelihood that a patient will heal. For venous ulcers, almost half of all patients heal within a few months of good standard care; for diabetic foot ulcers, the number is closer to one-third. The bulk of 'new' adjunctive medical therapies is targeted to the patients whose wounds fail to heal within this time frame.

References

1. Margolis DJ. Pentoxifylline in the treatment of venous leg ulcers. *Arch Dermatol* 2000;136: 1142–3
2. Falanga V, Fujitani RM, Diaz C, *et al*. Systemic treatment of venous leg ulcers with high doses of pentoxifylline: efficacy in a randomized, placebo-controlled trial. *Wound Repair Regen* 1999;7:208–13
3. Jull AB, Waters J, Arroll B. Oral pentoxifylline for treatment of venous leg ulcers. *Cochrane Database Syst Rev* 2000;2:000 75320
4. Dale JJ, Ruckley CV, Harper DR, Gibson B, Nelson EA, Prescott RJ. Randomised, double blind placebo controlled trial of pentoxifylline in the treatment of venous leg ulcers. *BMJ* 1999;319:875–8
5. Mandracchia VJ, Sanders SM, Frerichs JA. The use of becaplermin (rhPDGF-BB) gel for chronic nonhealing ulcers. A retrospective analysis. *Clin Podiatr Med Surg* 2001;18: 189–209
6. Ladin D. Becaplermin gel (PDGF-BB) as topical wound therapy. Plastic Surgery Educational Foundation DATA Committee. *Plast Reconstr Surg* 2000;105:1230–1
7. Smiell JM, Wieman TJ, Steed DL, Perry BH, Sampson AR, Schwab BH. Efficacy and safety of becaplermin (recombinant human platelet-derived growth factor-BB) in patients with nonhealing, lower extremity diabetic ulcers: a combined analysis of four randomized studies. *Wound Repair Regen* 1999;7:335–46

8. Lazarus GS, Cooper DM, Knighton DR, *et al.* Definitions and guidelines for assessment of wounds and evaluation of healing. *Arch Dermatol* 1994;130:489–93

9. Reiber GE, Lipsky BA, Gibbons GW. The burden of diabetic foot ulcers. *Am J Surg* 1998;176: 5S–10S

10. Chantelau E, Tanudjaja T, Altenhofer F, Ersanli Z, Lacigova S, Metzger C. Antibiotic treatment for uncomplicated neuropathic forefoot ulcers in diabetes: a controlled trial. *Diabet Med* 1996;13:156–9

11. Boyce ST, Warden GD, Holder IA. Cytotoxicity testing of topical antimicrobial agents on human keratinocytes and fibroblasts for cultured skin grafts. *J Burn Care Rehabil* 1995;16: 97–103

12. Holm J. Wound and graft infection. Clinical aspects and prophylaxis. *Acta Chir Scand Suppl* 1985;529:87–9

13. Larkin JM, Moylan JA. The role of prophylactic antibiotics in burn care. *Am Surg* 1976;42: 247–50

14. Leaper DJ. Prophylactic and therapeutic role of antibiotics in wound care. *Am J Surg* 1994;167: 15S–19S

15. Alvarez OM, Childs EJ. Pressure ulcers. Physical, supportive, and local aspects of management. *Clin Podiatr Med Surg* 1991;8:869–90

16. Lipsky BA, Berendt AR. Principles and practice of antibiotic therapy of diabetic foot infections. *Diabetes Metab Res Rev* 2000;16 (Suppl 1):S42–6

17. Temple ME, Nahata MC. Pharmacotherapy of lower limb diabetic ulcers. *J Am Geriatr Soc* 2000;48:822–8

18. O'Meara SM, Cullum NA, Majid M, Sheldon TA. Systematic review of antimicrobial agents used for chronic wounds. *Br J Surg* 2001;88: 4–21

19. Lipsky BA, Baker PD, Landon GC, Fernau R. Antibiotic therapy for diabetic foot infections: comparison of two parenteral-to-oral regimens. *Clin Infect Dis* 1997;24:643–8

20. Margolis DJ, Cohen JH. Management of chronic venous leg ulcers: a literature-guided approach. *Clin Dermatol* 1994;12:19–26

21. Margolis DJ, Lewis VL. A literature assessment of the use of miscellaneous topical agents, growth factors, and skin equivalents for the treatment of pressure ulcers. *Dermatol Surg* 1995;21:145–8

22. Brandrup F, Menne T, Agren MS, Stromberg HE, Holst R, Frisen M. A randomized trial of two occlusive dressings in the treatment of leg ulcers. *Acta Derm-Venereol* 1990;70:231–5

23. Margolis DJ, Berlin JA, Strom BL. Which venous leg ulcers will heal with limb compression bandages? *Am J Med* 2000;109:15–19

24. Agren MS, Franzen L, Chvapil M. Effects on wound healing of zinc oxide in a hydrocolloid dressing. *J Am Acad Dermatol* 1993;29:221–7

25. Becker L, Goodemote C. Treating pressure sores with or without antacid. *Am J Nurs* 1984; 84:351–2

26. Maass A, Grohe C, Oberdorf S, Sukhatme VP, Vetter H, Neyses L. Mitogenic signals control translation of the early growth response gene-1 in myogenic cells. *Biochem Biophys Res Commun* 1994;202:1337–46

27. Van Neste DJ, Rushton DH. Hair problems in women. *Clin Dermatol* 1997;15:113–25

28. Clement DL. Management of venous edema: insights from an international task force. *Angiology* 2000;51:13–17

29. Pedersen FM, Hamberg O, Sorensen MD, Neland K. Effect of O-(beta-hydroxyethyl)-rutoside (Venoruton) on symptomatic venous insufficiency in the lower limbs. *Ugeskr Laeger* 1992;154:2561–3

30. Nocker W, Diebschlag W, Lehmacher W. A 3-month, randomized double-blind dose-response study with O-(beta-hydroxyethyl)-rutoside oral solutions. *VASA J Vasc Dis* 1989; 18:235–8

31. Nocker W, Diebschlag W. Dose–response study with O-(beta-hydroxyethyl)-rutoside oral solution. *VASA J Vasc Dis* 1987;16:365–9

32. Bergqvist D, Hallbook T, Lindblad B, Lindhagen A. A double-blind trial of O-(beta-hydroxyethyl)-rutoside in patients with chronic venous insufficiency. *VASA J Vasc Dis* 1981;10:253–60

33. van Cauwenberge H. Double-blind study of the efficacy of a soluble rutoside derivative in the treatment of venous disease. *Arch Int Pharmacodyn Ther* 1972;196 (Suppl):122–30

34. Smith KW, Oden PW, Blaylock WK. A comparison of gold leaf and other occlusive therapy in the management of skin ulcers. *Arch Dermatol* 1967;96:703–7

35. Margolis DJ, Kantor J, Santanna J, Strom BL, Berlin JA. Effectiveness of platelet releasate for the treatment of diabetic neuropathic foot ulcers. *Diabetes Care* 2001;24:483–8

36. Kantor J, Margolis DJ. Treatment options for diabetic neuropathic foot ulcers: a cost-effectiveness analysis. *Dermatol Surg* 2001;27:347–51

37. Embil JM, Papp K, Sibbald G, *et al*. Recombinant human platelet-derived growth factor-BB (becaplermin) for healing chronic lower extremity diabetic ulcers: an open-label clinical evaluation of efficacy. *Wound Repair Regen* 2000;8:162–8

38. Margolis DJ, Kantor J, Berlin JA. Healing of diabetic neuropathic foot ulcers receiving standard treatment. A meta-analysis. *Diabetes Care* 1999;22:692–5

39. Rees RS, Robson MC, Smiell JM, Perry BH. Becaplermin gel in the treatment of pressure ulcers: a phase II randomized, double-blind, placebo-controlled study. *Wound Repair Regen* 1999;7:141–7

40. Edmonds M, Bates M, Doxford M, Gough A, Foster A. New treatments in ulcer healing and wound infection. *Diabetes Metab Res Rev* 2000;16 (Suppl 1):S51–4

41. Gough A, Clapperton M, Rolando N, Foster AV, Philpott-Howard J, Edmonds ME. Randomised placebo-controlled trial of granulocyte-colony stimulating factor in diabetic foot infection. *Lancet* 1997;350:855–9

42. de Lalla F, Pellizzer G, Strazzabosco M, *et al*. Randomized prospective controlled trial of recombinant granulocyte colony-stimulating factor as adjunctive therapy for limb-threatening diabetic foot infection. *Antimicrob Agents Chemother* 2001;45:1094–8

43. Veves A, Falanga V, Armstrong DG, Sabolinski ML. Graftskin, a human skin equivalent, is effective in the management of noninfected neuropathic diabetic foot ulcers: a prospective randomized multicenter clinical trial. *Diabetes Care* 2001;24:290–5

44. Eaglstein WH, Falanga V. Tissue engineering and the development of Apligraf, a human skin equivalent. *Cutis* 1998;62:1–8

45. Falanga V, Sabolinski M. A bilayered living skin construct (APLIGRAF) accelerates complete closure of hard-to-heal venous ulcers. *Wound Repair Regen* 1999;7:201–7

46. Dolynchuk K, Hull P, Guenther L, *et al*. The role of Apligraf in the treatment of venous leg ulcers. *Ostomy Wound Management* 1999;45:34–43

47. Eaglstein WH. Dermagraft treatment of diabetic ulcers. *J Dermatol* 1998;25:803–4

48. Bowering CK. Dermagraft in the treatment of diabetic foot ulcers. *J Cutan Med Surg* 1998;3 (Suppl 1):S1–32

49. Gentzkow GD, Iwasaki SD, Hershon KS, *et al*. Use of dermagraft, a cultured human dermis, to treat diabetic foot ulcers. *Diabetes Care* 1996;19:350–4

50. Allenet B, Paree F, Lebrun T, *et al*. Cost-effectiveness modeling of Dermagraft for the treatment of diabetic foot ulcers in the French context. *Diabetes Metab* 2000;26:125–32

51. Gould D. Wound management and pain control. *Nurs Stand* 1999;14:47–54

52. Emflorgo CA. The assessment and treatment of wound pain. *J Wound Care* 1999;8:384–5

53. Senecal SJ. Pain management of wound care. *Nurs Clin North Am* 1999;34:847–60

54. Rook JL. Wound care pain management. *Nurse Pract* 1997;22:122–6

55. Margolis DJ, Berlin JA, Strom BL. Risk factors associated with the failure of a venous leg ulcer to heal. *Arch Dermatol* 1999;135:920–6

56. Margolis DJ. Management of venous ulcerations. *Hosp Pract* 1992;27:32–4

57. Margolis DJ, Crombleholme T, Herlyn M. Clinical protocol: phase I trial to evaluate the safety of H5.020CMV.PDGF-B for the treatment of a diabetic insensate foot ulcer. *Wound Repair Regen* 2000;8:480–93

Compression for venous leg ulcer management

4

P. Vowden and K. R. Vowden

INTRODUCTION

The aim of this chapter is to discuss the science and practice of compression therapy as it applies to venous leg ulcer management. The data from venous ulcer studies have been examined and provide the evidence for change.

HISTORICAL BACKGROUND

Compression therapy has been used for the management of venous disease for many centuries, but compression is not, by itself, a cure for venous disease. The first known mention of leg ulcers is by Hippocrates who noted a relationship between leg ulcers and venous disorders[1]. The use of plasters and bandages to treat lower limb ulcers was suggested by Aurelius Celsus (25 BC – AD 50) and similar procedures were described by other later Roman physicians[1].

The concept of a compression garment or device developed in the late 17th century, with Richard Wiseman describing a laced stocking in 1676[2]. Wiseman observed the role of dependency and retrograde pressure in the development of lower limb ulceration. John Hunter noted the improvement in leg ulcers when patients were rested in the horizontal position[3]. Elasticated bandages were first introduced in the middle of the 19th century and there is now a wide range of products

available capable of delivering functional compression[4,5].

Contemporary use of compression therapy for venous disease dates from the recognition of the role of graduated compression in reversing the damage associated with chronic venous hypertension[6] and the identification of suitable compression levels to manage venous hypertension[7]. These, combined with improvements in material technology, have allowed the development of a number of compression bandages and other compression garments for the management of lower limb venous ulceration. Worldwide, a range of products or combination of products are used to generate compression. In the USA, for example, Unna's boot (a non-compliant, plaster-type bandage) is used, whilst, in mainland Europe and Australia, the inelastic, short-stretch bandage system is preferred[8]. In the UK, multi-layer elastic compression is widely employed using a four-layer bandage system based on the original Charing Cross four-layer treatment described by Blair[9]. Comparisons between compression systems are difficult as there is no internationally agreed performance standard or classification system for bandages or dressings, although a differing UK and European classification exists for hosiery. It is, however, clear that, for patients with venous disease, the application of graduated external compression can minimize, or in some patients reverse, the skin and vascular changes associated with chronic venous hypertension. It can also produce a fluid shift from the interstitial space back into the vascular and lymphatic compartments[10]. A list of the more commonly employed compression systems used for the treatment of venous leg ulcers is set out in Table 1.

Table 1 Commonly employed compression systems used for the treatment of venous leg ulcers. (Adapted from Thomas, 1995[5] and Cullum *et al.*, 2001[8])

Bandages:

Class	For	Function
1	Retention	To retain dressings
2	Support	To offer support for minor injuries such as sprains, e.g. crêpe. With particular application methods and frequent re-application, these bandages can apply low levels of compression, e.g. Elastocrepe (Smith and Nephew), Rosidal K (Lohman), Comprilan (Beiersdorf)
3a	Light compression	When applied in a simple spiral, these bandages provide 14–17 mmHg compression at the ankle, e.g. Elset (SSL), Litepress (Smith and Nephew), K-Plus (Parema)
3b	Moderate compression	When applied in a simple spiral, these bandages provide 18–24 mmHg compression at the ankle, e.g. Coban (3M), Co-plus (Smith and Nephew), Ko-Flex (Parema), Cofast (Robinson)
3c	High compression	When applied in a simple spiral, these bandages provide 25–35 mmHg compression at the ankle, e.g. Tensopress (Smith and Nephew), Surepress (Conva Tec), Setopress (SSL)
3d	Extra high compression	When applied in a simple spiral, these bandages provide up to 60 mmHg compression at the ankle, e.g. Blue line webbing

Compression systems:

Type	Constituents
Short stretch (inelastic)	Padding (orthopedic wool) plus short stretch bandages, e.g. Comprilan, Rosidal K, Actico (Activa)
Inelastic paste system	Paste bandage, e.g. Viscopaste (Smith and Nephew), Setopaste (SSL) plus support bandage
Three-layer elastic multi-layer	Padding (orthopedic wool) plus Class 3c bandage plus shaped tubular bandage, e.g. Shaped Tubigrip (SSL)
Four-layer elastic multi-layer	Padding (orthopedic wool) plus support bandage, e.g. crêpe, a Class 3a bandage and a cohesive moderate compression Class 3b bandage

Continued

Table 1 (continued)

Hosiery:

European standard	Compression rating	Use	Drug tariff equivalent
Class A	10–14 mmHg	Light compression only	
Class I (light support)	15–21 mmHg	Early varicose veins including those in pregnancy	14–17 mmHg
Class II (medium support)	23–32 mmHg	Moderate to severe varicose veins and the prevention of venous ulceration Also use to control mild edema	18–24 mmHg
Class III (strong support)	34–46 mmHg	Management of the post-phlebitic limb and the prevention of venous ulceration Also suitable to control moderate to severe edema	25–35 mmHg
Class IV (extra-strong support)	>49 mmHg	Control of lymphedema and congenital and acquired arteriovenous fistulae	None

*Commission Européenne de Normalisation[83]

EPIDEMIOLOGY

In a review of epidemiologic studies, Callam[11] concluded that:

> On the current available evidence, the best estimates for the whole adult population are a point prevalence for open leg ulceration of 0.15% with an open venous ulcer rate of 0.081 to 0.1%.

Local point prevalence studies confirmed this and identified over 500 active leg ulcers in a population of approximately 500 000[12,13]. The prevalence of venous ulceration is highest amongst women and increases with age.

ECONOMIC ASPECTS OF CARE

The annual cost of chronic lower limb venous ulceration to the National Health Service (NHS) was estimated to be approaching £400 million in 1991, i.e. 1–2% of the total health-care expenditure[14]. Estimates of treatment costs for a venous ulcer have been suggested to be between £1200 and £1400 per episode[15], although Moffatt and co-workers suggested the cost of treatment may be as high as £2500 per ulcer per patient per year[16]. Much of this expenditure and the associated nursing effort have, in the past, been directed towards unproven or ineffective treatments which impact adversely on the patient's quality of life[17]. UK National guidelines, published in 1998[18,19], aim to address this situation by providing a framework within which care should be provided.

QUALITY OF LIFE

Venous leg ulceration is a chronic, frequently recurrent, condition. Authors frequently report a high incidence of patients with recurrent ulceration, a typical example being the Lothian and Forth Valley trial in which 45% of patients reported recurrent ulceration extending over a 10-year period[20]. Walshe[21], in a phenomenologic study, concluded that venous ulceration is both a common and debilitating chronic problem that can impact significantly on a patient's quality of life and has an adverse effect on both body image and self-esteem which may result in isolation and depression. Chase and co-workers[22], in a similar phenomenologic study, identified four major themes from their analysis:

(1) 'A forever healing process' refers to the extended time over which healing occurs.

(2) 'Limits and accommodations' refers to the patterns of limitation related to mobility and activity restrictions due to pain and disfigurement.

(3) 'Powerlessness' describes the resignation about the inevitability of wound recurrence.

(4) 'Who cares?' refers to variation among the patients in assuming responsibility for managing their ulcer.

Care providers are able to work better when they empathize with patients' experiences. Patients can be encouraged to be active members of the treatment team and to assume responsibility for care and lifestyle choices. This is important as concordance with treatment is an aspect of care that requires consideration and is unfortunately frequently ignored, with a predictable deterioration in healing rates and an increase in treatment complications.

A satisfactory healing rate approaching 50% at 12 weeks and prevention of recurrence are therefore of significant advantage to the patient, as they reduce the impact of ulceration on the patient's lifestyle. They also potentially reduce the cost burden for leg ulcer care on the NHS.

VENOUS ANATOMY AND PATHOPHYSIOLOGY

The veins of the lower limb are classified into two groups: the superficial veins within the skin and subcutaneous tissues and the deep veins sited within the muscles. The two primary superficial venous systems are the long or greater and short or lesser saphenous veins and their tributaries. The long saphenous vein begins at the medial end of the dorsal venous arch of the foot and runs a course along the medial aspect of the calf and thigh to the groin, where it joins the deep venous system at the sapheno-femoral junction. The short saphenous vein starts at the lateral end of the dorsal venous arch of the foot; passing behind the lateral malleolus, it extends along the posterior aspect of the calf and joins the deep venous systems at the sapheno-popliteal junction behind the knee. The superficial venous network drains into the deep venous system through perforated or communicating veins. The deep veins which lie in the muscle compartment are either valveless sinuses or straight thin-walled channels with valves. The popliteal vein, which forms the outflow track for calf veins, is frequently referred to as the gatekeeper for the calf muscle pump.

Veins do not have an innate capacity to propel blood back to the heart. Venous return of blood to the heart largely depends on the competence of the valves, the function of the surrounding musculature and changes in the intra-abdominal and thoracic pressures. In the upright position, the compressive force exerted by the calf muscles during exercise (the calf muscle pump) and the compression of the venous plexus in the sole of the foot on weight-bearing set the blood in motion towards the heart. The one-way valves within the veins then prevent reflux of blood down into the limb, while valves within the communicating veins prevent reflux of blood from the deep to the superficial venous system during muscle contraction. As well as actively returning blood to the heart, exercise reduces the pressure in the distal venous system and, through the perforated veins, provides a means of emptying blood from the dermal venous plexus and the larger skin veins. The function of the calf muscle pump is dependent on two elements: mobility (of both the individual and the ankle) and a functioning set of venous valves. Without either, venous return will be compromised, leading to increased resting and ambulatory venous pressures. Elevation of the limb will restore venous return and reduce venous hydrostatic pressure. An association between reduced patient and ankle mobility and delayed leg ulcer healing is well recognized, reflecting the importance of the calf muscle pump in ulcer healing[23]. An association between popliteal venous valvular incompetence, as measured by duplex ultrasound, and increasing incidence of venous ulceration has been observed by Brittenden and co-workers[23], as has a link between popliteal reflux and ulcer healing[24].

Flow within the microcirculation depends upon the arterio-venous pressure difference, the vascular resistance, the viscosity of the blood and an intact arterio-venous response, that is a local sympathetic response mediated neurally that controls capillary flow by increasing the resistance of the pre-capillary sphincter. Venous hydrostatic pressure may rise either in the presence of venous outflow obstruction or when there is venous reflux in the deep or superficial systems. The overall effect is venous hypertension that disturbs the balance between osmotic and oncotic pressures within the capillary-venular bed, predisposing edema formation. Examination of the capillary bed in patients with venous hypertension reveals distortion of capillaries with elongation and tortuosity of individual capillary loops. Within these abnormal vessels, stasis and streaming occur with sequestration of white cells. This can give rise to white cell adhesion, activation and migration, the activated white cells releasing inflammatory mediators that will further increase vessel permeability.

These alterations within the capillary bed are partially responsible for the skin changes seen in chronic venous hypertension which include edema, brown skin discoloration, induration, lipodermatosclerosis, scarring and *atrophie blanche*[25] (Figures 4.1 and 4.2). There are a number of hypotheses which attempt to explain the link between high ambulatory venous pressure and the micro-circulatory changes that can result. These include stasis, arterio-venous shunting, tissue hypoxia, lymphatic obstruction, microangiopathy[26], the fibrin cuff theory[27] and white cell trapping[28]. The most likely explanation is that a combination of all these contribute to the skin changes associated with chronic venous hypertension (Figure 4.3). Chant[29] suggested that a number of mechanical factors come into play in the gaiter area and that these factors create an inevitable environment for ulceration and explain why the majority of venous ulcers occur in the gaiter area. The latter point of view fails to account for trauma, reported by many, as a trigger for skin breakdown. It is reasonable to conclude that the pathogenesis of venous ulcers remains unclear.

MODE OF ACTION OF COMPRESSION

There is considerable controversy over the mode of action of external compression. Compression treatment, whether by stockings or bandages, has been shown to improve venous hemodynamics[30]. This action may, at least in part, be due to a reduction in venous reflux and possibly a correction of venous valvular incompetence (Figure 4.4). Compression also increases pulsatile blood flow[31,32], which should increase capillary flow velocity and therefore decreased stasis and white cell marginalization[33,34]. Compression has also been shown to reverse the hypoxic state induced by high venous pressures and to promote more efficient absorption of perimalleolar extracellular fluid[30,35,36]. Edema control has been shown to be an important part of leg ulcer management and may in part explain the effectiveness of compression in healing venous leg ulceration[37]. There is, however, widespread acceptance of the benefits of this form of treatment. The suggested benefits of compression, brought about by reducing stasis, increasing venous velocity and decreasing white cell adhesion, may be reduced in the presence of calf muscle inactivity, as this will adversely affect calf pump function and limit any improvement in venous flow velocities.

One of the more striking findings in patients with severe lower limb venous disease is the presence of edema, although this may be masked by the presence of lipodermatosclerosis where scarring in the gaiter area may lead to the development of a classic champagne-bottle limb deformity (Figure 4.5). Alterations in limb shape, either due to scarring, obesity or edema, may cause significant technical problems when applying bandages (Figure 4.6).

Duby and co-workers[38], in a randomized controlled study, compared short-stretch, four-layer and elastic bandages in 67 ambulatory patients. They demonstrated that the reduction in limb volume was greater with four-layer and short-stretch than with elastic bandages and that the reduction in volume correlated with ulcer healing. These results suggest that edema reduction is an important element in ulcer healing and may be part of the mechanism by which compression therapy works.

OPTIMAL COMPRESSION LEVELS

Stemmer and Furderer[7] were able to identify the optimal compression level to reverse the effects of chronic venous hypertension. In this and in many subsequent studies[30,31,39–43], it has been demonstrated that the optimal compression value at the ankle is 40 mmHg, reducing sequentially to around 20 mmHg below the knee[44]. This, according to Laplace's Law (Box 1), is usually achieved due to the natural shape of the leg, which is wider at the calf than the ankle, when a bandage is applied at an equal tension from ankle to knee[45]. Debate continues as to how this formula should be modified to give a 'true' representation of the pressure profile, as Laplace's Law only applies to incompressible fluids[46]. Compression may be safely and effectively applied by elastic bandages, short-stretch bandages, multi-layer bandage systems or by compression hosiery[47,48]. These systems offer static compression; an alternative is to use dynamic compression by means of an intermittent pneumatic compression (IPC) device, either alone or in combination with a static compression system, to augment the effectiveness of the latter regime. A Cochrane review suggests the need for more randomized controlled trials[91].

Due to the shape of the limb, for any given bandage, greater pressure will be exerted at the ankle, the narrowest part of the limb, than the calf or knee. This, with even bandage application, will automatically generate graduated compression. Abnormal limb shape will change this relationship and affect the pressure profile.

Despite the evidence on compression levels, there is a paucity both of good quantitative and of qualitative research in the field of leg ulcer management. A systematic review published in the Effective Health Care Bulletin (EHCB) on 'compression therapy for venous leg ulcers'[47] revealed that only six randomized controlled trials addressed the question of whether compression is better than no compression[49–54]. These studies all conclude that compression improves significantly the healing rate of lower limb venous ulcer. Four other randomized controlled trials[20,38,55,56] have addressed the issue of high versus low compression. From these studies, it can be concluded:

(1) Healing rates are significantly improved with high compression when compared with low or no compression.

Box 1 Laplace's Law

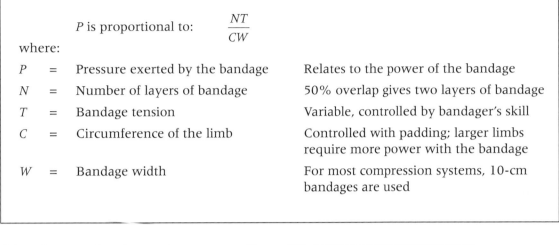

P is proportional to: $\dfrac{NT}{CW}$

where:

P	=	Pressure exerted by the bandage	Relates to the power of the bandage
N	=	Number of layers of bandage	50% overlap gives two layers of bandage
T	=	Bandage tension	Variable, controlled by bandager's skill
C	=	Circumference of the limb	Controlled with padding; larger limbs require more power with the bandage
W	=	Bandage width	For most compression systems, 10-cm bandages are used

(2) Compression therapy is more cost-effective because of improved healing rates.

Other forms of compression therapy have been advocated. These include the use of compression hosiery, both as primary treatment and to reduce ulcer recurrence[57], and the use of intermittent pneumatic compression, either in isolation or with a bandaging or hosiery regimen[58].

Since the publication of the EHCB, a number of other randomized controlled trials have been conducted. These include comparisons of long- and short-stretch bandages[55,59,60], short-stretch and four-layer bandaging[61,62] and the performance of various four-layer bandage regimens[63-65].

Lower limb ulceration may co-exist with lymphedema and, in such cases, management of the lymphedema can play an important part in the healing of the leg ulceration. This may require a modification of the standard below-knee compression systems employed for isolated venous ulceration, which may include the use of full leg bandaging, with digital compression and manual lymphatic drainage[66] and this is usually combined with an exercise program[67].

ELASTIC COMPRESSION BANDAGES

High compression elastic bandages (Type 3c e.g. Setopress, Surpress, Tensopress) are capable of delivering graduated compression with 40 mmHg at the ankle, irrespective of limb movement or position[68,69]. In practice, however, the pressure profile obtained from these bandages may not be maintained with continuous usage, as demonstrated by Sockalingham and co-workers[70], who continuously monitored ambulatory sub-bandage pressure for 1 week in a healthy subject and observed a decline in pressure profile down the limb.

SHORT-STRETCH BANDAGES

These bandages (e.g. Comprilan, Rosidal K, Actico), which are widely used throughout Europe for the management of venous disease, are inelastic, characterized by their inability to stretch. They act by forming a rigid containment around the leg, increasing the ejection force generated by the calf muscles during exercise[71]. The resting sub-bandage pressure is minimal as these are inelastic bandages[10,70,72] and patients must be mobile to achieve the maximum effectiveness from treatment[67]. This type of bandage may therefore be unsuitable for immobile patients. It is, however, the preferred form of treatment in patients with lymphedema as the intermittent increase in pressure associated with movement is more conducive to edema reduction[73,74]. Partsch and co-workers[62], in a randomized, multi-center trial, found no significant difference in the healing rates obtained with this form of bandaging and multi-layer (four-layer) bandaging. Scriven and co-workers[61], however, in an earlier study comparing short-stretch and four-layer bandaging, although able to demonstrate similar healing rates, found more treatment complications in the short-stretch group, perhaps indicating a greater safety margin for the multi-layer system.

MULTI-LAYER BANDAGING

Multi-layer bandage systems and in particular four-layer bandage systems (e.g. original Charing Cross four-layer bandage, Profore, Ultra four, K-four) are the most commonly used form of compression for the treatment of venous leg ulceration in the UK. The original four-layer compression system described by Blair and co-workers[9] consists of a combination of elastic compression bandages, crêpe and padding, the components varying with ankle circumference (Table 2). The effectiveness of this and similar multi-layer systems has been demonstrated in a number of clinical trials with 12-week healing rates reported to be in the order of 60%[9,75–79].

This bandage system has several advantages, one of which is that the elastic bandages form a rigid structure, maintained for 7 days, which enables the mobile patients to maintain high ejection force when walking, while maintaining an optimal therapeutic pressure at rest[80]. This maintained resting pressure is an advantage when treating an immobile patient.

A number of commercially available four-layer bandage systems are now available and comparison studies would seem to indicate that they are as effective as the original Charing Cross four-layer system[63–65].

COMPRESSION HOSIERY

Compression hosiery is used both to prevent ulcer relapse and as a treatment of frank ulceration[57]. Cowan[81] has reviewed the use and type of compression hosiery available. Moffatt[82] has looked specifically at the use of hosiery, including the measurement and fitting of stockings, in patients with active and healed venous ulceration. Part of the difficulty with compression hosiery, particularly in the age group at the highest risk of chronic lower limb venous ulceration, is the difficulty of application of the garment. A number of fitting aides are available including rubber gloves, Chinese slipper and the Medi Valet (Medi). Even with these, a number of patients are still unable to use the correct therapeutic grade of hosiery (usually Class II European classification 25–32 mmHg at the ankle) to achieve healing or prevent ulcer recurrence. An alternative is to provide the patient with two pairs of Class I hosiery and for them to wear two Class I stockings, one over the other, on the affected limb[82].

DYNAMIC COMPRESSION

The role of intermittent pneumatic compression (IPC) in the management of lower limb venous ulcer disease has been reviewed by Vowden[83]. Although the majority of the medical literature relates to the use of IPC in the prevention of deep vein thrombosis, there is some evidence that improvements in venous return resulting from the use of IPC may benefit the healing of venous ulceration. Eight small studies have been undertaken[58,84–90], the conclusions from which are that IPC may be of

Table 2 Components in the four-layer compression bandage system and how they vary according to ankle circumference

Ankle circumference	Bandage combination
Less than 18 cm	2 orthopedic wool layers – extra padding protects thin limbs
	1 cotton crêpe
	1 Class 3a – elastic (Elset)
	1 Class 3b – cohesive (Coban)
18–25 cm	1 orthopedic wool layer
	1 cotton crêpe
	1 Class 3a
	1 Class 3b
25–30 cm	1 orthopedic wool layer
	1 Class 3c – high compression bandage
	1 Class 3b
Greater than 30 cm	2 orthopedic wool bandages – necessary for extra length required
	1 Class 3a
	1 Class 3b
	1 Class 3c

Note effective compression will result in a decrease in edema and a reduction in ankle circumference. The limb should therefore be re-measured frequently and appropriate changes be made in the bandages used. For the majority of patients, the ankle circumference will be between 18 and 25 cm

benefit, particularly in conjunction with compression bandaging, but as yet there is no statistically significant evidence for its routine use[47,91]. From theoretic considerations alone, IPC would seem to be potentially valuable for the immobile patient with slow or non-healing ulcer disease[83].

ASSESSMENT OF THE PATIENT PRIOR TO THE APPLICATION OF COMPRESSION

The application of high compression to a limb carries with it a degree of risk. Patients should be fully assessed prior to treatment. The process of assessing a patient with lower limb ulceration has been set out on a number of publications[92–95] and features widely in the UK National Guidelines[18,19]. The assessment process should:

(1) Provide an accurate diagnosis.

(2) Identify factors likely to delay healing.

(3) Indicate the most appropriate treatment.

(4) Reveal potential dangers from high compression bandaging.

(5) Identify preventable factors likely to influence ulcer recurrence.

The most important factor in terms of initiating compression therapy is the identification of significant underlying arterial disease. The method of hand-held Doppler assessment of lower limb perfusion has been outlined by Vowden[96,97] and Stubbing and co-workers[98]. An ankle brachial pressure index (ABPI) less than 0.8 is an indication that the patient is unsuitable for high compression bandaging. An ABPI of 0.8 or greater does not always indicate that high compression bandaging can be undertaken safely and other factors may need to be considered, such as the skin condition, the shape of thc limb and the presence of neuropathy or cardiac failure.

THE APPLICATION OF BANDAGES

The correct application of high compression bandages requires both an understanding of the scientific principles behind their use and a practitioner skilled in their correct application. Incorrectly applied bandages and hosiery may not only be ineffective as they may actually lead to deterioration in the condition of the limb and may lead to amputation, particularly if used inappropriately on an ischemic limb[99]. Chan and co-workers[100] have recently described toe ulceration in association with compression bandaging, a condition that we have also observed.

The correct application of a graduated compression bandage demands a degree of technical skill that can only be acquired through training and maintained by regular practice[101]. Nelson confirmed this, using bandages marked with tension indicators[102]. Armstrong and co-workers[103], in a survey of leg ulcer care in Scotland, identified a deficiency in training for many leg ulcer practitioners. It has been suggested that the use of a sub-bandage pressure monitor may improve the effectiveness of training[104]. The widespread introduction of training days and leg ulcer management courses throughout the UK is intended to go a long way towards addressing these problems.

Regardless of the type of compression system chosen, it is important to identify areas at risk, such as bony prominences, prior to the application of bandages. Multi-layer bandage systems, which contain an orthopedic wool layer, are specifically designed to accommodate different sizes and shapes of limb and this can overcome the problems associated with applying excessive bandage tension and therefore pressure, when applying compression. To

avoid this problem, some bandages incorporate a symbol which allows the bandager to recognize the correct degree of extension for a particular bandage (Figure 4.7). The action of short-stretch bandages, for example, requires that the bandage be applied at 90% stretch. The key points to remember when applying any compression bandage and the method for applying these bandages are described and illustrated in Table 3 and its accompanying figures.

MONITORING SUB-BANDAGE PRESSURE

To be effective, compression bandaging must generate the correct pressure profile sustainable over a period of time. It would therefore seem to be of fundamental importance that a method of reliably measuring sub-bandage pressure should be readily available. This is in fact rarely the case[105], despite the fact that calibrated pressure recording devices have existed for some time[106,107] and commercial devices such as the Oxford Pressure Monitor (Talley Group Ltd) are available. Despite extensive research, doubt remains as to the most effective way of measuring a sub-bandage pressure[46,108] and few studies have been conducted evaluating sub-bandage pressure profiles under different bandaging systems over time[72,109,110].

HAZARDS AND COMPLICATIONS OF COMPRESSION THERAPY

Callam and co-workers[99] highlighted the risk of sub-bandage pressure complications associated with any form of compression therapy, including low level compression anti-embolism stockings. These risks are increased by poor patient assessment, inappropriate bandage selection and by poor bandaging technique. The 'at risk' areas are the malleoli, the area over the front of the ankle and dorsum of

Table 3 Application of compression bandages

For all limbs:
- Measure the ankle circumference and, where appropriate, adjust the system components
- Apply an appropriate wound dressing
- Keep the foot in a neutral position, i.e. at a 90° angle when applying padding or bandages

The method of application for short-stretch bandages:
- Apply orthopedic wool in a spiral from toe to knee and use additional padding to fill the area around the malleoli, especially if this is the site of ulceration, to ensure an equal distribution of pressure, and to compensate for abnormal limb contours (Figure 4.8)
- Start by applying two complete turns of the bandage at 50% extension around the foot
- Take the bandage around the heel with 50% above and 50% below the heel
- Take the next turn in a figure-of-eight pattern at 70–90% extension around the base of the foot ensuring that the foot, other than the toes, is now fully covered with bandage
- Follow this with a turn at 70–90% extension immediately above the heel
- Continue in a spiral pattern with 50% overlap and 70–90% extension to the knee (Figure 4.9a & b) finishing at the popliteal crease, ensuring that only two layers of bandage are in contact with any area of the leg
- As the number of layers of bandage affects the pressure, do not wrap excess bandage at the top as this will increase the pressure; simply turn the bandage back on itself and secure the turned-back edge with tape
- If a second bandage is required (due to the size of the limb) then it should be applied in the opposite direction to the first
- Finally check patient comfort. A correctly applied bandage can be left in place for up to 7 days, but may need to be changed more regularly during the initial period of treatment as the limb circumference decreases due to the removal of edema

The method of application for a four-layer bandage system (Charing Cross method)
- Apply orthopedic wool in a spiral from toe to knee and use additional padding to reshape the leg or if the ankle circumference is <18 cm or the leg misshapen
- Apply the 10 cm crêpe bandage in a spiral from toe to knee, finishing at the level of the popliteal crease
- Over this apply the 10 cm elastic Class 3a bandage (e.g. Litepress) in a figure-of-eight from toe to knee ensuring a 50% overlap (Figure 4.10) – when using reduced compression, this bandage is not used
- The fourth layer is a cohesive Class 3b bandage (e.g. Co-Plus), which is applied in a spiral at 50% stretch with 50% overlap (Figure 4.11), ensuring two layers of bandage at all levels. This applies additional pressure and stabilizes and supports the other layers. This maintains the integrity of the bandage for up to 7 days (Figure 4.12)

The method of application for elastic (long-stretch) bandages:
- Apply orthopedic wool in a spiral from toe to knee and use additional padding to reshape the leg or if the ankle is small
- Apply the Class 3c (Surepress) bandage in a spiral from toe to knee, keeping the bandage extended by 50% during application (Figure 4.13)
- Ensure a 50% overlap; more will increase the sub-bandage pressure, less will give sub-optimal compression and unevenness will produce pressure ridges
- Finish just below the knee at the popliteal crease and fix the bandage with tape
- If required, cover the bandage with a layer of stockinette or shaped Tubigrip

the foot, the bony prominence of the tibia, the area over the Achilles tendon and the outer border of the foot. Patients with a peripheral neuropathy, such as those with diabetes, are also at increased risk of complications with compression therapy. The heel area can be especially at risk in this patient group, particularly if they are bed-bound. Even when patients are correctly managed, there will always remain a risk that bandage damage will occur and this is frequently reflected in patient withdrawals from clinical trials[63,65]. The incidence of these complications would, however, appear to be lower with the four-layer system than other forms of compression[111].

Another potential complication associated with compression therapy relates to the fluid shift that may occur. This can precipitate cardiac failure and pulmonary edema in a few patients with severe underlying cardiac disease.

As with all skin contact therapies, particularly those where treatment may be prolonged, skin sensitivity may develop[112]. Care should be taken to use hypoallergenic products whenever possible to reduce this risk.

MIXED ULCERS

The prevalence of venous disease increases with age. Venous leg ulcers may co-exist with peripheral arterial disease, diabetes mellitus and rheumatoid arthritis. Nelzen and co-workers[113] found that the ABPI was 0.9 or less in 185 (40%) of ulcerated legs and that venous insufficiency was the dominating causative factor in 250 legs (54%), in 60% of which deep venous insufficiency was present either in isolation or in combination with superficial reflux. Arterial insufficiency was judged to be the possible dominant factor in 12% of cases, and in 6% of limbs the ulcer was clearly ischemic. Ghauri and co-workers[114] found a 17% incidence of co-existing arterial and venous disease, while Liew and Sinha[115] iden-

tified 13% and Scriven[116] 14% of patients with 'mixed' ulcers in their study populations. Is it correct to classify these patients with venous ulcers with concomitant arterial disease as having mixed ulcers? The term mixed ulcer implies that the ulcer has a dual etiology; however, the work of Simon and co-workers[117] would contradict this, suggesting that over time patients with a venous ulcer may have a slowly reducing ABPI, as they develop arterial disease. When reviewing patients with healed venous ulceration over a 12-month period, this group found that in 29% of patients the ABPI fell over time and that seven patients (9%) developed arterial insufficiency as defined by an ABPI of less than 0.8. This trend towards arterial insufficiency over time is recognized in the recommendations to reassess patients receiving any form of compression therapy at regular, 3-monthly intervals or earlier if symptoms change[18,19]. Fowkes and Callam[118], in a study comparing leg ulcer patients with age- and sex-matched controls, concluded that arterial disease was not found more frequently in patients than in controls, suggesting that arterial disease is not a risk factor for chronic venous ulceration.

The majority of patients defined as having mixed ulcers do not therefore have ulcers of mixed etiology, but in fact have ulcers of venous etiology. It is simply that the use of high compression bandaging is contra-indicated in this patient group. Figure 4.14 illustrates the therapeutic continuum that should be considered when treating patients with vascular lower limb ulceration. Over time, the ABPI will tend to fall with increasing age.

The transition zone for treatment of venous ulceration is usually taken to be an ABPI of 0.8[18]. Clearly, it is wrong to regard 0.8 as an absolute cut-off point as it neither defines the transition between venous and arterial ulceration nor takes into account differences in perfusion pressure between the three vessels at the ankle; a pressure difference of 15 mmHg or greater, for example, indicating a proximal stenosis or occlusion in the vessel with the lower pressure[119]. Such a pressure difference will increase the risk of skin damage in the zone of the calf supplied by the artery with the reduced perfusion pressure, irrespective of the calculated ABPI for the limb. Reliance on the ABPI also fails to take into consideration other factors which may increase the risk of bandage damage and be important when defining the level of compression to apply to any particular limb. These other factors include the limb shape, the presence of bony prominences, skin condition, the presence of other diseases and finally the patient's tolerance of compression.

In the group for whom high compression is considered inappropriate, the treatment options are:

(1)   To reduce the level of compression[114,120].

(2)   To correct the underlying arterial disease and then apply standard compression[114].

(3)   To use an alternative treatment such as intermittent pneumatic compression[88,121] or alternative bandage systems such as short-stretch on mobile patients[122].

REDUCED COMPRESSION

One of the advantages of the four-layer compression system is that it can be adjusted to accommodate patients with intolerance to full compression or a reduced ABPI. In these patients or in those where there is a concern over the immediate introduction of high compression, such as in a diabetic with a marked peripheral neuropathy, the use of three-layer compression, omitting the third Class 3a bandage from the standard four-layer system, offers an alternative. This is the method favored by Guest and co-workers[120] and we prefer this to the 'slack' four-layer system suggested by Ghauri and co-workers[114], which may compromise on the durability of the bandage system. Short-stretch bandages have also been advocated in this situation[122] but our experience suggests that the majority of these patients are less mobile and as such will not benefit fully from this form of compression. If even reduced compression is not tolerated, or the ulcer shows little or no sign of healing within 6 weeks, it would be prudent to image the peripheral circulation using color duplex arterial ultrasonography and/or arteriography with a view to angioplasty or surgery if feasible. Our basic management strategy for these patients is illustrated in Figure 4.15. This management strategy can be applied to the vast majority of patients with a reduced ABPI and we would only resort to further arterial investigations if the ulcer failed to respond to this treatment, the ABPI continued to fall or was below 0.5 at presentation, or the patient's symptoms, such as claudication or rest pain, required intervention in their own right. This is similar to the policy described in the Riverside study[75]. Patients presenting with primary lower limb ulceration and an ABPI of 0.5 or less, even if they have varicose veins or deep venous insufficiency, should be treated from the onset as if they have ischemic ulceration. In these patients, venous disease, especially if associated with lipodermatosclerosis or atrophy blanche, should be treated as a secondary event once the arterial insufficiency is corrected.

EXPECTED HEALING RATES

Data from existing clinical trials would suggest that healing rates for uncomplicated venous ulcers treated with effective high compression therapy should be above 60% at 12 weeks, rising to 85% at 24 weeks. In the Riverside study using the Charing Cross four-layer bandage system, Moffatt and co-workers[75], in community clinics, achieved complete healing in 318 (69%) venous ulcers by 12 weeks and 375 (83%) by 24 weeks, while, in 56 patients with a reduced ABPI treated with reduced compression, the healing rates were 24 (56%) at 12 weeks and 31 (75%) by 24 weeks, giving a figure for overall healing for all leg ulcers attending their community clinic of 351/550 (67%) at 12 weeks and 417/550 (81%) at 24 weeks. These results are similar to those obtained in the authors' secondary and tertiary referral clinics where healing rates of between 59% and 73% at 12 weeks and 76% and 83% at 20 weeks have been reported using a variety of four-layer bandage systems[64] (Figure 4.16). Not all centers have, however, reported such high healing rates[78] and it is not clear whether these variations in results reflect the patient population treated, the presence of known risk factors for delayed healing, the experience of the practitioners, or the type of care provided. Nelson[123] has reviewed a number of published studies on ulcer healing and these and further, more recent, studies have been reviewed in the EHCB[47] and in the latest Cochrane review[8]. These reviews have also examined other forms of compression therapy such as hosiery and IPC. Partsch and co-workers[62] have published data comparing healing with short-stretch (SSB) and four-layer compression (4LB) and were able to demonstrate similar healing rates over a treatment period up to a maximum of 16 weeks with both bandage systems (62% 4LB versus 73% SSB). It would therefore seem that it is the level of compression achieved, the quality of application of the bandage and the sustainability of the graduated compression that are important and not the compression system itself.

VARIABLES ADVERSELY AFFECTING THE HEALING OF VENOUS ULCERS

Franks and co-workers[124], using multivariate analysis, identified three major factors delaying ulcer healing; these were ulcer size, ulcer pre-treatment duration and limb mobility. These factors were also highlighted by Moffatt and co-workers[75] in an observational study on 475 patients with 550 ulcerated limbs attending community leg ulcer clinics. In the latter study, secondary analysis revealed that, in a sub-group of 209 immobile patients with severely limited mobility, defined as bed- or chair-bound, healing rates were reduced to 48% at 12 weeks and 70% at 24 weeks, compared with healing rates for mobile patients of 73% at 12 weeks and 86% at 24 weeks. We noted a similar difference in our hospital-based study where the equivalent results at 12 weeks were 50% for immobile and 68.6% for mobile patients[79]. Lambourne and co-workers[76], looking at the effect of ankle mobility on ulcer healing rate, identified a similar but more striking difference between patients with mobile (78% healing at 12 weeks) and fixed ankles (22% healing at 12 weeks). In a further study relating ulcer healing to a number of risk factors, we observed that poor ankle mobility, which adversely affects the efficiency of the calf muscle pump, had more effect on ulcer healing than the patient's general mobility[125].

Margolis and co-workers[126] have recently examined factors affecting healing and suggested a simple scoring system to predict ulcer healing. Barwell and co-workers[127] have also reviewed risk factors and have suggested that popliteal vein reflux is a further independent risk factor for delayed ulcer healing, their results paralleling the authors' observations[128] and those of Brittenden and co-workers[23] but are in contrast to those of Guest and co-workers[129] who suggest that this is not an important factor in ulcer healing.

COMPLIANCE WITH TREATMENT

A further factor that is recognized to influence treatment outcome is patient compliance or concordance. Even with the best possible treatment strategies based on reliable research evidence, many patients do not comply with recommended leg ulcer treatment and as a result have persistent non-healing ulceration[130]. Some of the reasons for this lack of concordance are discussed by House[131] and the literature on compliance with leg ulcer treatment has been reviewed by Erickson[132] and Tonge[133]. Both support the use of education and a holistic approach to care to aid compliance, noting that poor treatment compliance adversely affects both healing and ulcer recurrence. Compliance with leg ulcer treatment also depends on patient motivation. Motivation can be affected by factors such as social isolation or treatment discomfort, and House[131] emphasizes that nurses must enable patients to participate actively in their treatment. The importance of empowering or enabling patients to control their care has been explored by Buchmann[134] who established a link between self-efficacy and power which in turn leads to compliance. This is stated to be one advantage of IPC and hosiery as a means of delivering compression as the patient regains control over his/her treatment, a finding supported by Rowland[90] who noted a trend towards increased compliance with IPC therapy in a leg ulcer treatment population.

RECURRENCE RATES

Recurrence rates for venous leg ulcers remain depressingly high, Monk and Sarkany[135] reporting rates as high as 69% at 1 year. The Lothian and Forth Valley study found that over 60% of patients had a history of previous leg ulceration, 21% having had more than six episodes of ulceration[136]. The main use for compression hosiery is the prevention of ulcer recurrence[137]. The higher the level of compression the patient can tolerate, the lower the incidence of recurrence[138], although this does depend on the regular use and replacement of prescribed hosiery. Moffatt and Dorman[139]

identified, in a randomized controlled trial of 188 patients, factors that led to re-ulceration; these include history of a deep vein thrombosis, previous ulcer size and arterial hypertension. Patient immobility indirectly led to increased ulcer recurrence, as it affected the ability of the patient to apply the garments; 15% were unable to apply their own stockings and a further 26% had great difficulty in doing so and had to rely on support from relatives or the community nursing service. This results in a higher ulcer recurrence and less effective treatment in an immobile population. Even with effective hosiery management, high ulcer recurrence rates are reported but these may be improved by superficial venous surgery when this is appropriate. The role of surgery in both the healing and prevention of venous leg ulceration is yet to be established in a randomized controlled trial with long-term follow-up. Published results to date would, however, suggest that surgery reduces ulcer recurrence rates[24,140]. Barwell and co-workers[24] have demonstrated that recurrence rates for leg ulceration at 1, 2 and 3 years were 14%, 20% and 26% for legs benefiting from superficial venous surgery and 28%, 30% and 44% for those limbs receiving compression hosiery alone, these figures reaching significance.

COST ISSUES AND SERVICE MANAGEMENT

Effective leg ulcer care aims at the prompt restoration of the healed state and the maintenance of that state. Cost drivers for effective leg ulcer care are therefore based upon:

(1) Healing rates;

(2) Direct and indirect treatment costs;

(3) Ulcer recurrence rates.

These parameters have been applied in a Markov model[141] to analyze the effectiveness of compression[15]. The influence of care systems across health districts and their impact on cost and treatment outcome have also been studied[17] and have shown the advantages of high compression therapy within a structured service in the management of venous leg ulceration.

It is necessary to support guidelines by establishing the necessary infrastructure to enable care provision. Armstrong and co-workers[103] conclude that there are serious deficiencies in the support available for community care of leg ulcer patients, indicating that this situation requires to be remedied if more cost-effective outcomes for leg ulcer patients are to be achieved.

CONCLUSION

Thorough clinical assessment of the patient followed by compression therapy is an effective method of managing venous leg ulcers. The compression system itself is less important than the effectiveness with which the bandage is applied, sustained graduated compression being the key. If, however, used inappropriately or applied ineffectively, all compression systems can cause significant complications which may be limb-threatening. They will also fail to deliver expected healing rates. Compression, if used in isolation, is palliative and not curative. To prevent ulcer recurrence, patients require life-long compression therapy and/or an intervention to correct their underlying venous disease. This may be a key area for therapy as duplex studies indicate that up to 50% of patients with venous leg ulcers have isolated superficial venous reflux. Compression therapy will, however, along with rest and limb elevation, remain the mainstay for treatment and the prevention of recurrence. Given that the majority of patients with deep venous defects are unsuited for surgery, compression is of major importance.

References

1. Negus D. Historical background. In: *Leg Ulcers: A Practical Approach to Management*. Oxford: Butterworth–Heinemann, 1991: 3–10
2. Wiseman R. *Several Chirurgical Treatises*. London: Wilthoe and Knapton, 1676
3. Hunter J. Observation on the inflammation of the internal coats of veins (1775). In: Palmer JI, ed. *The Works of John Hunter*. London: Longman, Rees, Orme, Green and Longman, 1837:581–6
4. Thomas S, Nelson E. Compression therapy: a complete guide – types of compression bandage. *J Wound Care* 1998;7(Suppl 2):5–13
5. Thomas S. Bandages used in leg ulcer management. In: Cullum NA, Roe BH, eds. *Leg Ulcers: Nursing Management*. Harrow: Scutari, 1995
6. O'Donnell TF Jr, Rosenthal DA, Callow AD, Ledig BL. Effect of elastic compression on venous hemodynamics in postphlebitic limbs. *JAMA* 1979;242:2766–8
7. Stemmer R, Marescaux J, Furderer C. Compression treatment of the lower extremities particularly with compression stockings. *The Dermatologist* 1980;31:355–65
8. Cullum NA, Nelson EA, Fletcher AW, Sheldon TA. Compression for venous leg ulcers (Cochrane Review). In: *The Cochrane Library*. Oxford: Update Software, 2001
9. Blair SD, Wright DDI, Backhouse CD, Riddle E, McCollum CN. Sustained compression and healing of chronic venous ulcers. *BMJ* 1988; 297:1159–61
10. Thomas S, Nelson A. Graduated external compression in the treatment of venous disease. *J Wound Care* 1998;7(Suppl 2):1–4
11. Callam MJ. Leg ulcer and chronic venous insufficiency in the community. In: Ruckley CV, Fowkes FGR, Bradbury AW, eds. *Venous*

Disease: Epidemiology, Management and Delivery of Care. London: Springer-Verlag, 1999:15–25

12. Vowden KR. *Bradford Leg Ulcer Survey 1993: An Analysis of Prevalence and Treatment with Proposals for Possible Improvements in the Service*. Bradford: Bradford Health District, 1993

13. Baxter HS. *Prevalence Audit for the Management of Leg Ulcers*. Bradford: Bradford Health Authority, 1998

14. Bosanquet N. Cost of venous ulcers: from maintenance therapy to investment programmes. *Phlebology* 1992;(Suppl 1):44–6

15. Carr L, Philips Z, Posnett J. Comparative cost-effectiveness of four-layer bandaging in the treatment of venous leg ulceration. *J Wound Care* 1999;8:243–8

16. Moffatt C, Wright DD, Besley D, McCollum C, Greenhalgh RM. A new approach to chronic venous ulcers in the community. *Br J Surg* 1989;76:418

17. Simon DA, Freak L, Kinsella A, *et al.* Community leg ulcer clinics: a comparative study in two health authorities. *BMJ* 1996;312:1648–51

18. RCN. *The Management of Patients with Venous Leg Ulcers*. York: RCN Institute, 1998

19. SIGN. *The Care of Patients with Chronic Leg Ulcer*. Edinburgh: SIGN Secretariat, 1998

20. Callam MJ, Harper DR, Dale JJ, *et al.* Lothian and Forth Valley leg ulcer healing trial, Part 1: Elastic versus non-elastic bandaging in the treatment of chronic leg ulceration. *Phlebology* 1992;7:136–41

21. Walshe C. Living with a venous leg ulcer: a descriptive study of patients' experiences. *J Adv Nurs* 1995;22:1092–100

22. Chase SK, Melloni M, Savage A. A forever healing: the lived experience of venous ulcer disease. *J Vasc Nurs* 1997;15:73–8

23. Brittenden J, Bradbury AW, Allan PL, Prescott RJ, Harper DR, Ruckley CV. Popliteal vein reflux reduces the healing of chronic venous ulcer. *Br J Surg* 1998;85:60–2

24. Barwell JR, Taylor M, Deacon J, *et al.* Surgical correction of isolated superficial venous reflux reduces long-term recurrence rate in chronic venous leg ulcers. *Eur J Vasc Endovasc Surg* 2000;20:363–8

25. Vowden K. Lipodermatosclerosis and atrophie blanche. *J Wound Care* 1998;7:441–3

26. Leu AJ, Leu HJ, Franzeck UK, Bollinger A. Microvascular changes in chronic venous insufficiency – a review. *Cardiovasc Surg* 1995;3:237–45

27. Browse NL, Burnand KG. The cause of venous ulceration. *Lancet* 1982;8292:243–5

28. Cheatle TR, Scott HJ, Scurr JH, Coleridge Smith PD. White cells, skin blood flow and venous ulcers. *Br J Dermatol* 1991;125:288–90

29. Chant A. The biomechanics of leg ulceration. *Ann R Coll Surg Engl* 1999;81:80–5

30. Gaylarde PM, Sarkany I, Dodd HJ. The effect of compression on venous stasis. *Br J Dermatol* 1993;128:255–8

31. Mayrovitz H, Larsen P. Effects of compression bandaging on leg pulsatile blood flow. *Clin Physiol* 1997;17:105–17

32. Mayrovitz HN. Compression-induced pulsatile blood flow changes in human legs. *Clin Physiol* 1998;18:117–24

33. Bradbury AW, Murie JA, Ruckley CV. Role of the leucocyte in the pathogenesis of vascular disease. *Br J Surg* 1993;80:1503–12

34. Saharay M, Shields DA, Porter JB, Scurr JH, Coleridge Smith PD. Leucocyte activity in volunteers in response to experimental venous hypertension. *Phlebology* 1997;12:122–6

35. Puruhito. Pathophysiology of microcirculation in venous disease. *Clin Hemorheol Microcirc* 2000;23:239–42

36. Nehler M, Moneta CL, Woodard D, *et al.* Perimalleolar subcutaneous tissue pressure effects of elastic compression stockings. *J Vasc Surg* 1993;18:783–8

37. Cherry GW, Hofman D, Cameron J, Poore SM. Bandaging in the treatment of venous ulcers: a European view. *Ostomy Wound Management* 1996;42(Suppl):13S–18S

38. Duby T, Hoffman D, Cameron J, Doblhoff-Brown D, Cherry G, Ryan T. A randomized trial in the treatment of venous leg ulcers comparing short-stretch bandages, four layer bandage system, and a long stretch-paste bandage system. *Wounds: A Compendium of Clinical Practice and Research* 1993;5:276–9

39. Struckmann J. Compression stockings and their effect on the venous pump – a comparative study. *Phlebology* 1986;1:37–45

40. Abu-Own A, Scurr JH, Coleridge Smith PD. Effect of compression stockings on the skin microcirculation in chronic venous insufficiency. *Phlebology* 1995;10:5–11

41. Klopp R, Schippel W, Niemer W. Compression therapy and microcirculation: vital microscope investigations in patients suffering from chronic venous insufficiency before and after compression therapy. *Phlebology* 1996;11(Suppl 1):19–25

42. Veraart J, Neumann HAM. Interface pressure measurements underneath elastic and non-elastic bandages. *Phlebology* 1996;11(Suppl 1): 2–5

43. Jungbeck C, Thulin I, Darenheim C, Norgren L. Graduated compression treatment in patients with chronic venous insufficiency: a study comparing low and medium grade compression stockings. *Phlebology* 1997;12: 142–5

44. Alexander House Group. Consensus paper on venous leg ulcers. *Phlebology* 1992;7: 48–58

45. Moffatt C, Harper P. *Leg Ulcers*. New York: Churchill Livingstone, 1997

46. Melhuish JM, Clark M, Williams R, Harding KG. Physics of sub bandage pressure measurement. *J Wound Care* 2000;9:308–10

47. Baker S, Fletcher A, Glanville J, *et al.* Compression therapy for venous leg ulcers. *Effect Health Care* 1997;3:1–12

48. Fletcher A, Cullum N, Sheldon TA. A systemic review of compression treatment for venous leg ulcers. *BMJ* 1997;315:576–80

49. Eriksson G, Eklund A, Liden S. Comparison of different treatments of venous leg ulcers; a controlled study using stereophotogrammetry. *Curr Ther Res* 1984;35:678–84

50. Sikes E. Evaluation of a transparent dressing in the treatment of stasis ulcers of the lower limb. *J Enterostom Ther* 1985;12:116–20

51. Kikta MJ, Schuler JJ, Meyer JP, *et al.* A prospective, randomized trial of Unna's boots versus hydroactive dressing in the treatment of venous stasis ulcers. *J Vasc Surg* 1988;7: 478–83

52. Rubin JR, Alexander J, Plecha EJ, Marman C. Unna's boot vs polyurethane foam dressings for the treatment of venous ulceration. A randomized prospective study. *Arch Surg* 1990;125:489–90

53. Charles H. Compression healing of ulcers. *J Distr Nurs* 1991;4:6–7

54. Taylor AD, Taylor RJ, Marcuson RW. Prospective comparison of healing rates and therapy costs for conventional and four-layer high-compression bandaging treatments of venous leg ulcers. *Phlebology* 1998;13:20–4

55. Gould DJ, Campbell S, Newton H, Duffelen P, Griffin M, Harding EF. Setopress vs Elastocrepe in chronic venous ulceration. *Br J Nurs* 1998;7:66–70, 72–3

56. Northeast A, Layer G, Wilson N, *et al. Increased Compression Expedites Venous Ulcer Healing*. London: Royal Society of Medicine (Venous Forum), 1990

57. Keachie J. A cheaper alternative to the four-layer bandage system. *J Wound Care* 1993;2: 133

58. Coleridge Smith P, Sarin S, Hasty J, Scurr JH. Sequential gradient pneumatic compression enhances venous ulcer healing. *Surgery* 1990; 108:871–5

59. Moody M. Comparison of Rosidal K and SurePress in the treatment of venous leg ulcers. *Br J Nurs* 1999;8:345–55

60. Danielsen L, Madsen SM, Henriksen L. Venous leg ulcer healing: a randomized prospective study of long-stretch versus short-stretch compression bandages. *Phlebology* 1998;13:59–63

61. Scriven JM, Taylor LE, Wood AJ, Bell PR, Naylor AR, London NJ. A prospective randomised trial of four-layer versus short stretch compression bandages for the treatment of venous leg ulcers. *Ann R Coll Surg Engl* 1998;80:215–20

62. Partsch H, Damstra RJ, Tazelaar DJ, *et al.* Multicentre, randomised controlled trial of four-layer bandaging versus short-stretch bandaging in the treatment of venous leg ulcers. *Vasa* 2001;30:108–13

63. Moffatt CJ, Simon DA, Franks PJ, *et al.* Randomised trial comparing two four-layer bandage systems in the management of chronic leg ulceration. *Phlebology* 1999;14:139–42

64. Vowden KR, Mason A, Wilkinson D, Vowden P. Comparison of the healing rates and com-

plications of three four-layer bandage regimens. *J Wound Care* 2000;9:269–72

65. Vowden KR, Wilkinson D, Vowden P. The K-Four bandage system: evaluation of its effectiveness on recalcitrant venous ulcers. *J Wound Care* 2001;10:182–4

66. Cavezzi A, Michelini S. *Phlebolymphoedema: from Diagnosis to Therapy*. Bologna: PR Communications, 1998

67. Todd J. *Living with Lymphoedema*. London: Marie Curie Cancer Care, 1996

68. Thomas S. Bandages and bandaging: the science behind the art. *Care Sci Pract* 1990;8: 56–60

69. Thomas S. Bandages and bandaging. In: *Wound Management and Dressings*. London: The Pharmaceutical Press, 1990:88–98

70. Sockalingham S, Barbenel JC, Queen D. Ambulatory monitoring of the pressures beneath compression bandages. *Care Sci Pract* 1990;8:75–9

71. Charles H. Compression healing of venous ulcers. *Nurs Times* 1992;88:52

72. Partsch H, Menzinger G, Blazek V. Static and dynamic measurement of compression pressure. In: Blazek V, Schultz-Ehrenburg U, eds. *Frontiers in Computer-Aided Visualization of Vascular Functions*. Aachen: Verlag, 1997:145–52

73. Mortimer P. Managing lymphoedema. *Clin Exp Dermatol* 1995;20:98–106

74. Casley-Smith JR, Casley-Smith JR. *Compression Bandages in the Treatment of Lymphoedema*. 1995 Accessed: November 1999. www.lymphoedema.org.au/lymphoed.htm

75. Moffatt CJ, Franks PJ, Oldroyd M, *et al*. Community clinics for leg ulcers and impact on healing. *BMJ* 1992;305:1389–92

76. Lambourne LA, Moffatt CJ, Jones AC, Dorman MC, Franks PJ. Clinical audit and effective change in leg ulcer services. *J Wound Care* 1996;5:348–51

77. Stevens J, Franks PJ, Harrington M. A community/hospital leg ulcer service. *J Wound Care* 1997;6:62–8

78. Thomson B, Hooper P, Powell R, Warin AP. Four-layer bandaging and healing rates of venous leg ulcers. *J Wound Care* 1996;5: 213–16

79. Vowden KR, Barker A, Vowden P. Leg ulcer management in a nurse-led, hospital-based clinic. *J Wound Care* 1997;6:233–6

80. Partsch H. Compression therapy: is it worthwhile? In: Ruckley CV, Fowkes FGR, Bradbury AW, eds. *Venous Disease Epidemiology, Management and Delivery of Care*. London: Springer-Verlag, 1999:117–25

81. Cowan T. Compression hosiery. *Prof Nurse* 1997;12:881–6

82. Moffatt C, O'Hare L. Graduated compression hosiery for venous ulceration. *J Wound Care* 1995;4:459–62

83. Vowden K. The use of intermittent pneumatic compression in venous ulceration. *Br J Nurs* 2001;10:491–509

84. Pflug J. Intermittent compression in the management of swollen legs in general practice. *The Practitioner* 1975;215:69–76

85. Hazarika EZ, Wright DE. Chronic leg ulcers: the effects of pneumatic intermittent compression. *The Practitioner* 1981;225:189–92

86. Dillon RS. Treatment of resistant venous stasis ulcers and dermatitis with the end-diastolic pneumatic compression boot. *Angiology* 1986;37:47–56

87. Pekanmaki K, Kolari PJ, Kiistala U. Intermittent pneumatic compression for post-thrombotic leg ulcers. *Clin Exp Dermatol* 1987;12: 350–3

88. McCulloch JM, Marler KC, Neal MB, Phifer TJ. Intermittent pneumatic compression improves venous ulcer healing. *Adv Wound Care* 1994;7:22–4,26

89. Schuler JJ, Maibenco T, Megerman J, Ware M, Montalvo J. Treatment of chronic venous ulcers using sequential gradient intermittent pneumatic compression. *Phlebology* 1996;11: 111–16

90. Rowland J. Intermittent pump versus compression bandages in the treatment of venous leg ulcers. *Aust NZ J Surg* 2000;70:110–13

91. Mani R, Vowden K, Nelson EA. Intermittent pneumatic compression for the treatment of venous leg ulcers (Protocol for a Cochrane Review). In: *The Cochrane Library*. Oxford: Update Software, 2001

92. Morison M, Moffatt C. *A Colour Guide to the Assessment and Management of Leg Ulcers*. 2nd edn. London: Wolfe Publishing, 1994

93. Moffatt C. Issues in the assessment of leg ulceration. *J Wound Care* 1998;7:469–73

94. Vowden K, Vowden P. Vascular assessment in compression therapy. *Prof Nurse* 1997; 12(Suppl):S3–6

95. Ertl P. The multiple benefits of accurate assessment. Effective management of leg ulcers. *Prof Nurse* 1993;9:139–44

96. Vowden KR, Goulding V, Vowden P. Hand-held Doppler assessment for peripheral arterial disease. *J Wound Care* 1996;5:125–8

97. Vowden P, Vowden KR. *Doppler Assessment and ABPI: Interpretation in the Management of Leg Ulceration*. 2001 (Revision 1); Accessed: 2001(March). Internet Journal: www.world-widewounds.com

98. Stubbing NJ, Bailey P, Poole M. Protocol for accurate assessment of ABPI in patients with leg ulcers. *J Wound Care* 1997;6:417–18

99. Callam MJ, Ruckley CV, Dale JJ, Harper DR. Hazards of compression treatment of the leg: an estimate from Scottish surgeons. *BMJ* 1987;295:1382

100. Chan CLH, Meyer FJ, Hay RJ, Burnand KG. Toe ulceration associated with compression bandaging: observational study. *BMJ* 2001; 323:1099

101. Magazinovic N, Phillips-Turner J, Wison GV. Assessing nurses knowledge of bandages and bandaging. *J Wound Care* 1993;2:97–111

102. Nelson EA, Ruckley CV, Barbenel JC. Improvements in bandaging technique following training. *J Wound Care* 1995;4:181–4

103. Armstrong SH, Ruckley CV, Prescott RJ, Dale JJ, Nelson EA. Deficiencies in leg ulcer care: a national survey in Scotland. *Phlebology* 1998; 13:40–4

104. Taylor AD, Taylor RJ, Said SS. Using a bandage pressure monitor as an aid in improving bandaging skills. *J Wound Care* 1998;7:131–3

105. Williams RJ, Wertheim D, Melhuish J, Harding KG. How compression therapy works. *J Wound Care* 1999;8:297–8

106. Steinberg MD, Cooke ED. Design and evaluation of a device for measurement of interface pressure. *J Biomed Eng* 1993;15:464–8

107. Taylor RJ, Taylor AD. Construction and calibration of a low-cost bandage pressure monitor. *J Wound Care* 1998;7:125–8

108. Wertheim D, Melhuish J, Williams R, Harding K. Measurement of forces associated with compression therapy. *Med Biol Eng Comput* 1999;37:31–4

109. Danielsen L, Madsen M, Henriksen L, Sindrup J, Petersen L. Sub bandage pressure measurements comparing a long-stretch with a short-stretch compression bandage. *Acta Dermato-Venereol* 1998;78:201–4

110. Veraart JC, Pronk G, Neumann HA. Pressure differences of elastic compression stockings at the ankle region. *Dermatol Surg* 1997;23: 935–9

111. Scriven JM, Taylor LE, Wood AJ, Bell PRF, Naylor AR, London NJM. A prospective randomised trial of four-layer versus short stretch compression bandages for the treatment of venous leg ulcers. *Ann R Coll Surg Engl* 1998;80:215–20

112. Cameron J. The importance of contact dermatitis in the management of leg ulcers. *J Tiss Viab* 1995;5:52–5

113. Nelzen O, Bergqvist D, Lindhagen A. Leg ulcer etiology – cross sectional population study. *J Vasc Surg* 1991;14:557–64

114. Ghauri AS, Nyamekye I, Grabs AJ, Farndon JR, Poskitt KR. The diagnosis and management of mixed arterial/venous leg ulcers in community-based clinics. *Eur J Vasc Endovasc Surg* 1998;16:350–5

115. Liew I, Sinha S. A leg ulcer clinic: audit of the first three years. *J Wound Care* 1998;7:405–7

116. Scriven JM, Hartshorne T, Bell PR, Naylor AR, London NJ. Single-visit venous ulcer assessment clinic: the first year. *Br J Surg* 1997;84:334–6

117. Simon DA, Freak L, Williams IM, McCollum CN. Progression of arterial disease in patients with healed venous ulcers. *J Wound Care* 1994;3:179–80

118. Fowkes FGR, Callam MJ. Is arterial disease a risk factor for chronic leg ulceration? *Phlebology* 1994;9:87–90

119. Sumner DS. Non-invasive assessment of peripheral arterial occlusive disease. In: Rutherford KS, ed. *Vascular Surgery*, 3rd edn. Philadelphia: WB Saunders, 1989:61–111

120. Guest M, Williams A, Greenhalgh R, Davies A. Mixed leg ulcers. *Eur J Vasc Endovasc Surg* 1999;18:540–1

121. Smith PC, Sarin S, Hasty J, Scurr JH. Sequential gradient pneumatic compression enhances venous ulcer healing: a randomized trial. *Surgery* 1990;108:871–5

122. Hofman D. Leg ulceration with mixed arterial and venous disease. *J Wound Care* 1997;6:53–5

123. Nelson EA. Compression bandaging in the treatment of venous leg ulcers. *J Wound Care* 1996;5:415–18

124. Franks PJ, Moffatt CJ, Connolly M, *et al.* Factors associated with healing leg ulceration with high compression. *Age Ageing* 1995;24:407–10

125. Vowden KR, Goulden V, Wilkinson D, Vowden P. Venous disease in leg ulceration as revealed by duplex ultrasound: influence on healing and recurrence. *11th European Conference on Advances in Wound Management.* Dublin, Ireland, 17–19 May, 2001

126. Margolis DJ, Berlin JA, Strom BL. Which venous leg ulcers will heal with limb compression bandages? *Am J Med* 2000;109:15–19

127. Barwell JR, Ghauri ASK, Taylor M, *et al.* Risk factors for healing and recurrence of chronic venous leg ulcers. *Phlebology* 2000;15:49–52

128. Chetter I, Spark J, Goulding V, Vowden K, Wilkinson D, Vowden P. Is there a relationship between the aetiology and healing rates of lower limb venous ulcers? *Phlebology* 2001;16:47–8

129. Guest M, Smith JJ, Sira MS, Madden P, Greenhalgh RM, Davies AH. Venous ulcer healing by four-layer compression bandaging is not influenced by the pattern of venous incompetence. *Br J Surg* 1999;86:1437–40

130. Moffatt C, Franks P. The problem of recurrence in patients with leg ulceration. *J Tiss Viab* 1995;5:64–6

131. House N. Patient compliance with leg ulcer treatment. *Prof Nurse* 1996;12:33–6

132. Erickson CA, Lanza DJ, Karp DL, *et al.* Healing of venous ulcers in an ambulatory care program: the roles of chronic venous insufficiency and patient compliance. *J Vasc Surg* 1995;22:629–36

133. Tonge H. A review of factors affecting compliance in patients with leg ulcers. *J Wound Care* 1995;4:84–5

134. Buchmann WF. Adherence: a matter of self-efficacy and power. *J Adv Nurs* 1997;26:132–7

135. Monk BE, Sarkany I. Outcome of treatment of venous stasis ulcers. *Clin Exp Dermatol* 1982;7:397–400

136. Callam MJ, Ruckley CV, Harper DR, Dale JJ. Chronic ulceration of the leg: extent of the problem and provision of care. *BMJ* 1985;290:1855–6

137. Ellison DA, McCollum CN. Hospital or community: how should leg ulcer care be provided? In: Ruckley CV, Fowkes FGR, Bradbury AW, eds. *Venous Disease: Epidemiology, Management and Delivery of Care.* London: Springer–Verlag, 1999:222–9

138. Harper DR, Nelson EA, Gibson B, Prescott RJ, Ruckley CV. A prospective randomised trial of Class 2 and Class 3 elastic compression in the prevention of venous ulceration. *Phlebology* 1995;Suppl 1:872–3

139. Moffatt CJ, Dorman MC. Recurrence of leg ulcers within a community ulcer service. *J Wound Care* 1995;4:57–61

140. Ghauri AS, Nyamekye I, Grabs AJ, Farndon JR, Whyman MR, Poskitt KR. Influence of a specialised leg ulcer service and venous surgery on the outcome of venous leg ulcers. *Eur J Vasc Endovasc Surg* 1998;16:238–44

141. Sonnenberg FA, Beck R. Markov models in medical decision making: a practical guide. *Med Decis Making* 1993;13:322–8

The lessons learnt from wound healing in HIV-infected patients and the need for change of management

5

K. Jönsson and S. Mzezewa

INTRODUCTION

The prevalence of human immunodeficiency virus (HIV) infection in the adult population in the worst affected areas of the sub-Saharan Africa is at present higher than 25%. Wound healing is severely impaired, not only in patients with symptoms and signs of acquired immuno-deficiency syndrome (AIDS) but delayed healing has also been recorded in patients without clinical manifestations of HIV infection. Trauma, infections and complications of surgery in HIV-infected patients often result in difficult-to-heal wounds. It is therefore important to recognize clinical signs and symptoms of HIV infection in order to avoid or minimize surgery in non-emergency situations. Assessment with laboratory tests and serologic confirmation of HIV infection may facilitate surgical decision-making. Injuries and operations in HIV-infected patients seem to impair the immune system even further and result in clinical manifestations of immunodeficiency. Excision of anal fissures, implantation of foreign bodies (wires and sutures) and orthopedic implants should be avoided in HIV-infected patients, if possible. Split skin grafting for cover of large

tissue defects after necrotizing fasciitis or deep dermal burns in HIV-infected patients has to be planned very carefully because of the impaired graft survival in these patients often necessitating repeated procedures. In patients with manifest gangrene of the lower limbs, high amputations are recommended. Intestinal gangrene should be treated with resection and fashioning of a colostomy or ileostomy and mucus fistula for continued assessment of progression of gangrene, if this is possible. Basic surgical principles have to be evaluated in relation to the severity of the deficiency of the immune system. The impact of HIV infection on healing is often underestimated, resulting in chronic wounds.

Wound management in sub-Saharan Africa can at present only be discussed in a meaningful way in relation to the various manifestations of impaired immunity caused by HIV. Impaired healing of both acute and chronic wounds is often related to the presence of an ongoing HIV infection, *vide infra*. The highest prevalence of HIV infection in any population is found in sub-Saharan Africa where the infection probably has been present for more than half a century.

EPIDEMIOLOGY

Serologic evidence of HIV type 1 infection in Central Africa was noted in serum from patients collected in 1959 in the Congo and in 1973 in Uganda[1,2]. Central, East and Southern Africa has predominantly HIV type 1 infection, while HIV type 2 infection is found mainly in West Africa[3,4]. In Zimbabwe and Botswana, the countries with the highest rates of infection at present, more than one-quarter of the adult population is known to be infected. In hospital populations, this figure is even higher. The number of HIV-infected patients in a consecutive sample of 189 patients including children admitted to general surgery wards in Harare, Zimbabwe in 1995 was 24%[5]. In a similar study of adult patients admitted for abdominal surgery operations, the number of HIV-infected in 1998 was 34%[6].

Heterosexual transmission of the virus is the main mode of infection in adults in sub-Saharan Africa. Adults, as well as an increasing number of young children of infected mothers, succumb. The mother-to-child transmission of HIV in Africa has been reported to be 25–39%[7–10], while in Europe this figure is 14–20%[11–13]. In Europe this figure has been dramatically reduced after the introduction of anti-retroviral therapy, while in Africa it is still the same due to unaffordability of these drugs.

WOUNDS IN CHILDREN

The symptoms of HIV infection in children infected at birth or by breast feeding are usually first noted on the growth curve as a retarded weight gain, later on as frequent infections, diarrhea, malnutrition, pallor and thin, silky hair. The majority of wounds in need of hospital care in children below the age of 2 years are usually caused by burns. In a prospective study of patients admitted to the two burn units in Harare, one-third of all burns admitted was in children below the age of 2 years. In this group of patients under the age of 2 years, one-third of the burns was due to flame and two-thirds were caused by scalding[14].

Diarrhea and malnutrition are common symptoms in many African children. In children with concomitant burns, it is valuable to distinguish the etiology of these symptoms because aggressive treatment in the HIV-seronegative child has a favorable outcome in the long term if the burn injury is not too extensive. Surgical cover of a wound by split skin grafting has to be planned more carefully in the HIV-infected child because the failure rate of skin grafting is markedly increased in this group[15]. Testing for HIV is done in most places only after counseling and informed consent, very often by any of the newly introduced rapid tests. If the patient is seropositive for HIV, a second counseling takes place and the test is repeated, usually with an enzyme-linked immunosorbent assay (ELISA). In children under the age of 18 months, this test can read positive due to antibodies from the mother and may therefore not always indicate ongoing HIV infection.

Few centers in Africa have access to laboratory technology for direct testing of HIV-1 by polymerase chain reaction. This test provides the opportunity to diagnose HIV-infected patients who have not developed a serologic response. In clinical practice we mainly rely on symptoms and signs of HIV infections and less frequently on HIV testing. Therefore the situation where a child tests positive and its mother is unaware of her HIV infection is not often encountered. The mother is then offered tests, though some may refuse, fearful of a positive outcome.

The majority of burns are treated by topical application of silver sulfadiazine cream and covered by bandages in our unit. In burns affecting the distal parts of the extremities, we use long plastic gloves to cover the injuries. This type of wound cover will guarantee a moist wound environment and facilitate the work of the physiotherapists. The plastic gloves are cheap and easy to apply (Figure 5.1).

WOUNDS IN ADULTS

In adults, clinical signs of HIV infection are not always obvious, and so careful examination is essential. Reliable signs are temporal wasting, thin and silky hair, gray nails, target scars (i.e. scars with a lighter hyperkeratotic center), general lymphadenopathy, enlargement of especially epitrochlear lymph nodes and oral thrush (candidiasis). If a history of weight loss, night sweats and episodes of diarrhea and sometimes dysphagia is added to the signs mentioned, the correlation with an ongoing HIV infection is likely to exceed 80% in most areas of sub-Saharan Africa.

A wound in an immune-compromised patient has no specific features; instead it is the complete history and a careful physical examination of the whole patient which is important in order to obtain a correct diagnosis. On a number of occasions, we have noticed that large wounds, like deep burns in HIV-positive patients, look more pale than wounds in HIV-negative patients and formation of granulation tissue and wound contraction seem to progress at a slower rate. These impressions might be used to suspect HIV infection in patients with retarded rate of healing but are not specific for HIV infection *per se*. Additional signs, like herpes zoster scars observed in patients from sub-Saharan Africa, are in more than 90% correlated to the presence of an ongoing HIV infection[16].

A history of tuberculosis or ongoing treatment for tuberculosis is also highly correlated to HIV infection (Figure 5.2). In Lusaka, Zambia, 84% of patients with tuberculosis of the lymph nodes were found also to be infected with HIV[16]. In a prospective study at an infectious disease hospital in Harare, Zimbabwe, patients with pleural effusions containing acid-fast bacilli on aspiration or biopsy were found to be HIV-infected in 80% of the cases[17].

Oral lesions and healing

A complete physical examination also includes examination of the oral cavity and anus by inspection and palpation. In a study from Harare, the most common oral findings observed in immune-compromised patients were oral ulcers, candidiasis, gingivitis and Kaposi's sarcoma[18]. Oral Kaposi's sarcoma, noted as purple patches or purple tumors on the hard palate, is often asymptomatic and may therefore be the first sign of HIV infection in apparently healthy individuals[18–23] (Figure 5.3).

Kaposi's sarcoma

In Kaposi's sarcoma related to the HIV epidemic, male to female ratios of 3:1 have been noted, which is substantially higher than the ratios of 1.5:1 found in the classic endemic form described by Moritz Kaposi in 1872[22–26]. Soft tissue tumors of the distal parts of the lower extremities in elderly African men may occasionally represent the endemic form of Kaposi's sarcoma (Figure 5.4).

The overwhelming majority of the irregular hyperpigmented plaques seen on the skin related to HIV infection are often bilateral and are usually located to the proximal parts of the extremities. These tumors often have infiltrative growth associated with brawny edema. Early lesions may be difficult to diagnose and lesions of other diseases must be excluded. Differential diagnoses include pyogenic granuloma, angioma, glomus tumor, sarcoid nodule, malignant melanoma and lymphomatous nodules. In endemic areas, filariasis, Madura foot and Buruli ulcer caused by *Mycobacterium ulcerans* all need to be excluded. An excisional biopsy of the lesion for histologic examination, in combination with testing for HIV antibodies, is needed before treatment can be instituted. Kaposi's sarcoma was the leading cancer according to the National Cancer Registry for 1998 in black Zimbabwean men, accounting for 41% of all cases. It was also the leading tumor in children. The number of new cases diagnosed and treated in Harare increased from 192 in 1996 to 382 in the year 2000. In centers of sub-Saharan Africa, the mainstays of treatment are chemotherapy and radiation. In the Western world, topical therapies and interferon, in combination with anti-retroviral agents, are often added to chemotherapy and radiation.

ANAL LESIONS AND HEALING

Anal lesions are not so easy to detect on routine physical examination because a procto-scope and a good light source are necessary for inspection of the anal canal. However, simple external inspection and palpation of the anus and rectum will disclose the majority of important lesions such as condyloma acuminata and anal ulcers, which are the two most frequent manifestations correlated to HIV infection in patients from the Western world[27].

The most frequent etiology of anal ulcers in HIV-infected patients is related to concomitant herpes simplex virus infection followed by cytomegalovirus infection[27]. Anal fissures and anal abscesses are correlated to ongoing HIV infection in more than 90% of patients treated by surgeons in Zimbabwe[28]. Emergency surgical drainage of abscesses is needed in all patients in order to minimize infectious tissue destruction, but fissures are better treated non-operatively in sub-Saharan Africa until serologic tests have ruled out ongoing HIV infection. If the patient is HIV-infected, operative intervention is discouraged because of the very poor rate of healing in HIV-infected patients with chronic fissures[28-30]. Much of our knowledge on wound healing in the anal region has been accumulated in follow-up studies of patients undergoing hemorrhoid-ectomy. There seems to be impairment of the healing process in relation to progression of the infection. The rate of complete closure of surgical wounds in the anal region left open for healing by secondary intention was 69% in HIV-infected patients without symptoms of AIDS compared with only 26% in patients with AIDS[31]. These findings have recently been repeated and also extended to a group of HIV-infected patients without AIDS. In this prospective study of patients undergoing hemorrhoidectomy, delay in healing was noted, not only in AIDS patients but also in the HIV-infected group without symptoms of AIDS in comparison to non-infected control patients[32]. Some investigators have not found delayed healing of peri-anal wounds in patients without symptoms of immuno-suppression[33,34]. However, it seems reasonable to assume that there is a continuous impairment of wound healing in relation to progression of the deficiency of the immune system, and effort should be made to classify patients pre-operatively with white cell count[35-37] and T lymphocyte count of CD4-positive cells[29,30,32]. A white cell count of less than 3000 cells/mm³ and a CD4-positive lymphocyte count of less than 50/ml have both been related to impaired healing of peri-anal wounds[30,35]. These findings in patients are supported by earlier experimental studies in rats, indicating a positive correlation between the number of lymphocytes and the rate of wound healing[38,39]. In peri-anal ulcers of HIV-infected patients, aggressive diagnostic maneuvers in the form of cultures and biopsies for histologic examination have been advocated, in order to diagnose infection with cytomegalovirus, herpes simplex virus and acid-fast bacilli, as well as diagnosis of lymphoma and anal carcinoma, which are all correlated to HIV infection[40]. Cultures were found to be more helpful than biopsies to determine the etiology of these ulcers.

Aggressive diagnostic maneuvers, as indicated above, resulted in a healing rate of 68% of the ulcers. This was achieved after use of medical therapy in the form of transcriptase inhibitors, ganciclovir, broad-spectrum antibiotics and limited surgical procedures[40].

Aggressive diagnostic procedures, as indicated above, are however only meaningful and possible to use in the developed world where medical therapy is available and affordable. Few places in sub-Saharan Africa have the capacity to diagnose and treat anal ulcers in the way advocated above. The general consensus is to limit surgery as much as possible for anal conditions because of delayed wound healing in HIV-infected patients.

ABDOMINAL SURGERY AND HEALING

Delayed healing of peri-anal wounds in immune-compromised patients has been well documented[29,30,32,35]. Healing of laparotomy wounds has been less frequently studied. However, in some recent fairly large studies, an increased rate of infectious wound complications in HIV-positive patients after laparotomy has been noted[6,41]. In a prospective study of 82 HIV-infected patients undergoing laparotomy in Harare, Zimbabwe, pathology and outcome were compared with 160 non-infected patients with a similar magnitude of abdominal surgical disease. Two-thirds of the HIV-infected patients had signs of immunosuppression. The pathology in the HIV/AIDS group was noted as bowel perforations, bowel gangrene, primary peritonitis, acalculus cholecystitis, abdominal tuberculosis, Kaposi's sarcoma, non-Hodgkin's lymphoma and mycotic aortic aneurysm. This pathology was not observed in the HIV-seronegative control group. The final pathologic diagnosis was attributed to ongoing HIV infection in 61%. The total postoperative mortality in HIV-infected patients was six times higher and the overall morbidity was eight times higher than in the control group. The percentage of complications related to the surgical wound was 28% in the HIV/AIDS group compared to 4% in the control group. The complications were recorded as wound infections, wound dehiscence and fistula formation.

In a retrospective study in London over a 10-year period, 53 HIV-infected patients having laparotomies were included. The incidence of wound complications and wound breakdown in the HIV-infected group was found to be higher than in the HIV-seronegative matched control group[41]. In both the Harare and London studies it was demonstrated that HIV-infected patients had a higher incidence of wound breakdown[6,41]. The increased rate of wound infections in the HIV-infected patients in these two studies may explain the rate of wound dehiscence, but biomechanic testing of healed wounds of HIV-infected patients has shown that these wounds have lower resilience, toughness and maximum extension compared to wounds in control patients. The impaired strength of healed wounds in HIV-infected patients, as demonstrated by tensiometry, may be related to changes in collagen synthesis or maturation. The increased risk of wound dehiscence after laparotomy in HIV-infected patients may therefore be related to both increased breakdown of collagen due to infection and impaired or delayed gain of strength due to changes in synthesis or maturation of collagen, but this has to be evaluated in further studies.

In the developed world, surgical procedures in HIV-infected patients are performed less frequently for abdominal conditions than for anal[36]. The general consensus among surgeons attending the meeting of the Association of Surgeons of East Africa in Maputo, Mozambique in 2000 was to avoid surgery for anal conditions as much as possible because of the delayed wound healing after these operations in the HIV-infected population. There is usually very little opportunity to be restrictive with laparotomies in HIV-infected patients since these operations are performed mainly on patients presenting with symptoms and signs of acute abdomen[6]. The specific pathology and the impaired immunity are both contributors to the very high morbidity and mortality in HIV-infected patients undergoing surgery for procedures requiring laparotomy[6].

DENTAL SURGERY AND HEALING

The most frequent surgical procedure performed in HIV-infected patients is probably tooth extraction. In these patients, an increased number of post-extraction infectious complications and delayed healing have been reported[42–44]. Prophylactic antibiotics might reduce infectious complications in HIV-infected patients undergoing tooth extraction, but there is no uniform agreement of its clinical value[45,46]. The only predictive factor found for complications following tooth extractions in a prospective study was a low CD8 lymphocyte count[43]. However, in acute situations CD8 lymphocyte testing is not recommended since it will delay treatment and most of the complications were found to be minor[43].

GANGRENE ASSOCIATED WITH HIV INFECTION

Gangrene of limbs and healing of amputation stumps

Gangrene of the lower limbs has been noted with increasing prevalence of HIV infection in the population. In a retrospective study during the 2 years 1993 and 1994, a total of seven HIV-infected patients were amputated for gangrene of one or both lower limbs in a hospital-based study in Harare. In a prospective study conducted during the year 2000, a total of 19 patients were amputated of which 13 were HIV-infected. All but one were males in the age group of 20–55 years. A history of smoking

was recorded in two-thirds of our patients with HIV-associated lower limb gangrene. Thromboembolism, cytomegalovirus-associated vasculitis, *Pneumocystis carinii* infection and chemotherapy have all been proposed as contributing etiologic factors. Vasculitis has been noted on histopathologic examination in one study of amputated feet[47]. Gangrene of fingers has been related to vasculitis in an AIDS patient with a history of smoking[48]. *Pneumocystis carinii* infection and chemotherapy have both been associated with gangrene of fingers in HIV-infected men[49]. None of the patients in our two studies in Harare were found to have vasculitis on histologic examination of the amputated limbs and atherosclerosis was not observed in the HIV-infected group. Conservative amputations failed in most of our patients as a result of infection and progressive tissue necrosis (Figures 5.5 and 5.6).

Primary healing was achieved only after high amputations, as also noted and recommended by others[16] (Figure 5.7).

In order to increase the possibilities for primary healing and short hospital stay, lower limb gangrene associated with HIV infection should, if possible, be treated with high amputations. This was the general consensus at a recent meeting on AIDS and Surgery in Maputo, Mozambique. This recommendation is valid for treatment of HIV-infected patients in developing countries. Whether a more conservative approach can be taken in the developed world, with better diagnostic facilities, remains to be evaluated.

Gangrene of bowel and intestinal healing

Gangrene of limbs and gangrene of the bowel might have the same pathophysiology in HIV-infected patients. In a large prospective study of patients undergoing laparotomies, bowel gangrene and intestinal ischemia were found only in the HIV-infected group. The control group with twice the number of patients compared to the HIV-infected group had no bowel gangrene. Primary anastomosis after resection of the gangrenous bowel is discouraged, since it will result in a high rate of wound healing complications and high mortality[6]. Colostomy or ileostomy should be fashioned and the distal end should, if possible, be brought out as a mucus fistula. The stoma and the distal end can then be observed for progression of tissue necrosis and re-operation can be performed if necessary.

The increased rate of complications noted after laparotomies and intestinal resections in the HIV-infected patient and their weaker scars are important findings for surgeons when an intestinal anastomosis is considered in favor of a stoma[6,37,41]. However, these findings have to be added to the already well-established general and local factors known to affect healing in the gastrointestinal tract. The 'general factors' known to impair healing are advanced age[50–53], hypovolemia[54–58], hypoxia[59,60], uncontrolled diabetes mellitus[61,62], uremia[63,64], malnutrition[52,65,66] and steroid medication[67,68]. All these factors, except for age, can to a large extent be controlled by the surgeon.

The 'local factors' known to impair healing are infection and inflammation, i.e. peritonitis[51,69–74], bowel obstruction[75 83], fecal loading[52,84] and irradiation[51,84–88]. None of these factors, except for fecal loading, can be influenced by the surgeon. Prophylactic abdominal drains in the close proximity of an anastomosis are detrimental to anastomotic healing[89–94]. The drain is acting as a foreign body and increases the risk of infection, as will be discussed later.

Necrotizing fasciitis and Fournier's gangrene

Necrotizing fasciitis and Fournier's gangrene in the male usually have their origin in peri-anal and peri-urethral infections. In the female, necrotizing fasciitis often arises from the vulva and very often in association with septic abor-

tions. Aggressive resuscitation, together with broad-spectrum antibiotics with good anaerobic cover, should be instituted as soon as possible[16]. The subsequent surgical treatment recommended in the non-HIV-infected patient includes wide excision of all necrotic tissue including overlying skin, subcutaneous fat and fascia beyond the margin of infection. However, when clinical signs of immunosuppression are present, not all surgeons would agree to perform extensive surgery. A more limited surgical excision is often favored by surgeons who have to deal with patients in an advanced stage of immunosuppression (Figure 5.8).

Creation of large wounds without the possibility for intensive or high-care postoperatively may frequently lead to unsatisfactory situations for both patients and nursing staff. This has become even more evident after the findings of impaired split skin graft survival in HIV-infected patients[15] (Figures 5.9 and 5.10).

The limited resources in developing countries, the often limited experience of the surgeon and the impaired healing capacity, all have an impact on the possibilities for successful outcome of reconstructive surgery. The recommendations valid for non-HIV-infected patients are often controversial in patients with signs of immunosuppression in the setting of developing countries. Limited tissue-saving procedures, ending with hydrogen peroxide wash, repeated if necessary, during careful observation and frequent change of dressings, might be justified instead of very wide surgical excisions.

The optimum surgical treatment in immune-compromised patients presenting with symptoms and signs of necrotizing fasciitis is at present controversial and remains to be established.

THYROID ABSCESS

Inflammation of the thyroid gland, suppurative thyroiditis leading to abscess formation, is generally a very rare condition caused by bacteria. However, in the HIV-infected patient, this is a much more common finding. The presenting symptoms are usually neck pain and pain on swallowing in combination with fever. On palpation, the gland is extremely tender and a fluctuation or swelling only may be felt. During the last year, we treated four HIV-infected patients with thyroid abscess. Two had simple incision and drainage at the site of fluctuation in normal thyroid glands (Figure 5.11). The other two patients had symptoms of acute airway obstruction and large multinodular goiters on presentation. The diagnosis of thyroid abscess was difficult. Ultrasound scan was not attempted. Both had emergency intubation and, at operation, deep thyroid abscesses were found which could not be diagnosed by palpation. The abscesses were only diagnosed and drained when subtotal thyroidectomy was performed. Only one of the patients had fever on admission and she had clinical signs of immunosuppression. In the patient with immunosuppression, a tracheostomy had to be performed because of a hypoxic incident and subsequent failure to breathe spontaneously.

Very large goiters are common in the eastern parts of sub-Saharan Africa where the prevalence of HIV infection is also high. In patients with multinodular goiters in areas with high prevalence of HIV infection, who are presenting with acute onset of airway obstruction, a thyroid abscess must be suspected also without fever and signs of fluctuation on physical examination.

RESISTANCE TO WOUND INFECTION

Whether an operation will benefit an immune-compromised patient or not is very often dependent on the intrinsic ability of that particular patient to resist infection. Infectious complications and delayed healing account for the major increase in mortality and morbidity noticed both after major and minor surgical procedures in HIV-infected patients[6,28,30,32,41]. Decision-making is influenced by clinical symptoms and signs and a few laboratory tests. It is important to recognize anemia, leukocytopenia and thrombocytopenia before a decision to operate is made. Laboratory tests for these parameters are available in many hospitals in sub-Saharan Africa, but T lymphocyte count of CD4-positive cells is seldom available. The diagnosis of immunodeficiency, therefore, has to be made on clinical criteria, less often by HIV testing and lymphocyte count of CD4-positive cells. Most studies from Africa therefore lack the information on CD4 lymphocyte levels that is recommended as an important criterion by the Center for Disease Control (CDC) to classify patients with HIV infection.

The general risk factors of importance for predicting wound infection as recognized by the CDC are the following:

(1) The amount and type of microbial contamination of the wound;

(2) The condition of the wound at the end of the operation (vascular compromise, surgical technique);

(3) The susceptibility of the host or the intrinsic ability to deal with microbial contamination[95].

Microbial contamination

The amount of microbial contamination of a wound in a patient with HIV infection is not likely to differ from similar operations in the non-infected patient, since this is dependent on the procedure and the surgical technique. The types of bacteria found in HIV-infected patients are related to the pathology encountered[6].

Condition of the wound

The pathology found in patients undergoing laparotomy was in 61% directly related to the HIV infection[6]. Vascular compromise of a wound at the end of an operation for bowel gangrene, lower limb gangrene, necrotizing fasciitis and Fournier's gangrene may be difficult to assess. The likelihood of infection in these conditions is therefore increased and the need for prophylactic antibiotics or continued antibiotic treatment of the condition is not controversial.

Host susceptibility to infection

The intrinsic ability to deal with microbial contamination is related to factors like diabetes, uremia, malnutrition, steroid and anti-mitotic therapy[96]. These patient-dependent factors can and should as far as possible be controlled before surgery.

Other factors reducing host resistance such as advanced age, obesity, malignancy, liver cirrhosis and leukocytopenia due to HIV infection cannot be influenced by the surgeon.

There are, however, some factors determining resistance to infection or promoting infection which are under control of the surgeon. These are tissue oxygenation, foreign body implantation, hemostasis, blood transfusion, length of operation and pre-operative hospital stay. The level of tissue oxygen tension is correlated to infection[97–99]. Supplemental oxygen has been shown to decrease the extent of infectious tissue necrosis in animals undergoing surgery, with elevation of cutaneous and musculocutaneous flaps and inoculation with *Staphylococcus aureus* at the time of operation[99]. In patients it has been shown that measurements of tissue oxygen tension of a wound predicted the risk of wound infection and that these measurements were a better predictor of wound infection than any scoring system presently in use[100]. In a large recent randomized multicenter study of patients undergoing colorectal resections, it was found that supplemental oxygen at a concentration of 80% during operation and for 2 h postoperatively could reduce the number of wound infections by half, compared to a control group given oxygen at a concentration of 30% during the same period[101]. These experimental and clinical studies clearly indicate that it is possible to reduce wound infections by simple means such as perioperative supplemental oxygen administration. It has to be emphasized, though, that high tissue oxygen tensions can only be generated by administration of supplemental oxygen if the patients are well hydrated and well perfused[102]. Furthermore, optimal perfusion can only be guaranteed if perioperative normothermia prevails by adequate control and intervention[101]. The oxidative killing of bacteria in phagocytes is dependent on high tissue oxygen tensions for production of bactericidal superoxide radicals[103,104]. Molecular oxygen at a partial pressure of 5–250 mmHg is the substrate in this reaction[105]. Whether this defense mechanism is equally or more important in HIV/AIDS patients with relatively fewer phagocytes remains to be evaluated. It seems reasonable to assume that optimizing conditions for resistance to infection in the immune-compromised patient by increasing tissue oxygen tension might be of similar magnitude as in the normal patient in relation to the number of phagocytes available.

Foreign body implantation is correlated to an increased risk of infections. In experimental studies, it was shown that injection of *Staphylococcus aureus* at a concentration of 10^6/ml into the skin of the forearm produced little or no reaction but the concentration of 10^3/ml together with a silk suture resulted in formation of an abscess[106,107]. In HIV-infected patients, orthopedic implants are more likely to become infected than in non-HIV-infected patients. Patients who were HIV-infected at the time of joint arthroplasty had a 10 times higher risk of getting a bacterial infection compared to patients having non-arthroplasty procedures[108]. Mandibular fractures in HIV-infected patients treated by open reduction and internal fixation have an increased risk of becoming infected compared with those in HIV-seronegative patients[109,110]. Even if the implants are not contaminated at the time of surgery, there is an increased risk of later hematogenous infection from the frequent bacteriemias that immune-compromised patients experience[111,112]. If orthopedic implants are considered as the only successful method of treatment, it is recommended that the implants are removed at the earliest possible time in HIV-infected patients. The general consensus among orthopedic surgeons, in developing countries with high prevalence of HIV infection, is that, if possible, implants should be avoided or restricted to patients proven to be HIV-seronegative.

Hemostasis is usually not a major problem affecting HIV-infected patients undergoing surgical procedures even if a reduced number of platelets is found relatively early after infection with the human immunodeficiency virus. Only in AIDS patients with advanced disease and low or very low platelet counts has a surgically important impairment of hemostasis been noted. It is not only the number of platelets but also their capacity to function which are of importance for hemostasis. In a number of AIDS patients, we have observed an increased tendency to bleeding in wounds which have been left open for healing by secondary intention.

Blood transfusion reduces resistance to infection and results in higher postoperative rates of infection[113,114]. In developing countries, blood transfusions are almost always restricted to a minimum level due to the high cost and the relative unavailability of blood and blood products. Furthermore, most patients are relatively young and can tolerate low levels of hematocrit fairly well, as long as volume replacement with crystalloids and colloids is adequate. In HIV/AIDS patients with anemia who have to undergo operations or have to heal major wounds, the minimum level of hematocrit necessary for adequate tissue oxygenation and physiologically normal wound healing has to be obtained despite the negative effects of transfusion[113,114]. The minimum level of hematocrit needed for physiologically normal repair processes to take place has been found to be 15–18%[54,55].

Prolonged operation times are associated with a higher incidence of infection; prolonged preoperative hospitalization leads to colonization of the skin by organisms from the hospital environment which are more resistant to antibiotics[96]. These factors might be even more important in immune-compromised patients, but specific studies to this effect are at present lacking for this group of patients.

BURN INJURIES IN ADULTS

The prevalence of HIV infection in the adult population in sub-Saharan Africa is often more than 20% and even exceeds 25% in the most affected areas like Zimbabwe and Botswana. The majority of the population in most sub-Saharan countries use open fires for cooking meals. In Zimbabwe, 85% of the population use open fires when they are preparing food or warming water for bathing[15]. Most burns are sustained during preparation of meals either as scalding or open flame injury[15]. Treatment of burn wounds with split skin grafting was the most frequent procedure performed by general surgeons in Harare, Zimbabwe both in 1993 and 1998. At both periods investigated, one-third of all procedures performed at the tertiary referral centers were split skin grafting in order to cover burn wounds. Burn injuries in HIV-infected adults are common in most parts of sub-Saharan Africa where similar socioeconomic conditions and prevalence of HIV infection are found. In a major epidemiologic study involving 451 patients admitted to the two burn units in Harare, 71% had non-operative treatment while 26% had delayed split skin grafting and 3% early excision and split skin grafting[15]. Patients undergoing delayed split skin grafting have to wait for separation of necrotic and viable skin and formation of granulation tissue before grafting can take place. Impairment of their immunity has been recorded during this period. In earlier studies of animals subjected to burn injuries, a very high fatality rate after intraperitoneal bacterial injections was found in comparison to equal doses of bacteria injected into non-burnt animals, indicating a serious impairment of antibacterial defense mechanisms following burn injury[115]. Later studies in burn patients have shown impaired neutrophil leukocyte functions with maximum disturbances in the second week following burn injury. Chemotaxis and random migration of leukocytes were decreased and bactericidal capacity impaired[116]. The skin is a potent immunologic organ with a rich reservoir of lymphocytes, macrophages, neutrophils and dendritic cells. These play an important role in the immune response and are target cells of HIV infection. It is not known how the HIV-infected patient reacts immunologically to the delayed treatment of their burn injuries. However, the preferred method of treatment is early excision and split skin grafting. This method of treatment has been shown to reduce hospital stay by 60% in comparison to treatment by delayed split skin grafting of burns of equal size[14]. The outcome of treatment by early excision and split skin grafting of burns patients with HIV infection was recently compared to non-HIV-infected burn patients. It was found that split skin graft survival was only 23% in the HIV-infected patients compared with 79% in non-HIV-infected patients. The high failure rate among HIV-infected patients resulted in a doubling of their hospital stay[15]. The reason for the reduced graft survival in HIV-infected patients is not known, but our clinical impression seems to indicate that graft failure is noted at a later stage than graft failure due to bacterial infections in individuals without HIV infection. Therefore, we suspect that a mechanism other than bacterial infection may also be at play. In the case of autografting, as performed during split skin grafting, graft rejection implies a loss of tolerance. It is known that HIV infection changes the inflammatory cytokine response[117]. One might therefore speculate if cytokine imbalance contributes to the reduced graft survival observed. On several occasions, we have recorded signs of progressive impairment of the immunity in HIV-infected patients during treatment of major burns. Oral thrush, psychosis and herpes zoster have been noted in patients without any signs of impaired immunity on admission. Impaired immunity from HIV infection in combination with additional depression of the immune system by a major burn could be assumed to have an impact on infectious complications and outcome. Impaired graft survival has been noted, but mortality seems not to be affected, as indicated in a recent study of HIV-infected patients with moderate and severe burns compared to a non-infected control group[118].

References

1. Nahmias AJ, Weiss J, Yao X, *et al.* Evidence for human infection with an HTLV III/LAV-like virus in Central Africa, 1959. *Lancet* 1986;332:1279–80

2. Saxinger WC, Levine PH, Dean AG, *et al.* Evidence for exposure to HTLV-III in Uganda before 1973. *Science* 1985;227:1036–8

3. Kanki PJ, Barin F, M'Boup S, *et al*. New human T-lymphotropic retrovirus related to simian T-lymphotropic virus type III (STLV-IIIagm). *Science* 1986;232:238–43

4. Clavel F, Guétard D, Brun-Vézinet F, *et al*. Isolation of a new human retrovirus from West African patients with AIDS. *Science* 1986;233: 343–6

5. Girach A. A study of general surgical manifestations of AIDS and HIV. Thesis. University of Zimbabwe, Harare, 1995

6. Muchemwa FNM. Abdominal surgery in patients with HIV–AIDS. Indication, pathology, operative management and outcome. A prospective study in Zimbabwe. Thesis. University of Zimbabwe, Harare, 1998

7. Lepage P, Dabis F, Hitimana DG. Perinatal transmission of HIV-1: lack of impact of maternal HIV infection on characteristics of livebirths and on neonatal mortality in Kigali, Rwanda. *AIDS* 1991;5:295–300

8. Ryder RW, Nsa W, Hassig SE, *et al*. Perinatal transmission of the human immunodeficiency virus type 1 to infants of seropositive women in Zaire. *N Engl J Med* 1989;320:1637–42

9. Hira SK, Kamanga J, Bhat GJ, *et al*. Perinatal transmission of HIV-1 in Zambia. *Br Med J* 1989;299:1250–2

10. Lallemant M, Lallemant-Le Coeur S, Cheynier D, *et al*. Characteristics associated with HIV-1 infection in pregnant women in Brazzaville, Congo. *J Acquir Immune Defic Syndr* 1992;5: 279–85

11. Italian Multicenter Study. Epidemiology, clinical features and prognostic factors of paediatric HIV infection. *Lancet* 1988;334:1043–5

12. Blanche S, Rouzioux C, Guihard Moscato ML, *et al*. French Collaborative Study Group. A prospective study of infants born to women seropositive for human immunodeficiency virus type 1. *N Engl J Med* 1989;320:1643–8

13. European Collaborative Study. Children born to women with HIV-1 Infection: Natural history and risk of transmission. *Lancet* 1991;337: 253–60

14. Mzezewa S, Jönsson K, Aberg M, Salemark S. A prospective study on the epidemiology of burns in patients admitted to the Harare Burn Units. *Burns* 1999;25:499–504

15. Mzezewa S, Jönsson K, Åberg M, Salemark S. Healing of burn wounds after early excision and skin grafting in deep dermal burns in relation to HIV infection. *Eur Surg Res* 2001:33: 117–18

16. Bayley AC, Jellis JE, Watters DK. Surgery for HIV infected patients. In: Leaper DJ, Branicki FJ, eds. *International Surgical Practice*. Oxford, New York, Tokyo: Oxford University Press, 1992:65–93

17. Kadzirange G, Hakim J, Doherty T, Malin A, Mandisodza M. Tuberculous pleural disease in an HIV population in Harare. *University of Zimbabwe Proceedings: Annual Research Day* 1996:14

18. Jönsson N, Zimmerman M, Chidzonga MM, Jönsson K. Oral manifestations in 100 Zimbabwean HIV/AIDS patients referred to a specialist centre. *Cent Afr J Med* 1998;44:31–4

19. Greenspan D, Greenspan JS, Pindborg JJ, Schiodt M. *AIDS and the Dental Team*. Copenhagen: Munksgaard, 1986

20. Silverman S, Migliorati CA, Lozada-Nur F, Greenspan D, Conant MA. Oral findings in people with or at high risk of AIDS: a study of 375 homosexual males. *J Am Dent Assoc* 1986; 112:187–92

21. Schulten EAJM, TenKate RW, Van der Waal I. Oral manifestations of HIV infection in 75 Dutch patients. *J Oral Pathol Med* 1989;18:42–6

22. Reichart PA, Gelderblom HR, Becker J, Kuntz A. AIDS and the oral cavity. The HIV infection: virology, etiology, immunology, precautions and clinical observations in 110 patients. *Int J Oral Maxillofac Surg* 1987;16:129–53

23. Schiodt M, Pindborg JJ. AIDS and the oral cavity. Epidemiology and clinical oral manifestations of human immunodeficiency virus infection: A review. *Int J Oral Maxillofac Surg* 1987;16:1–14

24. Porter SR, Luker J, Scully C, Glover S, Griffith MJ. Oral manifestations of a group of British patients infected with HIV-1. *J Oral Pathol Med* 1989;18:47–8

25. Krizek TJ, Foster RS Jr. Skin and soft tissue. In: Davis JH, ed. *Clinical Surgery*. St Louis, Washington DC, Toronto: The CV Mosby Company, 1987;2369–2469

26. Kaposi M. Idiopatisches multiples Pigmentsarkom der Haut. *Arch Dermatol Syph* 1872;4: 265–73

27. Puy-Montbrun T, Denis J, Ganansia R, Mathoniere F, Lemarchand N, Arnous-Dubois N. Anorectal lesions in human immunodeficiency virus infected patients. *Int J Colorect Dis* 1992;7:26–30

28. Cotton MH. Etiology and treatment of anal fissure. *Br J Surg* 1997;84:279

29. Lord RV. Anorectal surgery in patients infected with human immunodeficiency virus: factors associated with delayed wound healing. *Ann Surg* 1997;226:2–9

30. Consten EC. Anorectal surgery in human immunodeficiency virus-infected patients. Clinical outcome in relation to immune status. *Dis Colon Rectum* 1995;38:1169–75

31. Safavi A, Gottesman L, Dailey TH. Anorectal surgery in the HIV+ patient: update. *Dis Colon Rectum* 1991;34:299–304

32. Morandi E, Merlini D, Salvaggio A, Foschi D, Trabucchi E. Prospective study of healing time after hemorrhoidectomy: influence of HIV infection, acquired immunodeficiency syndrome and anal wound infection. *Dis Colon Rectum* 1999;42:1140–4

33. Hewitt WR, Sokol TP, Fleshner PR. Should HIV status alter indications for hemorrhoidectomy? *Dis Colon Rectum* 1996;39:615–18

34. Burke EC, Orloff SL, Freisse CE, Macho JR, Schecter WP. Wound healing after anorectal surgery in human immunodeficiency virus-infected patients. *Arch Surg* 1991;126:1267–70

35. Nadal SR, Manzione CR, Galvao VM, Salim VR, Speranzini MB. Healing after anal fistulotomy: comparative study between HIV+ and HIV− patients. *Dis Colon Rectum* 1998;41:177–9

36. Wolkomir AF, Barone JE, Hardy HW III, Cottone FJ. Abdominal and anorectal surgery and the acquired immune deficiency syndrome in heterosexual intravenous drug users. *Dis Colon Rectum* 1990;33:267–70

37. Davis PA, Wastell C. A comparison of biomechanical properties of excised mature scar from HIV patients and non-HIV controls. *Am J Surg* 2000;180:217–22

38. Barbul A, Breslin RJ, Woodyard JP, Wasserkrug HL, Efron G. The effect of in vivo T helper and T suppressor lymphocyte depletion on wound healing. *Ann Surg* 1989;209:479–83

39. Fishel RS, Barbul A, Bisehorner WE, Wasserkrug HL, Efron G. Lymphocyte participation in wound healing: morphologic assessment using monoclonal antibodies. *Ann Surg* 1987;206:25–9

40. Schmitt SL, Wexner SD, Nogueras JJ, Jagelman DG. Is aggressive management of perianal ulcers in homosexual HIV-seropositive men justified? *Dis Colon Rectum* 1993;36:240–6

41. Davis PA, Corless DJ, Gazzard BG, Wastell C. Increased risk of wound complications and poor healing following laparotomy in HIV-seropositive and AIDS patients. *Dig Surg* 1999;16:60–7

42. Diz Dios P, Fernandez Feijoo J, Vasquez Garcia E. Tooth extraction in HIV sero-positive patients. *Int Dent J* 1999;49:317–21

43. Dodson TB. Predictors of postextraction complications in HIV-positive patients. *Oral Surg Oral Med Oral Pathol Oral Radiol Endod* 1997;84:474–9

44. Pankhurst CL, Lewis DA, Clark DT. Prophylactic application of an intra-alveolar socket medicament to reduce postextraction complication in HIV-seropositive patients. *Oral Surg Oral Med Oral Pathol* 1994;77:331–4

45. Porter SR, Scully C, Luker J. Complications of dental surgery in persons with HIV disease. *Oral Surg Oral Med Oral Pathol* 1993;75:165–7

46. Robinson PG, Cooper H, Hatt J. Healing after dental extractions in men with HIV infection. *Oral Surg Oral Med Oral Pathol* 1992;74:426–30

47. Berg RA, Belani A, Belani CP. Vasculitis in a suspected AIDS patient. *South Med J* 1986;79:914–15

48. Enelow RS, Hussein M, Grant K, *et al.* Vasculitis with eosinophilia and digital gangrene in a patient with acquired immunodeficiency syndrome. *J Rheumatol* 1992;19:1813–16

49. Davey RT, Margolis D, Kleiner D. Digital necrosis and disseminated *Pneumocystis carinii* infection after aerosolized pentamidine prophylaxis. *Ann Intern Med* 1989;111:681–2

50. Debas HT, Thomson FB. A critical review of colectomy with anastomosis. *Surg Gynecol Obstet* 1972;135:747–52

51. Schrock TR, Deveney CW, Dunphy JE. Factors contributing to leakage of colonic anastomoses. *Ann Surg* 1973;177:513–18

52. Irvin TT, Goligher JC. Aetiology of disruption of intestinal anastomoses. *Br J Surg* 1973;60: 461–4

53. Tagart REB. Colorectal anastomosis: factors influencing success. *J R Soc Med* 1981;74:111–18

54. Zederfeldt B. Studies on wound healing and trauma. *Acta Chir Scand* 1957;Suppl 224

55. Jönsson K, Jensen JA, Goodson WH III, *et al.* Tissue oxygenation anemia and perfusion in relation to wound healing in surgical patients. *Ann Surg* 1991;214:605–13

56. Hartmann M, Jönsson K, Zederfeldt B. Importance of dehydration for anastomotic and subcutaneous wound healing. An experimental study on rats. *Eur J Surg* 1992;158:78–82

57. Hartmann M, Jönsson K, Zederfeldt B. Effect of tissue perfusion and oxygenation on accumulation of collagen in healing wounds. Randomized study in patients after major abdominal operations. *Eur J Surg* 1992;158: 521–6

58. Hartmann M, Jönsson K, Zederfeldt B. Effects of Dextran and crystalloid on subcutaneous oxygen tension and collagen accumulation. A randomized study on surgical patients. *Eur Surg Res* 1993;25:270–7

59. Niinikoski J. Effect of oxygen supply on wound healing and formation of experimental granulation tissue. *Acta Physiol Scand* 1969; Suppl 334

60. Hunt TK, Niinikoski J, Zederfeldt B. Role of oxygen in repair processes. *Acta Chir Scand* 1972;136:109–10

61. Goodson WH, Hunt TK. Studies of wound healing in experimental diabetes mellitus. *J Surg Res* 1977;22:221–7

62. Gottrup F, Andreassen TT. Healing of incisional wounds in stomach and duodenum: the influence of experimental diabetes. *J Surg Res* 1981;31:61–6

63. Colin JF, Elliot P, Ellis H. The effect of uremia upon wound healing: an experimental study. *Br J Surg* 1979;66:793–7

64. Goodson WH III, Lindenfeld SM, Omachi RS, Hunt TK. Chronic uremia causes poor healing. *Surg Forum* 1982;33:54–6

65. Daly JM, Vars HM, Dudrick SJ. Effects of protein depletion on strength of colonic anastomoses. *Surg Gynecol Obstet* 1972;134:15–21

66. Irvin TT, Hunt TK. Reappraisal of the healing process of anastomoses of the colon. *Surg Gynecol Obstet* 1974;138:741–6

67. Ehrlich P, Hunt TK. Effects of cortisone and vitamin A on wound healing. *Ann Surg* 1968; 167:324–8

68. Gottrup F, Oxlund H. Healing of incisional wounds in stomach and duodenum: the effect of long-term cortisol treatment. *J Surg Res* 1981;31:165–71

69. Yamakawa T, Patin CS, Sobel S, Morgenstern L. Healing of colonic anastomoses following resection for experimental 'Diverticulitis'. *Arch Surg* 1971;103:17–20

70. Hawley PR. Causes and prevention of colonic anastomotic breakdown. *Dis Colon Rectum* 1973;16:272–7

71. De Haan BB, Ellis H, Wilks M. The role of infection on wound healing. *Surg Gynecol Obstet* 1974;138:693–700

72. Irvin TT. Collagen metabolism in infected colonic anastomoses. *Surg Gynecol Obstet* 1976; 143:220–4

73. Bucknall TE. The effect of local infection upon wound healing: an experimental study. *Br J Surg* 1980;67:851–5

74. Hesp FLEM, Hendiks T, Lubbers EJC, de Boer HHM. Wound healing in the intestinal wall. Effects of infection on experimental ileal and colonic anastomoses. *Dis Colon Rectum* 1984;27: 462–7

75. Dutton JW, Hreno A, Hampson LG. Mortality and prognosis of obstructing carcinoma of the large bowel. *Am J Surg* 1976;131:36–41

76. Irvin TT, Greaney MG. The treatment of colonic cancer presenting with intestinal obstruction. *Br J Surg* 1977;64:741–4

77. Kelly WE, Brown PW, Lawrence W Jr. Penetrating, obstructing and perforating carcinomas of the colon and rectum. *Arch Surg* 1981; 116:381–4

78. Öhman U. Prognosis in patients with obstructing colorectal carcinoma. *Am J Surg* 1982;143: 742–7

79. Wolmark N, other NSABP investigators. The prognostic significance or tumor location and bowel obstruction in Dukes B and C colorectal cancer. *Ann Surg* 1983:198:743–52

80. Barnett WO, Petro AB, Williamson JW. A current appraisal of problems with gangrenous bowel. *Ann Surg* 1976;183:653–9

81. Stewardson RH, Bombeck CT, Nyhus LM. Critical operative management of small bowel obstruction. *Ann Surg* 1978;187:189–93

82. Bizer LS, Liebling RW, Delany NM, Gliedman MD. Small bowel obstruction: the role of nonoperative treatment in simple intestinal obstruction and predictive criteria for strangulation obstruction. *Surgery* 1981;89:407–13

83. Ellis H. In: *Intestinal Obstruction*. New York: Appleton Century Crofts, 1982;1–9

84. Smith SRG, Connolly JC, Gilmore OJA. The effect of faecal loading on colonic anastomotic healing. *Br J Surg* 1983;70:49–50

85. De Cosse JJ, Rhodes RS, Wentz WB, Reagan JW, Dworken HJ, Holden WD. The natural history and management of radiation induced injury of the gastrointestinal tract. *Ann Surg* 1969;170:369–84

86. Swan RW, Fowler WC Jr, Boronow RC. Surgical management of radiation injury to the small intestine. *Surg Gynecol Obstet* 1976;142:325–7

87. Galland RB, Spencer J. Surgical aspects of radiation injury to the intestine. *Br J Surg* 1979;66:135–8

88. Murphy K, Frith C, Lang N, Westbrook KC. Effect of radiotherapy on healing of colonic anastomoses. *Surg Forum* 1980;31:222 3

89. Berliner SD, Burson LC, Lear PE. Intraperitoneal drains in surgery of the colon. *Am J Surg* 1967;113:646–7

90. Manz CW, LaTendresse C, Sako Y. The detrimental effects of drains on colonic anastomoses: a experimental study. *Dis Colon Rectum* 1970;13:17–25

91. Duthie HL. Drainage of the abdomen. *N Engl J Med* 1972;287:1081–3

92. Crowson WN, Wilson CS. An experimental study of the effects of drains on colon and anastomosis. *Am Surg* 1973;39:597–601

93. Ravitch MM, Brolin R, Kolter J, Yap S. Studies in the healing of intestinal anastomoses. *World J Surg* 1981;65:627–37

94. Smith SRG, Connolly JC, Crane PW, Gilmore OJA. The effect of surgical drainage materials on colonic healing. *Br J Surg* 1982;69:153–5

95. Simmons BP: CDC guidelines for prevention and control of nosocomial infections: guidelines for prevention of surgical wound infections. *Am J Infect Control* 1983;11:133–43

96. Taylor EW. Preventing surgical infection. In: Leaper DJ, Branicki FJ, eds. *International Surgical Practice*. Oxford, New York, Tokyo: Oxford University Press, 1992:40–64

97. Hunt TK, Linsey M, Sonne M, Jawetz E. Oxygen tension and wound infection. *Surg Forum* 1972;23:47–9

98. Knighton DR, Halliday B, Hunt TK. Oxygen as an antibiotic: the effect of inspired oxygen on infection. *Arch Surg* 1984;119:199–204

99. Jönsson K, Hunt TK, Mathes SJ. Oxygen as an isolated variable influences resistance to infection *Ann Surg* 1988;208:783–7

100. Hopf HW, Hunt TK, Blomquist P, *et al*. Assessment of wound infection risk by subcutaneous tissue oximetry. *Arch Surg* 1997;132:997–1004

101. Grief R, Akca O, Horn EP, Kurz A, Sessler D. Supplemental perioperative oxygen to reduce the incidence of surgical wound infection. *N Engl J Med* 2000;342:161–7

102. Jönsson K, Jensen JA, Goodson WH, Hunt TK. Assessment of perfusion in post-operative patients using tissue oxygen measurements. *Br J Surg* 1987;74:263–7

103. Mandell GL, Hook EN. Leucocyte bactericidal activity in chronic granulomatous disease: correlation of hydrogen peroxide production and susceptibility to intracellular killing. *J Bacteriol* 1969;100:531–2

104. Babior BM, Oxygen-dependent microbial killing by phagocytes. *N Engl J Med* 1978;298:659–68

105. Denison DM. Oxygen supply and uses in tissues. In: Reinhart K, Eyrich K, eds. *Clinical Aspects of Oxygen Transport and Tissue Oxygenation*. Berlin, Heidelberg, New York: Springer-Verlag, 1980:37–43.

106. Elek SD. Experimental staphylococcal infections in the skin of man. *Ann NY Acad Sci* 1956;65:85

107. Elek SD, Conen PE. The virulence of *Staphylococcus pyogenes* for man. A study of the problems of wound infection. *Br J Exp Pathol* 1957;38:573–86

108. Ragni MV, Crossett LS, Herndon JH. Postoperative infection following orthopaedic surgery

in human immunodeficiency virus-infected hemophiliacs with CD_4 counts $\leq 200/mm^3$. *J Arthroplasty* 1995;10:716–21

109. Schmidt B, Kearns G, Perrott D, Kaban LB. Infection following treatment of mandibular fractures in human immunodeficiency virus seropositive patients. *J Oral Maxillofac Surg* 1995;53:1134–9

110. Hoekman P, van-de Perre P, Nelissen J, Kwisanga B, Bogaerts J, Kanyangabo F. Increased frequency of infection after open reduction of fractures in patients who are seropositive for human immunodeficiency virus. *J Bone Joint Surg Am* 1991;73:675–9

111. Gold JWM. Clinical spectrum of infection in patients with HTLV III associated diseases. *Cancer Res* 1985(Suppl):4652

112. Sullivan PM, Johnston RC, Kelly SS. Late infection after total hip replacement caused by an oral organism after dental manipulation. *J Bone Joint Surg Am* 1990;72:121–3

113. Maetani S, Nishikawa T, Hirakawa A, Tobe T. Role of transfusion in organ system failure following major abdominal surgery. *Ann Surg* 1986;203,275–81

114. Jensen LS, Anderson A, Fristrup SL, *et al.* Comparison of one dose versus three doses of prophylactic antibiotics, and the influence of blood transfusion on infectious complications in acute and elective colorectal surgery. *Br J Surg* 1990;77,513–18

115. Liedberg CF. Antibacterial resistance in burns. The effect of intraperitoneal infection on survival and frequency of septicemia. An experimental study in the guinea pig. *Acta Chir Scand* 1960:120:88–94

116. Ransjö U, Forsgren A, Arturson G. Neutrophil leucocyte functions and wound bacteria in burn patients. *Burns* 1997;3:171–8

117. Casciato DA, Lowitz BB. *Manual of Clinical Oncology*, 4th edn. Philadelphia: Lippincott. 2000:686–8

118. Edge JM, van der Merwe AE, Pieper CH, Bouic P. Clinical outcome of HIV positive patients with moderate to severe burns. *Burns* 2001;27: 111–14

Changes in chronic wound management: perspectives from Tamil Nadu, India

6

C. V. Krishnaswami, N. S. Raji, K. M. Ramakrishnan and M. Babu

INTRODUCTION

Susruta (1000 BC), the great Hindu teacher and surgeon in India, introduced the concept of cosmetic surgery by reconstructing a chopped nose using a skin flap from the cheek. Wound healing was practiced by the Ayurvedic physicians (using the system of Indian medicine) starting from Charaka (500 BC)[1]; they used various herbal and plant products to accelerate healing of chronic wounds, mostly traumatic or surgical wounds. There are records of the usage of the powder of Sappan-wood, liquorica, barbery plant and cotton soaked in sesamum oil. Susruta's *Samhita* (compendium) mentions the use of black ants for suturing[2].

The aim of this chapter is to introduce some of the common denominators as well as changes related to chronic wound management in Chennai, Tamil Nadu, a south-eastern state in India.

DEFINITION AND NATURAL HISTORY

A wound is a break in the continuity of skin or mucous membrane. Wounds must be treated as individual entities since they may be acute or chronic, have different etiologies, be differently located or they may be infected.

The healing process will be adversely influenced by comorbid conditions, systemic deficiencies and environmental (external) factors.

Proper wound treatment requires knowledge both of the normal healing process and of the various factors influencing it. Treatment is often based on tradition and experience, though it ought to be evidence-based. It is difficult in India as elsewhere to adopt such an approach without local evidence. This chapter illustrates some evidence that could be influential in changing local concepts towards wound management.

The basic aspects of wound healing are similar in soft tissues. Continuity and strength are restored by formation of connective tissue and by epithelial overgrowth forming a fibrous scar. This is a continuous process, which for simplicity can be divided into three phases. The first phase is inflammation, also sometimes referred to as the lag phase; the second phase is proliferation, also sometimes referred to as the phase of fibroplasia; and the third phase is maturation.

The immediate response to wounding is vascular (briefly, initial vasoconstriction followed by vasodilatation, changes in capillary blood flow and permeability).

During the second phase, the inflammatory reaction merges into the proliferative phase leading to the formation of granulation tissue and collagen protein, which unites with fibers to form a scar. During the third phase of maturation, metabolism and blood flow in the area are still increased, lysis and remolding of collagen balance, and, at the end of the maturation phase, i.e. after about a year, the scar has almost but not quite reached the strength of the uninjured tissue. Surgical wounds and those caused by other trauma, including burns, are acute, usually following an acceptable course of healing. Occasionally, this healing course is disrupted by infection, comorbidity or other systemic or exogenous influences, leaving a chronic difficult-to-heal wound.

EPIDEMIOLOGY

Apart from non-healing surgical and post-traumatic sequelae, chronic wounds commonly seen in India include diabetic foot ulcers, burns and pressure ulcers, including those in patients with Hansen's disease. A recent large-scale field study by the Voluntary Health Services (VHS) diabetes department in collaboration with the National Institute of Epidemiology has shown the prevalence of non-insulin-dependent diabetes mellitus (NIDDM) in Chennai, Tamil Nadu, to be 2.9% for all ages and both sexes, increasing to 10.5% (95% CI, 9.8–11.2%) in individuals over 40 years of age[3]. This increase is worrying as it forecasts a large, growing burden on the local health-care system. Based on these figures, it is estimated that, in the southern parts of India, at least 60 million feet are at risk of a variety of injuries and infections, namely mechanical trauma, thermal injuries due to walking barefoot in tropical heat, anaerobic infections through the web space and trophic ulcers, nibbling of insensitive feet by rodents

while the person is asleep, fungal infections, filariasis, insect bites, etc.

In India, foot ulcers become infected, commonly leading to amputation and death even in the relatively young 40–60 years age group.

Peripheral occlusive vascular disease is uncommon relative to Western societies, less than 10% in the over 60 years age group. The management is medical, i.e. antibiotic therapy, and, when indicated, early surgical decompression of the infected diabetic foot using a technique pioneered by Murali[4].

Surgical decompression of the infected diabetic foot is indicated when pus and gas (in the presence of anaerobic infections) accumulate in the mid compartment of the sole between the plantar fascia and the fourth layer. This causes compression of the plantar vascular arch which in turn leads to distal digital ischemia and gangrene; proximal spread of the infection medially and upwards above the ankle (through the tarsal tunnel) to the soleal region causes thrombosis of the subsoleal venous plexus, arterial compression and systemic toxemia, very often resulting in major amputation of the limb. The decompression technique has yielded all-round improvement, preventing amputation in over 90% of the cases.

The flow chart in Figure 6.1[5] outlines the present approach to the management of the diabetic foot with ulceration/infection.

The technique of pulsed galvanic stimulation, reported by Kloth and Feeder[6] and Peters and co-workers[7], has been more used in pain relief and musculoskeletal injuries, particularly in athletes, but may have some potential benefit in wound healing. Two case reports of patients treated by one of the authors (C.V.K.) are presented.

Case 1

A 45-year-old woman from Singapore, a known diabetic for 14 years, NIDDM with polyneuropathy (diminished ankle jerks), preserved sensations of pain and vibration, heat, cold, full foot pulses present bilaterally, presented with a large 6.0 × 4.5 cm non-infected chronic ulcer and hypertrophied edges of more than 2 years' duration and failed skin grafting twice, as shown in Figure 6.2. She was treated with pulsed galvanic stimulation using silver-mesh stocking electrodes (Figure 6.3) 4–6 h as an outpatient procedure daily. Following initial success, defined by shrinkage of ulcer size in 4 weeks, the patient bought the equipment and started domiciliary self-application overnight (12 h). After 4 months, the ulcer reduced in size from 6.5 cm to 2.5 cm, as shown in Figure 6.4.

Case 2

A 55-year-old woman, diabetic for 17 years NIDDM (but presently insulin-requiring), had a severe degree of sensorimotor polyneuropathy and classical diabetic foot; both her foot pulses were present with good volume. She presented with acute thermal injury to the lateral three toes of the right foot (dorsal aspect). After 2 weeks of dressings and medication, skin grafting was considered to accelerate healing. This was unsuitable as she had cardiomyopathy and other problems; she did not want to undergo anesthesia and opted for the alternative modality of therapy. She responded well to daily application of the silver-mesh stocking electrodes with pulsed galvanic stimulation to the affected foot. The bluish coloration of the third digit, at presentation, improved in color with 1 week's therapy and the entire dorsal ulcers, which had exposed the tendons, epithelialized within 4–6 weeks (see Figure 6.5).

These case reports are evidence, albeit 'weak' by comparison with a full randomized controlled study. Nevertheless, these cases offer the basis for a full study of the potential benefits of this treatment option.

MANAGING BURNS

Burn injuries are common in India, occurring from accidental trauma caused by thermal, electric or chemical injuries through to domestic incidents. Burns management has been revolutionized over the last two decades, with better understanding of the process of burn wound healing and the availability of various kinds of biological dressing and skin replacement. One of the earliest events of burn injury in the tissue is the manifestation of the burn edema locally. This is the first manifestation of inflammatory response that occurs as part of the body response to the trauma. The inflammatory response to tissue injury is generally considered to be a protective mechanism by the host.

Today we know that the stages of inflammation are the deciding phase of the process of healing, as an important cascade of events occurs during this particular phase.

Certain pharmacologic agents are known today to modulate the physiologic factors responsible for inflammation and the effects can be channeled into beneficial actions by controlling the effects of inflammation.

The drugs that are used today are heparin, which is a glycosaminoglycan, triamcinolone acetate and enzyme; trypsin–chymotrypsin fibrinolysis is necessary to clear all the fibrin clots and erythrocyte sludge in the microcirculation, thereby restoring nutrients and oxygen for wound healing. This process is helped by the acute phase response that is evoked by the enzyme preparation.

It has been found that the increased secretion of the acute phase response reduces the level of liver enzymes and lysozyme enzymes. This reduction helps in reducing stress to the liver, by minimizing the degradative change.

Recent studies have shown that heparin (glycosaminoglycan) is very useful in burn wound healing when used systemically and topically. Collagen remodeling is accentuated by topical heparin and wound healing is hastened.

The relief observed in respiratory burns and acute respiratory distress syndrome in experimental animals is attributed to the antinitric oxide synthase activity of heparin.

Heparin has the capacity to reduce the inflammatory cytokine IL-6, which suggests the reason for heparin being a good anti-inflammatory agent in healing burn wounds.

BIOLOGICAL DRESSINGS

Prior to the development of synthetic dressing materials, biological dressings were exclusively used in burns. In developing nations, because of non-availability of synthetic skin replacements, biological dressings are still used effectively.

The native amniotic membrane is cost-effective and useful in the treatment of superficial burns and superficial partial thickness burns. However, viral infection transmission has raised doubts in this method. Commercially manufactured collagen membrane, derived from sheep's intestine, reconstituted bovine collagen membrane from the Achilles tendon of sheep, and reconstituted human amniotic collagen membrane, is used in superficial partial thickness burns as a biological dressing. Pictorial examples of some of these are shown in Figures 6.6–6.8.

Synthetic wound dressings, which are widely used, act only as temporary dressings and do not help in massive burn injuries; hence biological wound dressing materials, which are far superior to synthetic dressings, were developed. Among the biological dressings, collagen-based materials are found to be highly beneficial because of the important role played by collagen during wound healing. Despite advantages offered by collagen, the ideal treatment for large, full-thickness skin loss requires replacement both of the dermal and of epidermal components. This has led to the development of skin substitutes for immediate and permanent wound closure. The dermal components of the skin substitutes are based on bovine collagen and the epidermal component is provided by cultured epithelium developed from patient skin. Chakrabarty and colleagues developed the dermal component from reconstituted amniotic membrane collagen, which serves as a biocompatible scaffold for keratinocyte growth[8]. This cultured graft underwent limited clinical trials in burn patients and has proved to be effective. It is relevant and important to point out that bovine spongiform encephalitis or 'mad cow disease' has not been reported in India: this confers a degree of confidence on this product.

Babu and co-workers highlighted certain important aspects in chronic wound management in our country and the evidence that intervention by modulators in the form of drugs as well as application of dressing materials/cultured grafts accelerates healing[9–13].

DNA REPAIR AND WOUND HEALING

While the role of a balanced diet, high protein, certain amino acids and micronutrients such as zinc in helping the wound healing process are well documented, recent studies by Rao and Raji at Hyderabad, India[14,15] have highlighted the possible role played by low body mass index (BMI) and low calorie intake in improved DNA repair potential. These workers demonstrated that subjects with a low BMI (16–18.5), a consequence of chronic/prolonged reduced calorie intake, showed improved DNA repair mechanisms, also reflected in average telomeric length (ATL). These measurements were made on peripheral lymphocytes of the test subjects. Reduction in telomeric length has a direct bearing on the age of somatic cells and that of the donor. A positive correlation exists between telomeric length, the replicative capacity of a cell and the onset of senescence within the human. This study suggests further exploration in obesity and its effects on chronic wounds as well as on nutrition and retardation of the aging process at the molecular level in man.

THE ROLE OF INDIGENOUS MEDICINES AND HERBAL PREPARATIONS

Topical aloe vera facilitates wound healing. However, topical aloe vera gel was inferior to conventional management of surgical wounds[16]. A gotu kola extract can help heal infected wounds with no bony involvement[17,18] and in preventing and treating enlarged scars (keloids)[19]. Standardized extracts of gotu kola containing up to 100% total triterpenoids are generally taken, providing 60 mg once or twice per day. There are no known adverse reactions.

Horse chestnut contains a compound called aesculin that acts as an anti-inflammatory and reduces swelling with fluid following trauma, particularly sports injuries, surgery and head injury[20].

A topical preparation of chamomile combined with corticosteroids and antihistamines speeds wound healing in elderly people with venous stasis ulcers caused by inadequate circulation[21]. Topical use of chamomile ointment successfully treats mild stasis ulcers in elderly bedridden patients[22].

Topical application of honey has been used since antiquity to accelerate skin wound healing[23]. Honey has been shown to inhibit the growth of several organisms responsible for wound infections[24–26]. The use of honey to treat wounds should be under medical surveillance.

Used topically, arnica is considered to be among the best vulnerary (wound-healing) herbs available[27]. Arnica is poisonous if ingested. Calendula flowers were historically considered beneficial for wound healing, reducing inflammation and fighting infection as a natural antiseptic[28]. Echinacea[29] and calendula are used in treating poorly healing wounds[30]. Echinacea creams or ointments are applied several times a day to minor wounds.

Traditional herbalists sometimes recommend the topical use of herbs such as St. John's wort, calendula, chamomile and plantain, either alone or in combination, to speed wound healing. Clinical trials in humans have not yet validated this traditional practice.

Comfrey has anti-inflammatory properties that may decrease bruising when the herb is applied topically[31]. Comfrey is also widely used in traditional medicine as a topical application to help heal wounds[32]. Witch hazel can also be used topically to decrease inflammation and to stop bleeding[28]. Horsetail can be used both internally and topically to decrease inflammation and promote wound healing[33].

Chaparral has been used topically to decrease inflammation and pain and to promote healing of minor wounds[34]. Powdered chaparral can be applied directly to minor wounds, after they have been adequately cleansed.

Alginic acid is one of the main constituents in bladderwrack (*Fucus vesiculosus*), a type of brown algae (seaweed). Calcium alginate has shown promise as an agent to speed wound healing in animal studies[35], but has not been demonstrated to be effective in humans.

Modern herbalists recommend tea tree oil (at a strength of 70–100%) applied moderately in small areas, at least twice per day to the affected skin to treat cuts and skin infections[36]. For a variety of reasons, research confirms that tea tree oil should not be used to treat burns[37].

Ganesa Yogeeswaran has worked with indigenous Siddha and herbal phytochemicals on experimental burn wounds in mice and diabetic foot ulcers. The group has found the medicinal plant *Bryophyllum pinnata* ('Ranakalli' in the Tamil language and growing in humid parts of India and Sri Lanka) to be useful. They hypothesize that its terpenoid and flavinoid fractions promote better healing owing to increased and orderly formation of extracellular matrix substances in the wound (unpublished data, personal communication).

HANSEN'S ULCERATIONS AND CHANGES IN THERAPY

The estimated number of patients in India with Hansen's disease is approximately 4 million and the belt of high prevalence (about 5 per 1000) extends along the eastern coast of peninsular India, particularly Tamil Nadu, Andhra Pradesh, Orissa, Bihar and West Bengal, accounting for more than 60% of the total case load in the country[38]. Persons affected by lepromatous leprosy and unesthetic deformed limbs resulting in non-healing chronic ulcerations are still seen in some parts of India, particularly in Tamil Nadu (southern India).

The ulcers are classified into (1) plantar ulcers, (2) stasis ulcers and (3) lateral malleolus ulcers.

The treatment of uncomplicated ulcers consists of dressing and rest. This is difficult to achieve, for such problems are usually seen in the economically depressed persons who live in unhygienic conditions. Plaster of Paris (POP) casts that allow ambulation while taking the pressure off the affected area would be better to treat plantar ulcers in these patients. This is an effective and economic field treatment provided infection is adequately controlled and it protects the ulcers from repeated contamination and infection.

The treatment of a complicated ulcer is usually surgical after giving rest and antibiotics to control the infection. This work initiated by Dr Paul Brand three decades ago at the Christian Mission Hospital, Vellore, South India is continued through leprosy control programs available at the Schieffelin Leprosy Research and Training Centre, Karigiri, India[39] (personal communication and education handouts prepared by Schieffelin Leprosy Research and Training Centre, Karigiri 632 106, India, 1991).

DISCUSSION

The aim of this chapter is to illustrate some changes in chronic wound management in one large state in India, namely Tamil Nadu. This state has a growing burden of diabetic disease and with foot ulcers owing to the large number of people who walk barefoot, as well as problems from burns and Hansen's disease. To an extent, diabetic foot disease management in certain centers has developed well; it is planned that this will extend further with increasing resources and infrastructural development. Laboratory research and development have helped burn wound management. The most exciting in this context is the recent observation on low BMI and the capacity to improved DNA repair; this could have a profound influence on future thinking.

There is a great deal to be achieved, preferably through controlled studies on the use of therapeutic modalities including Indian medicines. The latter do not easily lend themselves to modern research assessment. The awareness of chronic wound problems is high in Tamil Nadu as well as in the rest of India.

ACKNOWLEDGEMENTS

We wish to express our sincere thanks to Mrs Lalitha Subramanian, Medical Secretary of the VHS Diabetes Department for enormous secretarial assistance during the preparation of this chapter and Dr N.S. Murali, Honorary Secretary of the Voluntary Health Services, for his continuing support of our academic and clinical research activities. Our thanks are due to the Council for Scientific and Industrial Research, India, for the research associateship of Dr N.S. Raji. We would also like to recognize the contribution of Dr V. Vijayalakshmi in organizing the pulsed galvanic stimulation therapy using the silver-mesh electrode in the wound healing process.

References

1. Sharma RK, Dash B. *Charaka Samhita*, vol. III. Varanasi, India: Chowkhamba Sanskrit Series Office, 1988
2. Udwadia FE. *Man and Medicine – A History*, New Delhi, India: Oxford University Press, 2000: 41–5
3. Asha Bhai PV, Murthy BN, Chellamariappan M, Gupte MD, Krishnaswamy CV. Prevalence of known diabetes in Chennai City. *J Assoc Physicians India* 2001;49:973–81
4. Lakshmi S, Murali NS, Badrinarayanan KR, Krishnaswami CV, Srivatsa A. Experience with NS Murali's plantar decompression surgery in diabetic foot infections in the last two years in South India. *The Diabetic Foot – Abstract Book of The Third International Symposium*. The Netherlands, 1999:128
5. *The Diabetic Foot*. www.diabetopaedia.com/foot.asp
6. Kloth LC, Feeder A. Acceleration of wound healing with high voltage monophasic, pulsed current. *J Am Phys Ther Assoc* 1988;68:503–7
7. Peters EJC, Armstrong DG, *et al*. The benefit of electrical stimulation to enhance perfusion in persons with diabetes mellitus. *J Foot Ankle Surg* 1998:396–400
8. Chakrabarty KH, Dawson RA, Harris P, *et al*. Development of autologous human epidermal/dermal composites based on sterilized human allodermis suitable for clinical use. *Br J Dermatol* 1999;141:811–23
9. Latha B, Ramakrishnan M, Jayaraman V, Babu M. Physiochemical properties of extra cellular matrix proteins in post-burn human granulation tissue. *Comp Biochem Physiol B* 1999;124: 241–9
10. Purna Sai K, Babu M. Traditional medicine and practices in burn care. Need for newer scientific perspectives. *Burns* 1998;24:387–8
11. Latha B, Ramakrishnan M, Jayaraman V, Babu M. Action of trypsin chemotrypsin (chemoral forte DS) preparation on acute phase proteins following burn injury in humans. *Burns* 1997; 23:S3–S7
12. Latha B, Ramakrishnan M, Jayaraman V, Babu M. Serum enzymatic changes modulated using trypsin chymotrypsin preparation during burn wounds in humans. *Burns* 1997;23:560–4
13. Babu M, Chandrakasam G, Ramakrishnan M. Biochemical studies on collagen from keloid tissues of South Indian patients. *Biomedicine* 1981;2:253
14. Subba Rao K, Raji NS. Dietary carbohydrates (calories) and longevity in Purushottam. In: Soni L, ed. *Trends in Carbohydrate Chemistry*, vol. 6, Dehradun (India): Surya International Publications, 2000:1–14
15. Subba Rao K, Ayyagari S, Raji NS, Murthy KJR. Under nutrition and aging: effects on DNA repair in human peripheral lymphocytes. *Curr Sci* 1996;71:464–9
16. Rodriguez-Moran M, Guerrero-Remero F. Low serum magnesium levels and foot ulcers in subjects with type 2 diabetes. *Arch Med Res* 2001;32:300–3
17. Schmidt JM, Greenspoon JS. Aloe vera dermal wound gel is associated with a delay in wound healing. *Obstet Gynecol* 1991;78:115–17
18. Morisset R, Cote NG, Panisset JC, *et al*. Evaluation of the healing activity of hydrocotyle tincture in the treatment of wounds. *Phytother Res* 1987;1:117–21
19. Kartnig T. Clinical applications of *Centella asiatica* (L) Urb. In: Craker LE, Simon JE, eds. *Herbs, Spices, and Medicinal Plants: Recent Advances in Botany, Horticulture, and Pharmacology*, vol. 3. Phoenix, AZ: Oryx Press, 1986: 145–73
20. Bossé JP, Papillon J, Frenette G, *et al*. Clinical study of a new antikeloid drug. *Ann Plastic Surg* 1979;3:13–21
21. Guillaume M, Padioleau F. Veinotonic effect, vascular protection, anti-inflammatory and free radical scavenging properties of horse

chestnut extract. *Arzneim-Forsch* 1994;44: 25–35

22. Nasemann T. Kamillosan therapy in dermatology. *Z Allg Med* 1975;25:1105–6

23. Glowania HJ, Raulin C, Swoboda M. The effect of chamomile on wound healing – a controlled, clinical, experimental double-blind trial. *Z Hautkr* 1987;62:1262–71

24. Forest RD. Development of wound therapy from Dark Ages to the present. *J R Soc Med* 1982;75:268–73

25. Cooper RA, Molan PC, Harding KG. Antibacterial activity of honey against strains of *Staphylococcus aureus* from infected wounds. *J R Soc Med* 1999;92:283–5

26. Khristov G, Mladenov S. Honey in surgical practice: the antibacterial properties of honey. *Khirurgiya* 1961;14:937–45

27. Obasieki-Ebor EE, Afonya TC, Onyekweli AO. Preliminary report on the antimicrobial activity of honey distillate. *J Pharm Pharmacol* 1983; 35:748–9

28. Weiss R. *Herbal Medicine*. Beaconsfield, UK: Beaconsfield Publishers Ltd, 1988:342

29. Leung A, Foster S. *Encyclopedia of Common Natural Ingredients Used in Food, Drugs and Cosmetics*, 2nd edn. New York: John Wiley & Sons, 1996: 113–14

30. Blumenthal M, Busse WR, Goldberg A, *et al.*, eds. *The Complete German Commission E Monographs: Therapeutic Guide to Herbal Medicines*. Boston: Integrative Medicine Communications, 1998:100

31. Hobbs C. Echinacea: a literature review. *Herbal Gram* 1994;30:33–48

32. Blumenthal M, Busse WR, Goldberg A, *et al. The Complete German Commission E Monographs. Therapeutic Guide to Herbal Medicines*. Austin, Texas: American Botanical Council, 1998: 115–16

33. Blumenthal M, Busse WR, Goldberg A, *et al. The Complete German Commission E Monographs. Therapeutic Guide to Herbal Medicines*. Austin, Texas: American Botanical Council, 1998:231

34. Blumenthal M, Busse WR, Goldberg A, *et al. The Complete German Commission E Monographs. Therapeutic Guide to Herbal Medicines*. Austin, Texas: American Botanical Council, 1998: 150–1

35. Kay MA. *Healing with Plants in the American and Mexican West*. Tucson: University of Arizona Press, 1996:178–81

36. Barnett SA, Varley SJ. The effects of calcium alginate on wound healing. *Ann R Coll Surg Engl* 1987;69:153–5

37. Carson CF, Riley TV. Antimicrobial activity of the essential oil of *Melaleuca alternifolia*: A review. *Lett Appl Microbiol* 1993;16:49–55

38. Faoagali J, George N, Leditschke JF. Does tea tree oil have a place in the topical treatment of burns? *Burns* 1997;23:349–51

39. Christian Epidemiology of Leprosy in Karigiri Leprosy Education Programme booklet on Epidemiology Sr No 12. Schieffelin Leprosy Research & Training Centre, Karigiri 632 106, India 1991: PP 11

Burn wound management: how to prevent a burn becoming a chronic wound

7

L. Téot and S. Otman

INTRODUCTION

Burns are wounds presenting special clinical features, both in the initial assessment and in the long-term tendency to develop pathologic scars. Long considered as chronic wounds, burns are in fact acute wounds that evolve, when poorly managed or in specific situations, into chronic wounds. A general consensus is that a burn wound has to be covered within a period of 2 weeks, a justification of the surgical approach popularized by US surgeons since the 1970s. Unfortunately, we still observe unhealed burn wounds after several weeks or months, due to skin graft infection or by ignoring some basic principles in local management. These can be considered as chronic wounds and several authors have focused on the high level of proteases observed in wounds after 3–4 weeks of non-healing.

New technologies have emerged over a decade, leading to a new armamentarium of therapeutic possibilities; among these, skin substitutes form a promising solution. Common dressings proposed for chronic wounds have been used in the last stage of minor burns, when skin grafting is unnecessary. Prevention of pathologic scars remains a challenge in burn wound management.

GENERAL CONSIDERATIONS INFLUENCING BURN WOUND MANAGEMENT

It seems difficult to think about burns without evoking a series of important considerations in the wound management. Skin lesions begin to appear after an exposure to heat: 45°C (1 h exposure) and 70°C (a few seconds exposure)[1]. The consequences of thermal burns were defined by Jackson[2] in three stages: coagulation, stasis and hyperemia.

Types of burns

The origins of burns can be thermal, electric or chemical. Thermal burns (scalds, fire) present a specific profile. They are considered not only as wounds but also as a general disease, having consequences on thermal regulation, glycemic control, immunologic status, myocardial function and pulmonary hypertension. The scars after thermal burns also present a tendency to develop hypertrophy and congestion, lasting for a longer period of time than in electric burns. Chemical burns often present a combination of chemical toxic effects on skin in addition to thermal consequences.

Influence of immediate care on the burn wound

The quality of immediate care has an important influence on the wound[3]. A superficial second-degree burn observed during the initial evaluation can turn into a deep second-degree burn the day after, either due to poor general management or because the general condition worsens in the resuscitation unit. Problems inherent to immediate burns care will not be developed in this chapter, but it is important to keep in mind the importance of adapted resuscitation management during the initial stage. Systemic antimicrobials are also of importance to consider when dealing with general infections arising from the burn wound.

BURN WOUND ASSESSMENT

Several key points have to be assessed, like the extent and depth of burns over the body surface and some other important factors such as age or pulmonary involvement. These points have to be checked as soon as possible in order to determine the gravity of the wound in terms of general prognosis, to establish a resuscitation plan as well as to choose adapted local management.

Extent of burns

The extent is evaluated according to charts derived from the Lund and Browder burn diagram, showing evolution of the respective volumes of the body from birth to adult or roughly using the rule of nines (Figure 7.1). Results are expressed in total body surface (TBS) involvement.

Estimation of burn depth

Traditionally, burn depth is defined in three degrees and clinical observation remains the main source of information for the clinician, even if some complementary examinations can be useful in determining the exact extent of deep burns. The surgical indication for excision and grafting depends in the majority of the cases on the visual evaluation of the wound. This part of burn assessment remains difficult and cannot be done with precision, even with experience, before the third day after injury. In second-degree burns, the first assessment has been estimated to be accurate in less than 70% of cases.

Clinical evaluation

The first-degree burn corresponds to a shallow wound. The aspect is red, the area is extremely painful, as the sensory endings remain intact. The typical example is sunburn. Only the superficial layer of the epidermis is involved. When the TBS is important, complications like cerebral edema can be encountered, but the wound remains easy to heal.

Superficial second-degree burns present usually as blisters, appearing some hours after the accident. Once the blister is removed, the wound can be observed (Figures 7.2 and 7.3). Redness is uniform, pain is extreme, rarely allowing the physician to touch the lesion. Healing time is short, usually within the first 2 weeks, without aesthetic sequelae. The superficial dermis is exposed, without involving the basal membrane, a guarantee that the superficial aspect of the skin will re-form quickly.

Deep second-degree burns present also as blisters, but, after removal the aspect is more white or patchwork-like (Figure 7.4). Sensitivity to touch is not as important as in more superficial lesions, due to a partial destruction of sensory endings. Blanching of the skin under digital pressure cannot be obtained. These burns have a tendency to heal spontaneously, except in critical general conditions or if burnt TBS is extensive; then the wound will stay unhealed or get worse and transform into a third-degree burn. Usually, healing can be observed within 2–3 weeks, but, as the deep dermis is exposed, a permanent scar will remain. These wounds can sometimes require excision and skin grafting.

The third-degree burns are deep burns involving subdermal structures. Extent in depth can be important, reaching aponeurosis or even bones. Lesions are sometimes circular on the limbs, a source of ischemia for the distal segments, necessitating emergency surgical procedures of discharge incisions in order to re-establish a normal distal blood flow. Lesions are white in color (Figure 7.5) and tissues are hard when touched. A black eschar will be observed after carbonization.

Complementary examinations

Some complementary examinations have been proposed to determine with more precision the exact depth of the burn:

(1) Near infrared spectroscopic assessment of hemodynamic changes has been proposed[4]. The principle is to check the tissue hemoglobin oxygen saturation, total hemoglobin and water content. Significant differences can be observed in the early post-burn period, (1–3 h after injury).

(2) Laser Doppler imaging was recently revisited by Pape and co-workers[5]. They found that accuracy in classifying lesions as superficial or deep was 97% compared to 60–70% for established clinical methods in 57 patients presenting with intermediate burns.

(3) Non-contact ultrasonography was proposed to determine burn depth. In 15 patients, Iraniha and associates[6] could evaluate the differences of ultrasonographic aspects on 78 burn sites compared to 42 normal skin areas, the probe being held 2.5 cm from the skin.

The overall accuracy was estimated to be 96% when predicting whether a wound would heal within a period of 3 weeks.

(a) A pyrophosphate nuclear scan can be considered as a complementary technique. Proposed by Affleck and colleagues[7], they investigated the technique in 11 patients. Eight had high-voltage electrical injury, one had severe frostbite and two had severe infections. Technetium-99m PyP scanning showed clear demarcation of viable and non-viable tissue, making it a key tool for decisions on amputation. The sensitivity was 94%, with a specificity of 100%.

(b) Diagnosis of burn depth using laser-induced indocyanine green fluorescence was proposed by Still and co-workers[8] in a preliminary clinical trial, where they could demonstrate the interest of the technique.

BURN WOUND MANAGEMENT

Several options concerning burn wound management have been proposed worldwide, from open exposure to early surgical excision, and coverage using skin substitutes to the systematic use of anti-infectious topical creams. Consensus is still lacking, except on the facts that burns are difficult to heal and there is a high risk of infection.

Concerning the immediate management, a consensus emerges on the immediate cooling of the burns using tap water at 15–18°C for a period of time varying from 5 to 15 min[9].

Pain has to be treated properly. Pain can be permanent or restricted to moments corresponding to the time of the dressing.

Treatment must be adapted to patient demand. Non-steroid anti-inflammatory drugs, morphine or equivalents are given orally or by injection before the dressing. In case of extensive burns, general anesthetic is sometimes proposed.

Skin substitutes

Skin substitutes represent the near future of burns coverage. Some products are already available on the market, but all of them have some limitations[10,11].

Temporary skin substitutes

(1) 'Allogenic skin' represents a living tissue, coming from cadavers and premortem situations. Legislation is not universally identical and in some countries this solution is not permitted. Allogenic skin can be used either as a fresh skin or as a cryoconserved skin tissue. Banking allows these products to freeze and be stored in adapted conditions. Usually, this skin is submitted to a rejection process, starting during the second week after application. Only the epidermal layer, presenting immunologically active cells, will be submitted to rejection. The dermis will adhere to the underlying wound and create a real mechanical support for any type of epidermal coverage. Usually, autologous keratinocyte cultures are used to cover this alloderm. Potentially, this cadaver allograft can transmit viral diseases.

(2) 'Other temporary skin replacement techniques' were recently developed. TransCyte® (Advanced Tissue Sciences) is produced by culturing fibroblasts on a vinyl mesh (Figure 7.6). Fibroblasts are secondarily extracted, but their local temporary 'production' of growth factors remains in the biomaterial. This skin substitute is therefore not cellularized, but contains products of allogenic cells. These cells come from neonates, whose contamination potential is severely controlled. TransCyte was used to cover excised wounds, but also as a temporary material for partial thickness burns[12–14]. Some studies have proven the efficacy of TransCyte over bacitracin alone[15] for standard therapy in children[16].

Artificial dermis

Several collagen-based artificial dermis products are available on the market:

(1) 'Alloderm' is based on cadaver skins, where the epidermal layer is removed, keeping intact the basal membrane. Engraftment of split-thickness meshed grafts is possible. Reports of improvement in cosmetic results were given. Alloderm was found useful when covering hand and foot burns[17]. In a control trial, Sheridan and co-workers did not find any statistical difference following the Vancouver scale test when using Alloderm and skin graft versus skin graft alone[18].

(2) 'Integra' is composed of bovine collagen type I cross-linked with glycosaminoglycans, covered with a silicone film acting as a temporary cover[19]. A multicenter study report of the use of Integra on recently burned patients concluded in the interest of the product[20]. The technique proposed is a two-step procedure. During the first stage, the burn wound is excised and covered with Integra (Figures 7.7 and 7.8). The second stage is performed after 3–4 weeks, and consists of peeling the silicone film and applying a very thin meshed autograft. Aesthetic results are improved, with a less prominent aspect of the mesh and a better pliability of the skin after a period of 1 year.

Other authors described the necessity to protect Integra from infection using a specific protocol including antiseptics applied on the edges of Integra during the revascularization time of the artificial dermis.

This technique has also been proposed for reconstructive surgery to resurface scarred areas[21]. The advantages for this are the use of thin split-thickness skin grafts, which are able to heal on the donor site area within a short period of time, giving a dermal support that increases the quality of the scar.

Cultured keratinocytes

Keratinocyte cultures were developed in the 1970s[22]. Application on burns was initiated by Gallico and associates[23] and several reports of a high rate of uptake can be found in the literature. Using Epicel, Odessey[24] reported an overall uptake close to 60%, but other authors consider the uptake to be dependent on the severity of burns[25]. Some have encouraged the preparation of the recipient bed using cadaver allografts[26], the epidermal layer being removed. The technique is demanding: harvesting several square centimeters of intact skin, sending them to the laboratory and then waiting 3 weeks for culture. During this time, excision of the burnt area is realized, preparation of the bed site needing the use of allogenic skin, its dermal component not being touched by the rejection process. The team must be familiar with the technique, numerous enough to realize long and difficult pre- and postgrafting dressings and the resuscitation team has to face the instability of the patient during this period of time. Used in children for extensive burns over 90% of TBS, keratinocyte cultures have proven to be a life-saving life solution[27].

Cosmetic results have been reported to be at least equivalent to meshed autografts, other reports signaling late severe contractures due to the lack of a dermal component.

Attempts to enhance the graft take and maturation have been proposed in different directions, such as modification of the support. Presently, the support has to be taken down some days after grafting keratinocyte cultures. To prevent this takedown, a source of possible trauma for the cells, resorbable supports were recently proposed (Figures 7.9 and 7.10) as well as cultivation of keratinocytes on spherical beads.

Despite serious interest in the development of cultured cells to cover large burns, these techniques remain reserved for highly specialized centers.

Anti-infectious topical creams

Local infection is characterized by growth and development of pathogen germs. Consequences of infection on the burn wound are important, the lesions being more pronounced and the healing delayed, transforming it into a chronic wound. The burn wound presents a permanent risk of infection, even if this risk is more pronounced during the initial stages. Therefore local antibacterial products are indicated at this initial stage. After obtaining a granulation tissue, especially in superficial second-degree burns, the wound can be managed using dressings having less action on infection and more effect on moist wound healing.

Prevention of infection is one of the most important criteria when treating a burn wound and, in most cases, a topical cream effective on different bacteria is proposed. Assessment of infection is another critical point. Clinical evaluation is required daily in order to identify signs of infection (color, odor, aspect, exudation). Bacteriologic counts are necessary to demonstrate the presence and virulence of pathogens; 10^5 pathogens/g of tissue, a result obtained by tissue biopsy, denotes the presence of infection. The specimen must be free from contamination by the normal flora and free of previous application of antiseptics.

Gram-positive (*Staphylococcus aureus*, *S. epidermidis*, *Streptococcus*) and Gram-negative (*Escherichia coli*, *Proteus*, *Pseudomonas aeruginosa*) bacteria are frequently observed on the burn wound. The consensus seems to be that a burn wound is not infected during the first 3 days. Topical anti-infectious creams should be prescribed immediately after the accident. Monafo and co-workers[28] recommend that topical antimicrobial therapy be started initially in order to delay and minimize wound infection. The best practices are to clean the wound, remove debris and necrotic parts, excise as soon as possible and cover the wound using skin grafts. Antimicrobial agents are used as part of this general principle. When a pathogen has been identified as responsible for a massive local infection, the topical antimicrobial agent to be applied must be specifically active on this germ.

Silver sulfadiazine is the most commonly used prophylactic topical cream. This white insoluble cream is composed of sodium sulfadiazine and silver nitrate. Painless to apply, this product causes a cooling sensation appreciated by the patient. This product is effective on *S. aureus*, *E. coli*, *Klebsiellae*, *P. aeruginosa*, *Enterobacter*, *Proteus* and *Candida albicans*, but penetrates poorly into the eschar. Used in a daily application, this topical cream has been observed to have some complications (cutaneous rash, methemoglobinemia and transient leukopenia)[29].

Cerium silver sulfadiazine, a modification consisting of the addition of 2% cerium nitrate to the original silver sulfadiazine, changes the behavior of the dressing. Confined to third-degree wounds, this product will create *de novo* a calcified crust over the burn eschar[30], which protects the area from contamination. Cerium sulfadiazine modifies the local aspect of the wound. Promoted by Wassermann in 1989[31] and used mainly in Europe, this product will actively promote spontaneous healing within a short period, preventing excessive excision and offers the possibility of sequentially grafting extensive burns, when harvesting of the few donor site areas must be repeated. However, Hadjiiski and co-workers[32] compared the respective effects of four different topical agents in four groups. The best effects were observed in those groups in which flammazine or flamm-

acerium were used, but the authors could not separate these two groups in term of results.

Silver nitrate solution (0.5%) is effective on *S. aureus* and *P. aeruginosa*, but even it does not penetrate into the burn eschar. This product causes hyponatremia and blackens linen and dressings. It is more commonly used after surgery to protect a skin graft from infection.

Mafenide acetate (Sulfamylon®) is effective on *P. aeruginosa*, *Clostridium* and a range of other micro-organisms[33]. This product penetrates well the wound eschar, but it was demonstrated to favor the appearance of *C. albicans* and to develop a metabolic acidosis if applied on large surfaces. Easy and painless to apply, this cream is used alone or in combination with others.

Povidone iodine has a large spectrum of activity on a series of germs and is also considered as an antifungal agent (10% solution). Problems due to cytotoxicity, pain and excessive absorption causing thyroid dysfunction limit povidone iodine to temporary use during wound dressing, the solution being washed away after a few minutes of application.

Bacitracin/polymixin, mupirocin, gentamicin sulfate, nitrofurantoin and nystatin have also been proposed as topical agents.

Acticoat

The silver delivery system is based upon a new technology, increasing the distance between the material and the wound. This nanocrystalline silver is placed on a bilayer of polyethylene, from which ionic silver and silver radicals are released in high concentrations when exposed to water. This system presents a higher bactericidal potential, without any described resistance. Some studies recently published demonstrated the value of such a product in the management of burn wounds[34–36]. However, this product has to be properly prescribed. In a recent study, Innes and co-workers[37] compared Allevyn® (Smith and Nephew) and Acticoat™ (Smith and Nephew) as dressings used for donor site coverage and Allevyn was superior to Acticoat in terms of rate of re-epithelialization and quality of scar. This new product must be restricted to prevention of sepsis in burn wounds.

Alternative solutions

Hydrocolloids are commonly used on minor burns, as well as hydrogels or hydrocellular dressings. When the problems of potential infection are overcome, it is possible to treat the burn wound as a simple loss of substance. Dressings promoting the moist wound healing principles can be used to aid granulation tissue formation.

However, hypergranulation can be observed using hydrocolloids after a period of 2 weeks. Usually, the keratinization process is better obtained using other local treatments, such as cortisone-based dressings or films. Experimentally, migration and multiplication of keratinocytes are favored when using films, compared to other types of dressings. No randomized control trials can be found in the literature, but most Burn Centers commonly use these types of dressings during the last stages of minor burn wound treatment.

Moist exposed burn ointment (MEBO) was described[38] as comparable to silver sulfadiazine in term of results on partial thickness burns of the face.

Negative pressure therapy, proposed by Morykwas and Argenta in 1997, can be used in two different applications on burn wounds:

(1) In acute burns, vacuum-assisted closure (VAC) has been proposed on deep second-degree burns following an experimental study on pigs. More recently, VAC was applied on third-degree burns that could not be immediately covered, after exposure of vascular pedicles, aponeurosis or nerves. This temporary covering allowed good healthy germ-free granulation tissue to be obtained within a period of 2 weeks[39,40]. VAC can also be used for a short period of time, as a tool for resorbing edema (Figures 7.11 and 7.12).

(2) VAC is more commonly used as a means of fixing a skin graft. In this indication, the pressure level must be low (about 55 mmHg). The machine is easy to use, options for the operator being the level of pressure and the mode of action, intermittent or continuous. Polyvinyl perforated pads are cut to the exact size of the area to be covered, fixed and secured using adhesive films[41].

Early surgical excision and skin grafting

Excision of the burn eschar

The first report of excision of living tissue followed by split skin grafting was provided by Janzekovic in 1970[42]. This tangential excision concept still remains the gold standard. Improvements in mortality rate observed since the 1950s are mainly due to the progress in resuscitation, but early excision and grafting represent an important step in reconstructive surgery for burns extending over 30% of TBS or less as this technique is commonly used for deep burns limited in surface.

The technique of eschar debridement is standardized. Tangential excision is usually realized using a special knife that provides the possibility of selecting the depth of tissue to be excised[43,44]. The appropriate depth is determined by obtaining a well-bled tissue. Excision will be done to the dermis for superficial excision and to subcutaneous tissue for more deep excisions. This technique involves bleeding, and preoperative applications of diluted epinephrine is highly recommended.

Complete excision of the eschar can be achieved when burns are very deep. The excision must in these cases be realized at the aponeurosis of the underlying muscles (fascial excision).

Skin grafting

Skin grafting can be done using different types of grafts, allografts coming from tissue banks or autologous skin grafts (partial thickness, expanded or not, full thickness):

(1) Allografts are skin substitutes (see above).

(2) Partial thickness skin grafts are harvested usually on a specific donor site area:

–   The skull represents the area to be used when possible. This technique hides the scar produced from harvesting inside the hair after regrowth. After shaving and injecting some inert liquid (sterile water) between the galea and the subcutaneous area, a thin piece of skin is harvested using a dermatome (0.2–0.4 mm).

–   When this zone cannot be used as a donor site, thigh, leg, abdomen or thorax can be used as the donor site area.

–   This graft can be used with or without skin expansion (×1.5, ×2, ×4) depending on the requirements of the recipient area and the surface of available donor site areas. For small surfaces, especially in children or women, a partial thickness skin graft from the skull is adapted. When dealing with very large surfaces, the 'sandwich technique', combining ×6 autografts and ×2 allografts can give satisfactory results in terms of graft uptake and coverage.

–   Complications are perioperative bleeding, secondary retractions due to the thinness of the skin graft and the low percentage of dermis it contains. Infection and itching in children are sources of loss of skin graft (Figure 7.13).

(3) Full thickness skin grafts can be harvested from selected areas where complete skin is present, i.e. the anterior folds of the groin area, elbow or knee. However, the amount of skin is limited. This type of skin graft, less subject to secondary retraction, will be promoted when grafting small areas located on mechanically demanding zones, like the feet and the hands.

(4) Color matching is very important. Brown skin should be analyzed with special care, the skin of the thigh presenting a color poorly compatible with the one of the face. It is preferable to use skin from an available area close to the recipient zone (the shoulder region is often used for the face).

PROBLEMS OF SKIN MATURATION

Clinical assessment strategy

The Vancouver scale was proposed in 1990 to rate burn scars[45]. Pigmentation, vascularity, pliability and scar height were assessed independently, with an increasing score being assigned to the greater pathologic condition. This scale has proven to be useful for burn scars and has been validated[43].

The main difficulty remains to determine as early as possible if a scar will become a source of pathologic problem and hence require an adapted treatment.

A regular assessment is useful during the first 3 months, the initial clinical evaluation being realized at the end of the first month after complete healing.

First month evaluation

Clinical assessment will determine the scar's general features, focusing on color and elevation. At this stage, color and vascularity seem to be the most important parameters to evaluate correctly. If a scar is red and hypervascular, there are risks of hypertrophic evolution.

Preventive measures such as silicone gel sheets are useful.

Laser Doppler evaluation can be proposed as a complementary technique to assess hypervascularization.

Second month evaluation

Clinically, changes in width, height and color are more easily observed. At this stage, redness is frequently accompanied by a moderate hypertrophy. A purple aspect will reflect an intense hypervascularization. Redness can change in intensity, depending on the anatomic location (more intense on limbs, close to the extremities), the muscular activity (more pronounced after movement) and the outside temperature. Itching is often present at this stage, with a maximum intensity when the patient is active and the scar is red. Pain is variable, reaching a peak on the lower leg scars during movement, generally appearing when standing up. Pain can considerably limit movement in post burns scars, largely those on the lower limbs. Local treatments can be indicated in the presence of hypertrophy, redness and increase in width. Laser Doppler evaluation can confirm the scar hypervascularization.

Third month evaluation

Signs are generally evident. Hypertrophy is visible, problems with pliability and texture are patent (Figure 7.14).

Prevention

Two types of prevention must be distinguished, prevention of burns themselves, a very large politico-social problem depending on the quality of life evolution in each country, and the technical management of freshly epithelialized skin surface in order to prevent a pathologic evolution towards hypertrophy of keloids.

Epidemiology

In children, prevention remains linked to the causes of burns and to the sociocultural environment. In Malta, fireworks represent the highest cause of burns. In most countries, the rate of burns is linked to the socioeconomic level and the typical profile of burns in children is a 3-year-old child, a boy, inside the house, the mother or guardian being present, occupied, with two or three other children. Burns occur in the kitchen or the bathroom, the mean TBS being smaller than in adults. Scalds remain the principal cause of burns.

Faadak[46] studied a population of burned children seen for post-burn retractile scars operated on in four cities in Yemen. His conclusions are that efficient education (on-site conferences, symposia and training programs, local personnel to visit burn centers overseas, burn research and prevention activities, and epidemiological studies) can improve burn management. Delgado[47] analyzed the occurrence of burns in a developing country, as a basis for future prevention programs, using a questionnaire administered to all consenting guardians of children admitted to hospital during a period of 14 months; 740 cases and controls were enrolled. Altogether, in 77.5% of the cases, burns occurred in the patient's home, with 67.8% in the kitchen; 74% were due to scalding. Most involved children younger than 5 years. Lack of water supply and low income were associated with an increased risk. The presence of a living room and better maternal education were protective factors.

Hippisley-Cox and colleagues[48] compared the socioeconomic level with the rate of child admissions to hospital in the Trent Area in Northern England. In terms of injury mechanisms, the steepest socioeconomic gradients were for pedestrian injuries (adjusted rate ratio 3.65), burns and scalds (adjusted rate ratio 3.49), and poisoning (adjusted rate ratio 2.98).

Anlatica and colleagues[49] studied a population in Turkey of more than 1000 patients admitted for burn injuries; these were more common in winter and spring, and most occurred at home. There was a predominance of male patients (71.9%) in the study population, but the proportions of children and adults were equal. Almost half of the males and the majority of the females were children/students. More than half of the patients suffered second-degree burns, and the others all had deeper burn injuries. Causes were predominantly flame, scalding, and electrical burns. There were no differences between the sexes regarding depth of burn, whereas the percentage of total burned surface area was higher in females. Children had a lower mean TBSA and lower rate of third-degree burns. The mortality rate of the study population was 33.5%.

In the elderly, prevention of burns remains difficult, even if the outcomes of the treatment are improving for mild surface areas. Burns in the elderly are commonly considered as having a poor prognosis. In fact, due to advances in resuscitation and the positive effects of surgical and topical management, the Rule of Baux[50] (sum of the age and surface not exceeding the number 100) can be exceeded slightly. The prognosis of burns in aged patients has moved from a systematic very poor prognosis to better outcomes. It is now possible to consider that a patient aged 70, in good health, reacts to burns as any other adult patient. A mild predominance of females affected by burns is a reflection of the male-female ratio at this age.

Barillo and colleagues[51] found a 17% rate in the UK. Iliopolou[52] in Greece reported a 33% rate, in France Dhennin[53] a 44% rate, Stella[54] in Italy a 45% rate. These variations are more due to differences in age in the populations than to differences in burn management. If we segment this analysis by age, we can assess that mortality is low between the ages of 65 and 75, it triples between 75 and 80, and is quadrupled after 80 (difficulties in escaping from a dangerous situation, poor general health, polypathology).

Cadier[55] reported that, at the mean age of 84, the mean surface of burns is 9.6% and the corresponding mortality is 26%; 98% of burns are house burns, by contact (27%), scalding (34%) or flame (25%), by immersion (8%), boiling oil (1%), or electrical contact (2%). This large variety in the origin of burns is also dependent on culture and mode of daily life.

In Greece[52], 63% are due to flames. In Scotland[56] only 25% are due to the same agent. For Langley[57], 17% of the patients presented a stroke before being burnt, but 48% of the burnt patients were considered at high risk of stroke; 67% of these aged patients lived alone.

Harper[58] reported that patients burned at home had a poorer death prognosis than the same population living in a community.

In the Barillo series[51], most of the deaths were observed after a period of resuscitation between 21 and 29 days, after a pulmonary complication being found in 42% at the origin of death.

Prevention of evolution of pathologic scar

One of the main preventive measures remaining is the clinical evaluation of scars at regular intervals. Simply defining problematic from normal scarring could be beneficial for the patients. Painful, hypertrophic or retractile scars observed after several months of evolution could have been easier to manage if seen at an early stage.

An early clinical assessment strategy can be considered as a good preventive measure to control any pathologic evolution of scars, whatever the origin of the scar and the intensity of the pathologic process. The absence of validated tools concerning assessment and clinical measurement of scars must lead to clinical research, in order to quantify the different pathologic aspects, focusing on redness and elevation. Profiles of evolution are more important than one single assessment. In the mind of many specialists, two successive evaluations, carried out after the first month and after the second month post complete healing are necessary to prevent transformation into problematic hypertrophy. Early determination of a keloid profile can be a determinant to propose and undertake appropriate therapeutic measures.

Proof of the efficacy of silicone gel sheeting and of corticosteroid injections is statistically established. An early management of very active scars will be beneficial to the patient.

Burns can be considered as a reflection of the socioeconomic status of human activities. The rate can be improved when using adapted educational programs. Burn management good practices are well-defined, based on a combination of resuscitation measures and a surgical approach to the deep burns. Prevention of pathologic scar can be improved, but real effectiveness of the presently proposed techniques has to be confirmed by evidence.

References

1. Moritz AR, Henriques FC. Studies of thermal injuries. II. The relative importance of time and surface temperature in the causation of cutaneous burns. *Am J Pathol* 1947;23:695–720

2. Jackson DM. The diagnosis of the depth of burning. *Br J Surg* 1953;40:588–96

3. Kim DE, Phillips TM, Jeng JC, *et al.* Microvascular assessment of burn depth conversion during varying resuscitation conditions. *J Burn Care Rehabil* 2001;22:406–16

4. Sowa MG, Leonardi L, Payette JR, Fisch JS, Mantsch HH. Near infrared spectroscopic assessment of hemodynamic changes in the early post-burn period. *Burns* 2001;27:241–9

5. Pape SA, Skouras CA, Byrne PO. An audit of the use of laser Doppler imaging (LDI) in the assessment of burns of intermediate depth. *Burns* 2001;27:233–9

6. Irahina S, Cinat ME, VanderKam VM, *et al.* Determination of burn depth with noncontact ultrasonography. *J Burn Care Rehabil* 2000;2: 333–8

7. Affleck DG, Edelman L, Morris SE, Saffle JR. Assessment of tissue viability in complex extremity injuries: utility of the pyrophosphate nuclear scan. *J Trauma* 2001;50: 263–9

8. Still JM, Law EJ, Klavuhn KG, Island TC, Holtz JZ. Diagnosis of burn depth using laser-induced indocyanine green fluorescence; a preliminary clinical trial. *Burns* 2001;27: 364–71

9. Jandera V, Hudson DA, de Wet PM, Innes PM, Rode H. Cooling the burn wound: evaluation of different modalities. *Burns* 2000;26:265–70

10. Van Zuijlen, Vloemans JF, van Trier AJ, *et al.* Dermal substitution in acute burns and reconstructive surgery: a subjective and objective long-term follow-up. *Plast Reconstr Surg* 2001; 108:1938–46

11. Boyce ST, Kagan RJ, Yabukoff KP, *et al.* Cultured skin substitutes reduce donor skin harvesting for closure of excised, full-thickness burns. *Ann Surg* 2002;235:269–79

12. Hansbrough JF, Mozingo DW, Kealey GP. Clinical trials of a biosynthetic temporary skin replacement, Dermagraft-Transitional Covering™ compared with cryopreserved human cadaver skin for temporary coverage of excised burn wounds. *J Burn Care Rehabil* 1997;18: 43–51

13. Purdue GF, Hunt JL, Still JM. A multicenter clinical trial of a biosynthetic skin replacement, Dermagraft-TC, compared with cryopreserved human cadaver skin for temporary coverage of excised burn wounds. *J Burn Care Rehabil* 1997;18:52–7

14. Noordenhbos J, Doré C, Hansbrough JF. Safety and efficacy of Dermagraft-TC for treatment of partial thickness burns. *J Burn Care Rehabil* 1999;20:275–81

15. Demling RH, DeSanti L. Management of partial thickness facial burns (comparison of

topical antibiotics and bio-engineered skin substitutes). *Burns* 1999;25:256–61

16. Lukish JR, Eichelberger MR, Newman KD, *et al.* The use of a bioactive skin substitute decreases length of stay for pediatric burn patients. *J Pediatr Surg* 2001;36:1118–21

17. Lattari V, Jones LM, Varcelotti J, Late'nser BA, Sherman HF, Barette RR. The use of a permanent dermal allograft in full-thickness burns of the hand and foot: a report of three cases. *J Burn Care Rehabil* 1997;18:147–55

18. Sheridan R, Choucair R, Donelan M, Lydon M, Petras L, Tompkins R. Acellular allodermis in burn surgery: 1-year results of a pilot trial. *J Burn Care Rehabil* 1998;19:528–30

19. Yannas IV. Studies on the biological activity of the dermal regeneration template. *Wound Repair Regen* 1998;6:518–24

20. Heimbach D, Luterman A, Burke J, *et al.* Artificial dermis for major burns. A multicenter randomized clinical trial. *Ann Surg* 1988;208: 313–20

21. Dantzer E, Braye FM. Reconstructive surgery using an artificial dermis (integra): results with 39 grafts. *Br J Plast Surg* 2001;54:659–64

22. Rheinwald JG, Green H. Serial cultivation of strains of human epidermal keratinocytes: the formation of keratinizing colonies from single cells. *Cell* 1975;6:448–51

23. Gallico GG, O'Connor NE, Compton CC, Kehind O, Green H. Permanent coverage of large burn wounds with autologous cultured human epithelium. *N Engl J Med* 1984;311: 448–51

24. Odessey R. Multicenter experience with cultured epidermal autografts for treatment of burns. *J Burn Care Rehabil* 1992;13:174–80

25. Compton CC, Hickerson W, Nadire K, Press W. Acceleration of skin regeneration from cultured epithelial autografts by transplantation to homograft dermis. *J Burn Care Rehabil* 1993; 14:653–62

26. Hefton JM, Madden MR, Finkelstein JL, Shires GT. Grafting of patients with allografts of cultured cells. *Lancet* 1983;2:428–30

27. Sheridan TL, Tompkins RG. Cultured autologous epithelium in patients with burns of ninety percent or more of the body surface. *J Trauma* 1995;38:48–53

28. Monafo WW, West MA. Current treatment recommendations for topical burn therapy. *Drugs* 1990;40:364–73

29. Thomson PD, Moore NP, Rice TL, Prasad JV. Leukopenia in acute thermal injury: evidence against topical silver sulfadiazine as the causative agent. *J Burn Care Rehabil* 1989;10: 418–20

30. Koller J, Orsag M. Our experience with the use of cerium sulphadiazine in the treatment of extensive burns. *Acta Chir Plast* 1998;40:73–5

31. Wassermann D, Schlotterer M, Lebreton F, Levy J, Guelfi MC. Use of topically applied silver sulfadiazine plus cerium nitrate in major burns. *Burns* 1989;15:257–60

32. Murphy RC, Kucan JO, Robson MC, Heggers JP. The effect of 5% mafenide acetate solution on bacterial contamination of infected rat burns. *J Trauma* 1983;23:878–81

33. Hadkiiski OG, Lesseva MI. Comparison of four drugs for local treatment of burn wounds. *Eur J Emerg Med* 1999;6:41–7

34. Yin HG, Langford R, Tredget EE, Burell RE. Effect of Acticoat antimicrobial barrier dressing on wound healing and graft take. *J Burn Care Rehabil* 1999;20:S231

35. Burell RE, Heggers JP, Davis GJ, Wright JB. Efficacy of silver coated dressings as bacterial barriers in a rodent burn sepsis model. *Wounds* 1999;11:64–71

36. Tredget EE, Shankowsky HA, Groenveld A, Burell R. A matched-pair, randomized study evaluating the efficacy and safety of Acticoat silver-coated dressing for the treatment of burn wounds. *J Burn Care Rehabil* 1998;19: 532–7

37. Innes ME, Umraw N, Fish JS, Gomez M, Cartotto RC. The use of silver coated dressings on donor site wounds: a prospective, controlled matched pair study. *Burns* 2001;27: 621–7

38. Ang ES, Lee ST, Gan CS, *et al.* The role of alternative therapy in the management of partial thickness burns of the face – experience with the use of moist exposed burn ointment (MEBO) compared with silver sulfadiazine. *Ann Acad Med Singapore* 2000;29:7–10

39. Téot L, Otman S, Giovannini U. The use of negative pressure therapy in managing wounds. ETRS Annual meeting. Satellite sym-

posium Cardiff, UK, Sept 2001. Springer-Verlag (in press)

40. Webb LX, Schmidt U. Wound management with vacuum therapy. *Unfallchirurg* 2001;104:918–26

41. Chang KP, Tsaii CC, Lin TM, Lai CS, Lin SD. An alternative dressing for skin graft immobilization: negative pressure dressing. *Burns* 2001;27:839–42

42. Janzekovic Z. A new concept in the early excision and immediate grafting of burns. *J. Trauma* 1970;10:1103–8

43. Sachs A, Watson J. Four years experience at a specialized burns centre. *Lancet* 1969;1:718–21

44. Lagrot F, Micheau P, Costagliola M, Castaigne J. Value of excision–homograft in burned patients. *Ann Chir* 1973;27:191–202

45. Sullivan T, Smith J, Kermode J, McIver E, Courtemanche DJ. Rating the burn scar. *J Burn Care Rehab* 1990;11:256–61

46. Fadaak H. The management of burns in a developing country: an experience from the republic of Yemen. *Burns* 2002;28:65–9

47. Delgado J, Ramirez-Cardich ME, *et al.* Risk factors for burns in children: crowding, poverty, and poor maternal education. *Inj Prev* 2002;8:38–41

48. Hippisley-Cox J, Groom L, Kendrick D, *et al.* Cross sectional survey of socioeconomic varia-tions in severity and mechanism of childhood injuries in Trent 1992–7. *BMJ* 2002;324:1132

49. Anlatici R, Ozerdem OR, Dalay C, *et al.* A retrospective analysis of 1083 Turkish patients with serious burns. *Burns* 2002;28:231–7

50. Baux S, Mimoun M, Saade H, *et al.* Burns in the elderly. *Burns* 1989;15:239

51. Barillo DF, Goode R. Fire fatality study: demography of fire victims. *Burns* 1996;22:85–8

52. Iliopolou E, Lochaitis A, Kalophonou M, *et al.* Senility and burns – a four year experience. *Ann Burns Fire Dis* 1995;8:203–6

53. Dhennin C, Vesin N. Mortalité chez las patients agés. Abstracts of 1st Italo-French Burns Meeting 1992:69

54. Stella M. Il paziente anziano ustionato: strateggie chirurgiche. Abstracts of 1st Italo-French Burns Meeting 1992:69

55. Cadier MA, Shakespeare PG. Burns in octogenarians. *Burns* 1995;21:200–4

56. Sarhadi NS, Kinsaid R, MacGregor JC, *et al.* Burns in the elderly in South East of Scotland. *Burns* 1995;21:91–5

57. Langley J. Death to the elderly in residential institutions due to major fires. *N Engl Med J* 1989;102:419

58. Harper RD, Dickson H. Reducing the burn risk to elderly persons living in residential care. *Burns* 1995;21:205–8

Changes in diabetic foot ulcer management

8

M. Edmonds and A. Foster

INTRODUCTION

Major advances have taken place in the last decade and this has led to improved outcomes in ulcer healing and a reduced number of amputations[1]. There has been increased interest in the diabetic foot, resulting in systematic reviews[2-4], guidelines[5] and consensus development[6,7]. These reports have stressed the importance of early recognition of the at-risk foot, the prompt institution of preventive measures and the provision of rapid and intensive treatment of foot infection in multidisciplinary foot clinics. Such measures can reduce the number of amputations in diabetic patients.

This chapter outlines a simple classification of the diabetic foot into the neuropathic and neuroischemic foot and then describes a simple staging system of the natural history of the diabetic foot and a treatment plan for each stage, within a multidisciplinary framework[8]. Successful management of the diabetic foot needs the expertise of a multidisciplinary team, which should include physician, podiatrist, nurse, orthotist, radiologist and surgeon working closely together, within the focus of a diabetic foot clinic.

CLASSIFICATION

An important prelude to proper management of the diabetic foot is the correct diagnosis of its two main syndromes: the neuropathic foot, in which neuropathy predominates but the major arterial supply to the foot is intact; and the neuroischemic foot, where both neuropathy and ischemia, resulting from a reduced arterial supply, contribute to the clinical presentation[9]. The significance of structural abnormalities of the skin microcirculation is not fully understood, although there are numerous functional abnormalities that may be important. These include increased blood flow, widespread vascular dilation, increased vascular permeability, impaired vascular activity and limitation of hyperemia[10].

Infection is rarely a sole factor but often complicates neuropathy and ischemia and is responsible for considerable tissue necrosis in the diabetic patient. In diabetes, deficiencies in neutrophil chemotaxis, phagocytosis, superoxide production, respiratory burst activity and intracellular killing have all been described[11].

Neuropathic foot

This is a warm, well-perfused foot with sensory deficit and autonomic dysfunction leading to arteriovenous shunting and distended dorsal veins. Peripheral autosympathectomy damages the neurogenic control mechanisms that regulate capillary and arteriovenous shunt flow and loss of pre-capillary vasoconstriction[10]. The pulses are palpable. Sweating is diminished and the skin may be dry and prone to fissuring. Motor neuropathy also plays a role, with paralysis of the small muscles contributing to structural deformities such as a high arch and claw toes. This leads to prominence of the metatarsal heads. It has two main complications, the neuropathic ulcer and the neuropathic (Charcot) foot.

Neuroischemic foot

This is a cool, pulseless foot with poor perfusion. It also has neuropathy. Ischemia results from atherosclerosis of the leg vessels. This is often bilateral, multisegmental and distal, involving arteries below the knee. Intermittent claudication and rest pain may be absent because of co-existing neuropathy and the distal distribution of the arterial disease to the leg. Ulcers in the neuroischemic foot develop on margins of the foot at sites made vulnerable, by underlying ischemia, to the moderate but continuous pressure often from poorly fitting shoes.

THE NATURAL HISTORY OF THE DIABETIC FOOT

The natural history of the diabetic foot can be divided into six stages[8]:

(1) The foot is normal and not at risk. The patient does not have the risk factors that render him vulnerable to foot ulcers. These are neuropathy, ischemia, deformity, callus and edema;

(2) High-risk foot. The patient has developed one or more of the risk factors for ulceration of the foot;

(3) Foot with ulcer. Ulceration is on the plantar surface in the neuropathic foot and on the margin in the neuroischemic foot;

(4) Foot with cellulitis. The ulcer has developed infection with the presence of cellulitis which can complicate both the neuropathic and the neuroischemic foot;

(5) Foot with necrosis. In the neuropathic foot, infection is usually the cause. In the neuroischemic foot, infection is still the most common reason, although severe ischemia can directly lead to necrosis;

(6) The foot cannot be saved and will need a major amputation.

Every diabetic patient can be placed into one of these stages and the appropriate management then carried out. In stages (1) and (2), the emphasis is on prevention of ulceration. In stage (3) the presentation and management of foot ulceration are discussed. Finally, stage (4) and (5) address complications of foot ulceration, notably, cellulitis and necrosis.

THE MANAGEMENT OF THE DIABETIC FOOT

At each stage, it is necessary to take 'control' to prevent further progression of diabetic foot disease, and management will be considered under the following headings:

- Wound control
- Microbiologic control
- Mechanical control
- Vascular control
- Metabolic control
- Educational control

Metabolic control is important at every stage. Tight control of blood glucose, blood pressure and blood cholesterol and triglycerides should be followed to preserve neurologic and cardiovascular function. Advice should be given to stop smoking. In stages (4) and (5), considerable metabolic decompensation may occur in the presence of infection and full metabolic resuscitation is often required[8].

STAGE 1: NORMAL FOOT

Presentation

By definition, the foot does not have the risk factors for foot ulcers, namely, neuropathy, ischemia, deformity, callus and swelling and the diagnosis of stage 1 is made by screening patients and excluding these five risk factors.

Neuropathy

A simple technique for detecting patients with loss of protective pain sensation is to use a nylon monofilament which, when applied perpendicular to the foot, buckles at a given force of 10 g. The filament should be pressed against several sites including the plantar aspect of the first toe, the first, third and fifth metatarsal heads, the plantar surface of the heel and the dorsum of the foot. The filament should not be applied at any site until callus has been removed. If the patient cannot feel the filament at any of these tested areas, then significant neuropathy is present and protective pain sensation is lost[12].

Ischemia

The most important maneuver to detect ischemia is the palpation of the foot pulses, namely the dorsalis pedis pulse and the posterior tibial pulse. If either of these foot pulses can be felt, then it is highly unlikely that there is significant ischemia. A small hand-held Doppler can be used to confirm the presence of pulses and to calculate the pressure index, which is the ratio of ankle systolic pressure to brachial systolic pressure (ABPI). In normal subjects, the pressure index is usually greater than 1, but in the presence of ischemia is less than 0.8. Thus, absence of pulses and a pressure index of less than 0.8 confirms ischemia.

Many diabetic patients have medial arterial calcification, giving an artificially elevated systolic pressure and therefore falsely high ABPI, even in the presence of ischemia. It is thus difficult to assess the diabetic foot when the pulses are not palpable, but the pressure index is less than 1. It is then necessary to use other methods to assess flow in the arteries of the foot, such as examining the pattern of the Doppler arterial waveform and imaging the arterial tree using Duplex ultrasonography or measuring transcutaneous oxygen tension or toe systolic pressures[13].

Deformity

Deformity often leads to bony prominences, which are associated with high mechanical pressures on the overlying skin. This leads to ulceration, particularly in the absence of protective pain sensation and when shoes are unsuitable. Common deformities are claw toes, pes cavus, hallux valgus, hallux rigidus, hammer toe and nail deformities and Charcot foot (see below).

Callus

This is a thickened area of epidermis which develops at sites of high pressure and friction. It should not be allowed to become excessive as this can be a forerunner of ulceration in the presence of neuropathy.

Edema

Edema is a major factor predisposing to ulceration by reducing skin oxygenation. It is often exacerbated by poorly fitting shoes.

Management

This stage by definition does not have any evidence of skin breakdown or ischemia. However, mechanical and educational control are important to prevent development of ulceration.

Mechanical control

Mechanical control is based upon wearing sensible footwear. Shoes should have broad rounded or square toes, adequate toe depth, low heels to avoid excessive toe pressure on the forefoot and lace-up, Velcro or buckle straps to prevent movement within the shoe[14].

Educational control

Advice on basic foot care, including nail cutting techniques, the treatment of minor injuries and the purchase of shoes, should be given. Educational programs involving behavioral contracts and organizational intervention for health-care providers have shown a significant reduction in foot ulceration at 1-year follow-up[15].

STAGE 2: THE HIGH-RISK FOOT

Presentation

The foot has developed one or more of the risk factors for ulceration: neuropathy, ischemia, deformity, callus and edema. It is important to detect these by a regular screening examination. Referral of such patients at risk to a multidisciplinary program of care has been shown to reduce amputations[16].

The Charcot foot is a particularly devastating deformity which needs prompt diagnosis and treatment and is described at the end of this section.

Management

Mechanical, vascular and educational control are important.

Mechanical control

Deformity must be accommodated and callus, dry skin, fissures and edema must be treated.

Deformities

Deformities in the neuropathic foot tend to render the plantar surface vulnerable to ulcers, requiring special insoles, whereas in the neuroischemic foot, the margins need protection and appropriately wide shoes should therefore be advised.

Footwear can be divided into three broad types: sensible shoes (from high street shops) for patients with minimal sensory loss; ready-made stock (off the shelf) shoes for neuroischemic feet that need protection along the margins of the foot but that are not greatly deformed; and customized or bespoke (made-to-measure) shoes containing cradled, cushioned insoles. These are necessary to redistribute the high pressures on the plantar surface of the neuropathic foot.

Callus

Patients should never cut their callus off or use callus removers. It should be removed regularly by sharp debridement.

Dry skin and fissures

Dry skin should be treated with an emollient such as E45 cream or calmurid cream.

Edema

Edema may complicate both the neuropathic and the neuroischemic foot. Its main cause will be impaired cardiac and renal function, which should be treated accordingly. Edema may rarely be secondary to neuropathy. It responds to ephedrine, starting at a dose of 10 mg three times a day and increasing up to 30–60 mg three times a day.

Vascular control

Patients with absent foot pulses should have the ABPI measured to confirm ischemia and to provide a baseline, so that subsequent deterioration can be detected. If the patient has rest pain, disabling claudication or the ABPI is below 0.5, then he/she already has severe ischemia and should be referred for a vascular opinion. All diabetic patients with evidence of peripheral vascular disease may benefit from anti-platelet agents: 75 mg aspirin daily or, if this cannot be tolerated, clopidrogel 75 mg daily.

Educational control

Patients have lost protective pain sensation and therefore need advice to protect their feet from mechanical, thermal and chemical trauma. They should establish a habit of regular inspection of the feet so that problems can be detected quickly and they seek help early.

Charcot foot

The term Charcot foot refers to bone and joint destruction that occurs in the neuropathic foot[17]. It can be divided into three phases:

(1) Acute onset;

(2) Bony destruction/deformity;

(3) Stabilization.

Acute onset

The foot presents with unilateral erythema, warmth and edema. There may be a history of minor trauma. About 30% of patients complain of pain or discomfort. X-ray at this time may be normal. However, a technetium-99m diphosphonate bone scan will detect early evidence of bony destruction. Cellulitis, gout and deep vein thrombosis may masquerade as a Charcot foot. Initially the foot is immobilized in a non-weight-bearing cast to prevent deformity. After 1 month, a total contact cast is applied and the patient may mobilize for brief periods. However, the patient is given crutches and encouraged to keep his walking to a minimum. An alternative is the Aircast, but a cradled moulded insole should protect the sole. Such treatment, if given early, should help to prevent the second phase, that of bony destruction and deformity. Bisphosphonates may be helpful in the initial treatment of the Charcot foot[18].

Bony destruction

Clinical signs are swelling, warmth and deformities that include the rocker bottom deformity and the medial convexity. X-ray reveals fragmentation, fracture, new bone formation, subluxation and dislocation. The aim of treatment is immobilization until there is no longer evidence on X-ray of continuing bone destruction and the foot temperature is within 2°C of the contralateral foot. Deformity in a Charcot foot can predispose to ulceration, which may become infected and lead to osteomyelitis. This may be difficult to distinguish from neuropathic bone and joint change, as on X-ray, bone scan or magnetic resonance imaging, appearances may be similar. However, if the ulcer can be probed to bone, osteomyelitis is the more likely diagnosis.

Stabilization

The foot is no longer warm and red. There may still be edema but the difference in skin temperature between the feet is less than 2°C. X-ray shows fracture healing, sclerosis and bone remodeling. The patient can now progress from a total contact or Aircast to an orthotic walker, fitted with cradled moulded insoles. However, too rapid mobilization can be disastrous, resulting in further bone destruction. Extremely careful rehabilitation should be the rule. Finally, the patient may progress to bespoke footwear with moulded insoles.

The rocker bottom Charcot foot with plantar bony prominence is a site of very high pressure. Regular reduction of callus can prevent ulceration. If ulceration does occur, an exostectomy may be needed. The most serious complication of a Charcot foot is instability of the hind foot and ankle joint. This can lead to a flail ankle on which it is impossible to walk. Reconstructive surgery and arthrodesis, with a long-term ankle foot orthosis, have resulted in high levels and limb salvage[19].

STAGE 3: THE ULCERATED FOOT

Presentation

It is essential to differentiate between ulceration in the neuropathic foot compared with that in the neuroischemic foot.

Neuropathic ulcer

Neuropathic ulcers result from mechanical, thermal or chemical injuries that are unperceived by the patient because of loss of pain sensation. The classical position is under the metatarsal heads, but it is more frequently found on the plantar aspects of the toes. Direct mechanical injuries may result from treading on sharp objects, but the most frequent cause of ulceration is the repetitive mechanical forces of gait, which result in callosity formation, inflammatory autolysis and subkeratotic hematomas. Tissue necrosis occurs below the plaque of callus resulting in a small cavity filled with serous fluid, which eventually breaks through to the surface with ulcer formation.

Neuroischemic ulcer

Ulceration in the neuroischemic foot usually occurs on the margins of the foot and the first sign of ischemic ulceration is a red mark which blisters and then develops into a shallow ulcer with a base of sparse pale granulations or yellowish, closely adherent slough. Although ulcers occur on the medial surface of the first metatarso-phalangeal joint and over the lateral aspect of the fifth metatarso-phalangeal joint, the most common sites are the apices of the toes and also beneath the nails if allowed to become overly thick.

Management

Mechanical, wound, microbiologic, vascular and educational control are important.

Mechanical control

In the neuropathic foot, the aim is to redistribute plantar pressures, while in the neuroischemic foot, it is to protect the vulnerable margins of the foot.

Neuropathic foot

The most efficient way to redistribute plantar pressure is by the immediate application of some form of cast[20]. Various casts are available and include the Aircast, total contact cast and Scotchcast boot.

The Aircast[21] is a removable bivalved cast and the halves are joined together with Velcro strapping. It is lined with four air cells which can be inflated with a hand pump through four valves to ensure a close fit. The total contact cast[22] should be reserved for plantar ulcers that have not responded to other casting treatments. It is a close-fitting plaster of Paris and fiberglass cast applied over minimum padding. The Scotchcast boot[23] is a simple removable boot made of stockinette, felt and fiberglass tape which is effective in redistributing plantar pressure. If casting techniques are not available, temporary ready-made shoes with a plastozote insole such as a Drushoe can off-load the site of ulceration.

The 5-year cumulative rate of ulcer recurrence is 66%[24]. In the long term, cradled or moulded insoles are designed to redistribute weight-bearing away from the vulnerable pressure areas and prevent recurrence. In a controlled trial of therapeutic shoes compared with the patient's own shoes, the risk of ulcer recurrence at 1 year was 27% in the intervention group and 58% in the control group[25].

Neuroischemic feet

Ulcers in neuroischemic feet are often associated with tight shoes which lead to frictional forces on the vulnerable margins of the foot. A high street shoe that is sufficiently long, broad and deep and fastens with a lace or strap high on the foot may be sufficient. Alternatively, a ready-made stock shoe which is wide fitting may be suitable.

Wound control

Wound control consists of three parts: debridement, dressings and stimulation of wound healing.

Debridement

Debridement is the most important part of wound control and is best carried out with a scalpel. It allows removal of callus and devitalized tissue and enables the true dimensions of the ulcer to be perceived. It reduces the bacterial load of the ulcer even in the absence of overt infection, restores chronic wounds to acute wounds and releases growth factors to aid the healing process[8]. It also enables a deep swab to be taken for culture. The larvae of the green bottle fly are sometimes used to debride ulcers, especially in the neuroischemic foot[26].

Dressings

Sterile, non-adherent dressings should cover all ulcers to protect them from trauma, absorb exudate, reduce infection and promote healing. There is no evidence to support a particular dressing[3]. The following dressing properties are essential for the diabetic foot: ease and speed of lifting, ability to be walked on without disintegrating and good exudate control. Dressings should be lifted every day to ensure that problems or complications are detected quickly, especially in patients who lack protective pain sensation.

Stimulation of wound healing

Techniques to stimulate wound healing include Regranex (platelet-derived growth factor), Dermagraft, Apligraf, Hyaff, Promogran and the Vacuum-Assisted Closure® (VAC) technique. VAC is a trademark of KCI, San Antonio, USA.

REGRANEX® (ORTHO-MACNEILL PHARMACEUTICALS). Platelet-derived growth factor (Regranex) stimulates fibroblasts and other connective tissue cells located in the skin and is beneficial in enhancing wound healing processes of cell growth and repair. It is applied once daily. A multicenter, double-blind, placebo-controlled study of 118 patients demonstrated that Regranex gel 30 µg/g healed significantly more chronic diabetic ulcers compared with placebo gel (48% versus 25%, $p = 0.016$) and also decreased healing times by 9 weeks compared with placebo gel[27]. A pivotal study in 382 patients demonstrated that Regranex gel 100 µg/g healed 50% of chronic diabetic ulcers which was significantly greater than 35% healed with placebo gel. Regranex gel 100 µg/g also significantly decreased time to healing by 6 weeks[28].

DERMAGRAFT® (SMITH & NEPHEW). Dermagraft is an artificial human dermis manufactured through the process of tissue engineering. Human fibroblast cells obtained from neonatal foreskin are cultivated on a three-dimensional polyglactin scaffold. As fibroblasts proliferate within the scaffold, they secrete human dermal collagen, growth factors and other proteins, embedding themselves in a self-produced dermal matrix. This results in a metabolically active dermal tissue with the structure of a papillary dermis of newborn skin. A randomized, controlled, multicenter study of 281 patients with neuropathic foot ulcers demonstrated that, at 12 weeks, 50.8% of the Dermagraft group experienced complete wound closure which was significantly greater than in the controls, of whom 31.7% healed. Furthermore, at week 32, Dermagraft patients still had a statistically significant higher number of healed ulcers, 58% compared with 42% in controls[29].

APLIGRAF® (NOVARTIS). Apligraf consists of a collagen gel seeded with fibroblasts and covered by a surface layer of keratinocytes. A recent randomized, controlled study was carried out at 24 centers with 208 patients. At 12 weeks, 38% of the controls achieved wound closure while 56% of subjects treated with Apligraf had healed ($p = 0.0042$). Average time to healing was 90 days in the control group and 65 days in the Apligraf group ($p = 0.0026$)[30].

HYAFF® (HYALOFILL CONVATEC). Hyaff is an ester of hyaluronic acid, which is a major component of the extra cellular matrix[31]. Hyaluronic acid is polysaccharide that facilitates growth and movement of fibroblasts but is unstable when applied to tissues. When it is esterified, it becomes more stable and, when in contact with wound exudate, produces a hydrophilic gel which covers the wound. This creates a hyaluronic acid–rich tissue interface which promotes granulation and healing.

A pilot study of 30 diabetic patients randomized to treatment with Hyaff or standard care showed promising results in the treatment of neuropathic foot ulcers, especially those with sinuses. Recently, Hyaff has been used to treat 30 diabetic patients with indolent neuropathic ulcers in a randomized, controlled study. Fifteen patients were treated with Hyaff plus standard treatment (active group) and 15 received standard treatment alone (controls). In the active group, there were 13 ulcers with sinuses and 13 with bone exposed. In the control group, there were nine ulcers with sinuses and nine with bone exposed. In the active group, 12 of 13 sinuses healed compared with one of nine in the control group ($p < 0.01$). In the active group, ten of the 15 ulcers healed, compared with three out of 15 in the control group ($p < 0.05$). Thus, Hyaff application resulted in a higher degree of closure of sinuses and improved healing of indolent neuropathic ulcers[32].

PROMOGRAN® (JOHNSON AND JOHNSON). Promogran inhibits protease activity in wound exudate, binds growth factors and re-delivers growth factors into the wound in an active state. It consists of collagen and oxidized regenerated cellulose. Collagen attracts granulocytes and fibroblasts, reduces wound contractions and enhances deposition of collagen fibers. Oxidized cellulose stimulates cell proliferation.

In a 12-week study of 184 patients, 37% of Promogran-treated patients healed compared with 28% of saline gauze-treated patients (in ulcers of less than 6 months' duration, leaking was 45% in Promogran-treated patients and 33% in saline gauze-treated patients, $p = 0.056$).

VACUUM-ASSISTED CLOSURE (VAC)® (KCI, SAN ANTONIO, US). In this technique, the VAC pump applies gentle negative pressure to the ulcer through a tube and foam sponge which are applied to the ulcer over a dressing and sealed in place with a plastic film to create a vacuum. Exudate from the wound is sucked along the tube to a disposable collecting chamber. The negative pressure improves the vascularity and stimulates granulation of the wound.

Microbiologic control

When the skin of the foot is broken, the patient is at great risk of infection as there is a clear portal of entry for invading bacteria. At every patient visit, the foot should be examined for local signs of infection, cellulitis or osteomyelitis. If these are found, antibiotic therapy is indicated.

However, uniform agreed practice on the place of antibiotics in the clinically non-infected ulcer has not been established. In a recent investigation, 32 patients with new foot ulcers were treated with oral antibiotics and 32 patients without antibiotics[33]. In the group with no antibiotics, 15 patients developed clinical infection compared with none in the antibiotic group ($p < 0.001$). Seven patients in the non-antibiotic group needed hospital admission and three patients came to amputation (one major and two minor). Seventeen patients healed in the non-antibiotic group compared with 27 in the antibiotic group ($p < 0.02$). When the 15 patients who developed clinical infection were compared to 17 patients who did not, there were significantly more ischemic patients in the infected group. Furthermore, out of the 15 patients who became clinically infected, 11 had positive ulcer swabs at the start of the study compared with only one patient out of 17 in the non-infected group ($p < 0.01$). From this study, it was concluded that diabetic patients with clean ulcers associated with peripheral vascular disease and positive ulcer swabs should be considered for early antibiotic treatment. Thus, for the neuropathic ulcer, at the first visit, if there is no cellulitis, discharge or probing to bone (indicative of osteomyelitis – see below), then debridement, cleansing with saline, application of dressing and daily inspections will suffice.

For the neuroischemic ulcer, at the initial visit, if the ulcer is superficial, oral amoxycillin 500 mg three times a day and flucloxacillin 500 mg four times a day may be prescribed (if the patient is penicillin-allergic, prescribe erythromycin 500 mg four times a day or cephadroxyl 1 g twice daily). If the ulcer is deep, extending to the subcutaneous tissue, trimethoprim 200 mg bd and metronidazole 400 mg three times a day may be added[8].

The patient is reviewed, preferably at 1 week, together with the result of the ulcer swab. If the ulcer shows no sign of infection and the swab is negative, treatment is continued without antibiotics. However, in the cases of severe ischemia (pressure index < 0.5), antibiotics may be prescribed until the ulcer is healed. If either the neuropathic or neuroischemic ulcer has a positive swab, the patient may be treated with the appropriate antibiotic according to sensitivities, until the repeat swab, taken at weekly intervals, is negative.

Vascular control

If an ulcer has not responded to optimum treatment within 6 weeks and ABPI is less than 0.5 and the Doppler waveform is monophasic, i.e. damped, or transcutaneous oxygen is less than 30 mmHg or toe pressure is less than 30 mmHg, then, ideally, angiography should be carried out.

This can be performed by a Duplex examination, which combines the features of Doppler waveform analysis with ultrasound imaging to produce a picture of arterial flow dynamics and morphology[8]. Alternatively, transfemoral angiography can be performed, together with digital subtraction angiography to assess the distal arteries.

Angioplasty is a valuable treatment to improve arterial flow in the presence of ischemic ulcers and is indicated for the treatment of isolated or multiple stenoses as well as short segment occlusions less than 10 cm in length[34]. If lesions are too widespread for angioplasty, then arterial bypass may be considered. However, this is a major, sometimes lengthy, operation, not without risk and is more commonly reserved to treat the foot with severe tissue destruction which cannot be managed without the restoration of pulsatile blood flow.

Educational control

Patients should be instructed on the principles of ulcer care, stressing the importance of rest, footwear, regular dressings and frequent observation for signs of infection.

STAGE 4: FOOT ULCER AND CELLULITIS

Presentation

Infection is caused by bacteria which invade the ulcer from the surrounding skin. Staphylococci and streptococci are the most common pathogens[35]. However, infection due to Gram-negative and anaerobic organisms occur in approximately 50% of patients and often infection is polymicrobial[36]. The most common manifestation is cellulitis. However, this stage covers a spectrum of presentations, ranging from local infection of the ulcer to spreading cellulitis, sloughing of soft tissue and finally, vascular compromise of the skin, seen as a blue discoloration when there is an inadequate supply of oxygen to the soft tissues.

Infected ulcer

Local signs that an ulcer has become infected include color change of the base of the lesion from healthy pink granulations to yellowish or gray tissue, purulent discharge, unpleasant smell and the development of sinuses with undermined edges or exposed bone. There may also be localized erythema, warmth and swelling. In the neuroischemic foot, it may be difficult to differentiate between the erythema of cellulitis and the redness of ischemia. However, the redness of ischemia is usually cold although not always so and is most marked on dependency, whereas the erythema of inflammation is warm.

Cellulitis

When infection spreads, there is widespread intense erythema and swelling and lymphangitis, regional lymphadenitis, malaise, 'flu-like' symptoms, fever and rigors may develop. In the presence of neuropathy, pain and throbbing are often absent, but, if present, usually indicate pus within the tissues. Palpation may reveal fluctuation suggesting abscess formation, although discrete abscesses are relatively uncommon in the infected diabetic foot. Often, there is a generalized sloughing of the ulcer and surrounding subcutaneous tissues, which liquefy and disintegrate. Subcutaneous gas may be detected by direct palpation of the foot and the diagnosis is confirmed by the appearance of gas in the soft tissue on the radiograph. Although clostridial organisms have previously been held responsible for this presentation, non-clostridial organisms are more frequently the offending pathogens. These include *Bacteroides*, *Escherichia coli* and anaerobic streptococci. Only 50% of episodes of severe cellulitis will provoke a fever or leukocytosis[37]. A substantial number of patients with a deep foot infection do not have severe symptoms and signs indicating the presence of deep infection. However, when increased body temperature or leukocytosis is present, it usually indicates a substantial tissue damage[38].

Osteomyelitis

If a sterile probe inserted into the ulcer reaches bone, this strongly suggests the diagnosis of osteomyelitis. In the initial stages, plain X-ray may be normal and localized loss of bone density and cortical outline may not be apparent until at least 14 days later. The radionuclide bone scan using technetium-99m diphosphonate is very sensitive but not specific for osteomyelitis. Gallium or indium scans may improve specificity but magnetic resonance imaging may be most helpful in demonstrating loss of bony cortex[39]. Chronic osteomyelitis of a toe has a swollen, red, sausage-like appearance[40].

Management

Infection in the diabetic foot needs full multidisciplinary treatment. It is vital to achieve microbiologic, wound, vascular, mechanical and educational control, for, if infection is not controlled, it can spread with alarming rapidity, causing extensive tissue necrosis and taking the foot into stage 5.

Microbiologic control

General principles

At initial presentation, it is impossible to predict the organisms from the clinical appearance. Thus, it is important to prescribe wide-spectrum antibiotics and to take cultures without delay in all stage 4 patients. Deep swabs or tissue should be taken from the ulcer after initial debridement and, if the patient undergoes operative debridement, then deep tissue should also be sent. Ulcer swabs should be taken at every follow-up visit. It is possible that bacterial species that are usually not pathogenic can cause a true infection in a diabetic foot when part of a mixed flora. As there is a poor immune response of the diabetic patient to sepsis, even bacteria regarded as skin commensals may cause severe tissue damage. This includes Gram-negative organisms such as Citrobacter, Serratia, Pseudomonas and Acinetobacter. When Gram-negative bacteria are isolated from an ulcer swab, they should not be automatically regarded as insignificant. Blood cultures should also be sent, if there is fever and systemic toxicity. Close contact with the microbiologist is advised and it is helpful to do laboratory bench rounds to discuss management.

Antibiotic treatment

Infection in the neuroischemic foot is often more serious than in the neuropathic foot which has a good arterial blood supply; therefore a positive ulcer swab in a neuroischemic foot has serious implications and this influences antibiotic policy.

Antibiotic treatment is discussed both as initial treatment and at follow-up: dosage should be determined by the level of renal function and serum levels when available. Clinical and microbiologic response rates have been similar in trials of various antibiotics and no single agent or combination has emerged as most effective[3]. Chantelau randomized patients with neuropathic ulcers (some of which had cellulitis) to oral amoxycillin plus clavulinic acid or matched placebo. At 20 days follow-up, there was no significant difference in outcome[41]. Lipsky randomized 56 patients with an infected lesion to oral clindamycin or oral cephalexin in an outpatient setting and at 2 weeks there was no difference in treatment[42]. Grayson randomized 93 patients to intravenous imipenem/cilastatin or intravenous ampicillin/sulbactam and, after 5 days, cure had been effected in 60% of the ampicillin/sulbactam group and 58% of the imipenem/cilastatin group[36].

The following regime has been developed and is based on many years of treating the diabetic foot and significantly reducing amputations.

LOCAL SIGNS OF INFECTION IN THE ULCER OR MILD CELLULITIS – Initial treatment:

- Give amoxycillin, flucloxacillin, metronidazole and trimethoprim orally. If the patient is allergic to penicillin, substitute erythromycin for flucloxacillin.
- Cellulitis, on the borderline of mild to severe, can be treated with ceftriaxone i.m.

Follow-up plan (with reference to previous visit's swab):

- If no signs of infection and no organisms isolated – stop antibiotics; but if the patient is severely ischemic with a pressure index below 0.5, consider continuing antibiotics until healing.
- If no signs of infection are present but organisms are isolated, focus antibiotics and review in 1 week.
- If signs of infection are present but no organisms are isolated, continue the antibiotics as above.
- If signs of infection are still present and organisms are isolated, focus antibiotic regime according to sensitivities.
- If methicillin-resistant *Staphylococcus aureus* (MRSA) is grown, but there are no local or systemic signs of infection, use topical mupirocin 2% ointment (if sensitive).
- If MRSA is grown, with local signs of infection, consider oral therapy with two of the following: sodium fusidate, rifampicin, trimethoprim and doxycycline, according to sensitivities, together with topical mupirocin 2% ointment.

FOOT WITH SEVERE CELLULITIS – Initial treatment:
- If admission is not possible, then give ceftriaxone i.m. and metronidazole orally. On review as an outpatient, if cellulitis is controlled, continue ceftriaxone i.m. and metronidazole orally and review 1 week later.
- If cellulitis is increasing, then admit for intravenous antibiotics. Quadruple therapy is indicated: amoxycillin, flucloxacillin, metronidazole and ceftazidime. If patient is allergic to penicillin, replace amoxycillin and flucloxacillin, with erythromycin or vancomycin (with doses adjusted according to serum levels). On admission, the foot should be urgently assessed as to the need for surgical debridement (see Wound Control).

Follow-up plan:
- The infected foot should be inspected daily to gauge the initial response to antibiotic therapy.
- Appropriate antibiotics should be selected when sensitivities are available. If an infection responds well to the initial antibiotics but the swabs suggest that these antibiotics are resistant to the isolated organisms, it is best to change the antibiotics according to sensitivities, although this is not universal practice.
- If no organisms are isolated and yet the foot remains severely cellulitic, then a repeat deep swab should be taken, but the quadruple antibiotic therapy, as above, should be continued.
- If MRSA is isolated, give vancomycin (dosage to be adjusted according to serum levels) or teicoplanin. These antibiotics may need to be accompanied by either sodium fusidate or rifampicin orally. Intravenous antibiotic therapy can be changed to the appropriate oral therapy when the signs of cellulitis have resolved.

OSTEOMYELITIS – Initial treatment:
- At first, antibiotics will be given for the associated infected ulcer and cellulitis as above.

Follow-up plan:
- On review, antibiotic selection is guided by the results of deep swabs, but it is useful to choose antibiotics with good bone penetration, such as sodium fusidate, rifampicin, clindamycin and ciprofloxacin. Antibiotics should be given for at least 12 weeks.
- Such conservative therapy is often successful and is associated with resolution of cellulitis and healing of the ulcer. However, if after 3 months treatment, the ulcer persists, with continued probing to bone, which is fragmented on X-ray, then

in the neuropathic foot, resection of the underlying bone is probably indicated.

Wound control

Diabetic foot infections are almost always more extensive than would appear from initial examination and surface appearance.

It is wise to perform an initial debridement so that the true dimensions of the lesion can be revealed and samples obtained for culture. Often callus may be overlying the ulcer and this must be removed to reveal the extent of the underlying ulcer and allow drainage of pus and removal of infected sloughy tissue.

Cellulitis should respond to intravenous antibiotics, but the patient needs daily review to ensure the erythema is resolving. In severe episodes of cellulitis, the ulcer may be complicated by extensive infected subcutaneous soft tissue. At this point, the tissue is not frankly necrotic but has started to break down and liquefy. It is best for this tissue to be removed operatively. The definite indications for urgent surgical intervention are a large area of infected sloughy tissue, localized fluctuation and expression of pus, crepitus with gas in the soft tissues on X-ray and purplish discoloration of the skin, indicating subcutaneous necrosis.

The role of hyperbaric oxygen in the management of wounds is not yet established but two small randomized, controlled trials found that systemic hyperbaric oxygen reduced the absolute risk of foot amputation in people with severely infected ulcers compared with routine care[3].

Vascular control

It is important to explore the possibility of revascularization in the infected neuro-ischemic foot. Improvement of perfusion will not only help to control infection but will also promote healing of wounds if operative debridement is necessary.

Mechanical control

Patients should be on bedrest with heel protection using foam wedges.

Educational control

The patient should be advised of the importance of rest in severe infection. If the patient has mild cellulitis and is treated at home, he should understand the signs of advancing and progressing cellulitis so as to return early to clinic. Patient education provided after the management of acute foot complications decreases ulcer recurrences and major amputations[43].

STAGE 5: FOOT ULCER AND NECROSIS

Presentation

This stage is characterized by the presence of necrosis. It is classified as either wet necrosis due to infection or dry necrosis due to ischemia. In wet necrosis, the tissues are gray or black, moist and often malodorous. Adjoining tissues are infected and pus may discharge from the ulcerated demarcation line between necrosis and viable tissue. Dry necrosis is hard, blackened, mummified tissue and there is usually a clean demarcation line between necrosis and viable tissue.

Necrosis presents in both the neuropathic and the neuroischemic foot and the management is different in both.

Neuropathic foot

In the neuropathic foot, necrosis is invariably wet and is usually caused by infection complicating an ulcer and leading to a septic vasculitis of the digital and small arteries of the foot. The walls of these arteries are infiltrated by polymorphs, leading to occlusion of the lumen by septic thrombus.

Necrosis can involve skin, subcutaneous and fascial layers. In the skin, it is easily evident but in the subcutaneous and fascial layers it is not so apparent. Often the bluish-black discoloration of skin is the 'tip of an iceberg' of deep necrosis which occurs in subcutaneous and fascial planes, so-called necrotizing fasciitis.

Neuroischemic foot

Both wet and dry necrosis can occur in the neuroischemic foot. Wet necrosis is also caused by a septic vasculitis. However, reduced arterial perfusion to the foot resulting from atherosclerotic disease of the leg arteries is an important predisposing factor.

Dry necrosis is usually secondary to a severe reduction in arterial perfusion and occurs in three circumstances: severe chronic ischemia, acute ischemia and emboli to the toes.

Severe chronic ischemia

A gradual but severe reduction in arterial perfusion results in vascular compromise of the skin, leading to blue toes, which usually become necrotic unless the foot is revascularized.

Acute ischemia

Blue discoloration leading to necrosis of the toes is also seen in acute ischemia. It presents as a sudden onset of pain in the leg associated with pallor of the foot, quickly followed by mottling and slate-gray discoloration.

Emboli to the toes

Emboli to the digital circulation result in a bluish or purple discoloration which is quite well demarcated but which quickly proceeds to necrosis. If it escapes infection, the toe will dry out and mummify. Microemboli present with painful petechial lesions in the foot that do not blanch on pressure.

Digital necrosis in the patient with renal impairment

Digital necrosis is a relatively common problem in patients with advanced diabetic nephropathy. It may result from a septic neutrophilic vasculitis but can occur in the absence of infection. It may be precipitated by trauma.

Management

Patients should be admitted for urgent investigations and multidisciplinary management. It is important to achieve wound, microbiologic, vascular, mechanical and educational control.

Wound control

Neuropathic foot

Operative debridement is almost always indicated for wet gangrene. It is important to remove all necrotic tissue, down to bleeding tissue, as well as opening up all sinuses. Deep necrotic tissue should be sent for culture immediately. Although necrosis in the diabetic foot may not be associated with a definite collection of pus, the necrotic tissue still needs to be removed. In the neuropathic foot, there is good arterial circulation and the wound always heals as long as infection is controlled. Wounds should not be sutured. Skin grafting may be the best way to accelerate healing of large tissue deficits. When there is extensive loss of tissue, modern reconstructive surgical techniques have recently proved useful[44].

Neuroischemic foot

In the neuroischemic foot, wet necrosis should also be removed when it is associated with severe spreading sepsis. This should be done whether pus is present or not.

In cases where the limb is not immediately threatened and the necrosis is limited to one or two toes, it may be possible to control infection with intravenous antibiotics and proceed to urgent revascularization and at the same operation, perform digital or ray amputation. Wounds in the neuroischemic foot may be slow to heal even after revascularization and wound care needs to continue as an outpatient in the diabetic foot clinic, but with patience outcomes may be surprisingly good.

If revascularization is not possible for digital necrosis, then a decision must be made to either amputate the toe in the presence of ischemia or allow the toe, if infection is controlled, to convert to dry necrosis and autoamputate. Surgical amputation should be undertaken if the toe is painful or if the circulation is not severely impaired, that is, a pressure index greater than 0.5 or a transcutaneous oxygen tension greater than 30 mmHg[8].

Microbiologic control

Wet necrosis

When the patient initially presents, wound swabs and tissue specimens should be sent for culture. Deep tissue taken at operative debridement must also go for culture. Intravenous antibiotic therapy (amoxycillin, flucloxacillin, metronidazole and ceftazidime) should be given. However, if the patient is allergic to penicillin, then erythromycin or vancomycin (dosage adjusted according to serum levels) may be used instead of amoxycillin and flucloxacillin. Intravenous antibiotics can be replaced with oral therapy after operative debridement and when infection is controlled. When the wound is granulating well and swabs are negative, then the antibiotics may be stopped.

Dry necrosis

When dry necrosis develops secondary to ischemia, antibiotics should be prescribed if discharge is present or the wound swab is positive and continued until there is no evidence of clinical or microbiologic infection.

Vascular control

After operative debridement of wet necrosis, revascularization is often essential to heal the tissue deficit. In dry necrosis, which occurs in the background of severe macrovascular disease, revascularization is necessary to maintain the viability of the limb. When dry necrosis is secondary to emboli, a possible source should be investigated.

In some patients, increased perfusion following angioplasty may be useful. However, unless there is a very significant localized stenosis in iliac or femoral arteries, angioplasty rarely restores to the foot the pulsatile blood flow which is necessary to keep the limb viable in severe ischemia or restore considerable tissue deficits secondary to necrosis. This is best achieved by arterial bypass.

Peripheral arterial disease is common in the tibial arteries, and distal bypass with autologous vein has become an established method of revascularization, in which a conduit is fashioned from either the femoral or popliteal artery down to a tibial artery in the lower leg or the dorsalis pedis artery on the dorsum of the foot. Patency rates and limb salvage rates after revascularization do not differ between diabetic patients and non-diabetic patients and a more aggressive approach to such revascularization procedures should be promoted[45].

Mechanical control

During the peri- and postoperative period, bed rest is essential with elevation of the limb to relieve edema and afford heel protection. After operative debridement in the neuroischemic foot, non-weight-bearing is advised until the wound is healed, especially when revascularization has not been possible. In the neuropathic foot, non-weight-bearing is advisable initially and then off-loading of the healing postoperative wound may be achieved by casting techniques. If necrosis is to be treated conservatively, by autoamputation, which can take several months, then the patient needs a wide-fitting shoe to accommodate the foot and dressings.

Educational control

For patients in hospital, advice is similar to that given for severe cellulitis.

For patients undergoing autoamputation at home, it is important to rest the foot and keep it dry and covered with a dressing and bandage. Patients should be advised to return to the clinic immediately if the foot becomes swollen, painful, develops an unpleasant smell or discharges pus.

CONCLUSION

This chapter has outlined a simple classification of the diabetic foot into the neuropathic and neuroischemic foot and defined six specific stages in its natural history. It has described a simple plan of management for each stage that requires a well-organized multidisciplinary approach that provides continuity of care between primary and secondary sectors[46].

Secondary care should be focused on a diabetic foot clinic to which rapid referrals should be possible. Such clinics have reported a reduction in amputations, a major welcome change, and should be available to all diabetic patients[47].

References

1. Edmonds ME. Progress in care of the diabetic foot. *Lancet* 1999;354:270–2
2. Mason JM, O'Keefe C, McIntosh A, Hutchinson A, Booth A, Young R. A systematic review of foot ulcer in patients with Type 2 diabetes mellitus. I: Prevention. *Diabet Med* 1999;16:801–12
3. Mason JM, O'Keefe C, Hutchinson A, McIntosh A, Young R, Booth A. A systematic review of foot ulcer in patients with Type 2 diabetes mellitus. II: Treatment. *Diabet Med* 1999;16: 889–909
4. Hunt D, Gerstein H. Foot ulcers in diabetes. *Clinical Evidence* 1999;2:231–7
5. Pinzur MS, Slovenkai MP, Trepman E. Guidelines for diabetic foot care. *Foot Ankle Int* 1999; 20:695–702
6. International Consensus on the Diabetic Foot 1999. The International Working Group on the Diabetic Foot
7. Consensus Development Conference on Diabetic Foot Wound Care. American Diabetes Association. *Diabetes Care* 1999;22:1354–60
8. Edmonds ME, Foster AVM. *Managing the Diabetic Foot*. Oxford: Blackwell Science, 2000
9. Edmonds ME, Foster AVM. Classification and management of neuropathic and neuroischaemic ulcers. In: Boulton AJM, Connor H, Cavanagh PR, eds. *The Foot in Diabetes*, 2nd edn. Chichester: John Wiley & Sons Ltd, 1994
10. Flynn MD. The diabetic foot. In: Tooke JE, ed. *Diabetic Angiopathy*. London: Arnold, 1999
11. Johnston CLW. Infection and diabetes mellitus. In: Pickup J, Williams G eds. *Textbook of Diabetes*, Vol 2. Oxford: Blackwell Science, 1997:70.1–14
12. Rith-Najarian SJ, Stolusky T, Godhes DM. Identifying diabetic patients at risk for lower extremity amputation in a primary healthcare setting. *Diabetes Care* 1992;15:1386–9

13. Hurley JJ, Woods JJ, Hershey FB. Non-invasive testing: practical knowledge for evaluating diabetic patients. In: Levin MF, O'Neal LW, Bowker JH, eds. *The Diabetic Foot*. St Louis: Mosby Year Book, 1993:321-40

14. Tovey FI. The manufacture of diabetic footwear. *Diabet Med* 1984;1:69–71

15. Litzelman DK, Slemenda CW, Langefield CD, *et al*. Reduction of lower extremity clinical abnormalities in patients with non-insulin dependent diabetes mellitus. *Ann Intern Med* 1993;199:36–41

16. McCabe CJ, Stevenson RC, Dolan AM. Evaluation of a diabetic foot screening and protection programme. *Diabet Med* 1998;15:80–4

17. Sanders LJ, Frykberg RG. Diabetic neuropathic osteoarthropathy: the Charcot foot. In: Frykberg RG, ed. *The High Risk Foot in Diabetes*. New York: Churchill Livingstone, 1991: 227–38

18. Jude EB, Selby PL, Burgess J, *et al*. Bisphosphonates in the treatment of Charcot neuroarthropathy: a double-blind randomised controlled trial. *Diabetologia* 2001;44:2032–7

19. Papa J, Myerson MS, Girard P. Salvage with arthrodesis in intractable diabetic neuropathic arthropathy of the foot and ankle. *J Bone Joint Surg* 1993;75a:1056–66

20. Armstrong DG, Lavery LA. Evidence based options for off loading diabetic wounds. *Clin Podiatr Med Surg* 1998;15:95–104

21. Kalish SR, Pelcovitz N, Zawada S, Donatelli RA, Wooden MJ, Castellano BD. The Aircast walking brace versus conventional casting methods. *J Am Podiatr Med Assoc* 1987;77:589–95

22. Armstrong DG, Nguyen HC, Lavery LA, van Schie CH, Boulton AJ, Harkless LB. Off-loading the diabetic foot wound: a randomized clinical trial. *Diabetes Care* 2001;24:1019–22

23. Burden AC, Jones GR, Jones R, Blandford RL. Use of the 'Scotchcast boot' in treating diabetic foot ulcers. *Br Med J* 1983;286:1555–7

24. Apelqvist J, Larsson J, Agardh C.-D. Long term prognosis for diabetic patients with foot ulcers. *J Int Med* 1993;233:485–91

25. Uccioli L, Aldeghi A, Faglia E, *et al*. Manufactured shoes in the prevention of diabetic foot ulcers. *Diabetes Care* 1995;18:1376–8

26. Rayman A, Stansfield G, Woollard T, Mackie A, Rayman G. Use of larvae in the treatment of the diabetic necrotic foot. *Diabet Foot* 1998;1: 7–13

27. Steed DL and the Diabetic Ulcer Study Group. Clinical evaluation of recombinant human platelet-derived growth factor for the treatment of lower extremity diabetic ulcers. *J Vasc Surg* 1995;21:71–81

28. Wieman TJ, Smiell JM, Su Y. Efficacy and safety of a topical gel formulation of recombinant human platelet derived growth factor – BB (Becaplermin) in patients with non-healing diabetic ulcers: a phase III, randomized, placebo-controlled, double-blind study. *Diabetes Care* 1998;21:822–7

29. Naughton G, Mansbridge J, Gentzkow G. A metabolically active human dermal replacement for the treatment of diabetic foot ulcers. *Artificial Organs* 1997;21:1203–10

30. Pham HT, Rosenblum BI, Lyons TE, *et al*. Evaluation of Graftskin (Apligraf R), a human skin equivalent for the treatment of diabetic foot ulcers. *Diabetes* 1999;48(Suppl 1):A18

31. Chen WYJ, Abatangelo G. Functions of hyaluronan in wound repair. *Wound Repair Regen* 1999;7:79–89

32. Foster AM, Bates M, Doxford M, Edmonds ME. The treatment of indolent neuropathic ulceration of the diabetic foot with Hyaff. *Diabet Med* 1999; S94

33. Foster A, Mccolgan M, Edmonds M. Should oral antibiotics be given to clean foot ulcers with no cellulitis? *Diabet Med* 1998;15(Suppl 2):S10

34. Edmonds ME, Walters H. Angioplasty and the diabetic foot. *Vasc Med Rev* 1995;6:205–14

35. Lipsky BA. A current approach to diabetic foot infections. *Curr Infect Disease Rep* 1999;1: 253–60

36. Grayson ML. Diabetic foot infections: antimicrobial therapy. In: Eliopoulos GM, ed. *Infectious Disease Clinics of North America*. Philadelphia: WB Saunders, 1995:143–62

37. Armstrong DG, Lavery LA, Sariaya M, Ashry H. Leukocytosis is a poor indicator of acute osteomyelitis of the foot in diabetes mellitus. *J Foot Ankle Surg* 1996;4:280–3

38. Eneroth M, Apelqvist J, Stenstrom A. Clinical characteristics and outcome in 223 diabetic

patients with deep foot infections. *Foot Ankle Int* 1997;18:716–22

39. Longmaid III HE, Kruskal JB. Imaging infections in diabetic patients. In: Eliopoulos GM, ed. *Infectious Disease Clinics of North America*. Philadelphia: WB Saunders, 1995:163–82

40. Rajbhandari S, Sutton M, Davies C, Tesfaye S, Ward JD. Sausage toe: a reliable sign of underlying osteomyelitis. *Diabet Med* 2000;17:74–7

41. Chantelau E, Tanudjaja T, Altenhofer F, Ersanili Z , Lacigova S, Metzger C. Antibiotic treatment for uncomplicated neuropathic forefoot ulcers in diabetes: a controlled trial. *Diabet Med* 1996;13:156–9

42. Lipsky BA, Pecoraro RE, Larson SA, Hanley ME, Ahroni JH. Outpatient management of uncomplicated lower-extremity infections in diabetic patients. *Arch Intern Med* 1990;150: 790–7

43. Malone JM, Snyder M, Anderson G, Bernhard VM, Holloway GA, Bunt TJ. Prevention of amputation by diabetic education. *Am J Surg* 1989;158:520–4

44. Armstrong MD, Villalobos RE, Leppink DM. Free tissue transfer for lower extremity reconstruction in the immunosuppressed diabetic transplant recipient. *J Reconstr Microsurg* 1997; 13:1–5

45. Pomposelli FB, Marcaccio EJ, Gibbons GW, *et al*. Dorsalis pedis arterial bypass: durable limb salvage for foot ischaemia in patients with diabetes mellitus. *J Vasc Surg* 1995;21:375–84

46. Edmonds M, Boulton A, Buckenham T, *et al*. Report of the diabetic foot and amputation group. *Diabet Med* 1996;13:S27–42

47. Larsson J, Apelqvist J, Agardh CD, Stenstrom A. Decreasing incidence of major amputation in diabetic patients: a consequence of a multidisciplinary foot care team approach? *Diabet Med* 1995;12:770–6

Pressure ulcer studies: reasons to change

9

M. Romanelli, D. Mastronicola, A. Magliaro and S. Siani

INTRODUCTION

Pressure ulcers represent a major health problem causing a considerable amount of suffering for patients and a high financial burden for health-care systems. The geriatric population with an increased risk of pressure ulcer development is increasing steadily due to chronic degenerative diseases which can lead to prolonged immobilization and poor nutrition. Evidence clearly indicates that preventive measures are essential to reduce the prevalence rates of pressure ulcers, and therefore health-care professionals must be able to identify the appropriate strategies to adopt, in order to meet the individual patient's requirements. Over the last decade, there has been an increase in new therapeutic options for the management of pressure ulcers. The introduction of advanced medical devices and new concepts on systemic treatment have led to a better understanding of the mechanism of tissue repair in pressure ulcers, aided by the delivery of standardized guidelines of prevention and treatment. The aim of this chapter is to review the latest technologic advances in local and systemic treatment for pressure ulcers.

DEFINITION

Pressure ulcers are defined as areas of localized damage to the skin and underlying tissue caused by pressure, shear, friction and/or a combination of these[1]. The above is a working definition. New theories are being developed but further work is required before they can be included in an accepted definition. Although the term 'pressure ulcer' is the most widely accepted, because it clearly describes the nature of this lesion, over the years several terms have been used to describe pressure ulcers, such as bedsore, decubitus and pressure sore.

NUTRITION AND PRESSURE ULCERS

Even though the type of wound, timing of wound closure and wound care techniques may vary, the process of healing and the factors influencing the healing process are basically the same for all types of wounds. In the healing process, there are three major interrelated and overlapping components: (1) inflammation and hemostasis, (2) proliferation and (3) wound contraction and remodeling. All these phases require energy, protein and anabolic stimulus.

The concept that nutritional status dramatically influences the healing process is a relatively new and now proven concept, but we have to consider that immobility, fecal and urinary incontinence and altered mental state are other important associated risk factors in elderly patients or in individuals with spinal cord injuries, traumatic brain injuries and neuromuscular disorders[2,3]. Nutrition plays a fundamental role in the treatment and healing of pressure ulcers; a well-balanced, nutritionally adequate diet should be a priority for all patients at risk of pressure ulcers. Nutrition and hydration are fundamental components in maintaining the normal integrity of tissues and promoting the healing process. Any alteration of the nutritional state, associated with low body weight, induces tissue damage. Dehydration represents a risk factor because it leads to low volume and subsequent changes in the peripheral circulation, with a reduction in tissue nutrients and oxygen. Anemia is the cause of reduced oxygenation of fibroblasts and the result is a slower synthesis of collagen and a modification of the healing process. The low levels of serum albumin and hypoproteinemia result in edema with a lack of cutaneous elasticity, as well as some important changes in microcirculation and subsequent delay in wound closure[4].

Studies performed by Henderson[5] have shown that hypocholesterolemia is also an important associated risk factor, because cholesterol builds up the plasmatic wall of the cells and its deficiency can slow the healing process. There are some nutrients that require more attention such as proteins, vitamins, minerals. Proteins play a very important role in pressure ulcers, being the rate-limiting factor in the tissue repair process. Healing cannot occur unless there is an adequate protein intake to make new tissue. It is estimated that at least 1 g/body-kg is needed to achieve nitrogen equilibrium. It is largely accepted that patients at risk of pressure ulcers have to take a daily dose of multivitamins: vitamin C (ascorbic acid) is necessary for the formation of hydroxyproline from proline; hydroxyproline is an essential constituent of collagen. In a prospective double-blind study[6] of the supplementation of ascorbic acid (1 g per day) in 20

patients, the group which received placebo had a reduction in pressure sore area of 43% over 1 month. The group which received ascorbic acid had much higher tissue levels and had a reduction in pressure sore area of 84%. Vitamin B complex is necessary for energy metabolism, vitamin A is an essential nutrient for many physiologic reactions, such as the synthesis of new tissue, and vitamin D plays an important role in wound healing and immune responses. But the causal relationship between pressure ulcer development, inadequate healing and nutritional impairment has not yet been established exactly.

A connection has been found in several cases between some features of nutritional risk, such as low serum albumin or low dietary intake and pressure ulcers[7]. On the other hand, less convincing is the association between a reduced body weight and the increased risk of pressure ulcer. Therefore, only the decreased incidence of pressure ulcers in response to improvement of any nutritional impairment would provide real evidence for this. Thus, the first goal in patients at risk of pressure ulcer development is to improve their nutritional status. For this purpose, the usual anorexia encountered in at-risk patients must be overcome. The use of a special diet or commercially available oral nutritional supplementation seems to be effective in improving the caloric and protein intake of anorexic patients, but the total amount of food actually ingested obviously remains below the needs of these subjects. Whereas the improvement of nutritional status and particularly of anthropometric features is not immediate, the risk of pressure ulcer begins on the first day of immobilization and requires early prevention. Finally, when pressure ulcers are constituted, anorexia and hypercatabolism are maintained, particularly in stage 3 or in more serious ulcers.

Oral supplementation should therefore be useful in the prevention of pressure ulcers, owing to the immediate improvement of dietary intake and not to significant changes in global nutritional status. Because the observed improvement in nutritional intake is minimal when using oral supplementation, the expected beneficial effect is not spectacular. Trials investigating the effects of oral nutritional intervention should show an improvement in nutritional intake specifically due to supplementation and thus should demonstrate why this improvement has an independent protective effect on pressure ulcer development and healing[8,9]. The logical consequence of this reasoning is to propose the giving of artificially controlled amounts of calories, proteins or other potentially protective compounds so as to obtain the expected protection. This led to implementing enteral or parenteral nutrition in patients at risk of pressure ulcers in order to promote ulcer healing. Unfortunately, the results of the published studies are disappointing. The lack of success in attempts to date could be partly due to the increase in immobility associated with artificial nutrition or at least to the difficulties associated with active mobilization of patients receiving artificial support. Furthermore, subjects who are offered such nutritional support are likely to be chronically immobilized and this is a major risk factor for pressure ulcers. On the other hand, both parenteral and enteral nutrition can lead to adverse effects that may counteract any beneficial effects on pressure ulcer outcome.

Improvement in function and particularly mobility is another means to limit the pressure ulcer risk. This can be promoted by nutritional support, because of the expected increase in muscle strength. However, this potential effect of nutritional support needs at least a few days or weeks to be felt. Furthermore, muscle strength increase does not seem to be achievable using nutritional support only, but in combination with reconditioning. This could be beneficial in a long-term care setting but is unlikely to play a significant role during the acute phase of a disease. Interventional data regarding the benefit of nutrition or pharmaconutrients on pressure ulcer healing are very scarce, because of the many complications involved in staging such clinical trials, such as the fact that the patients' underlying conditions are decisive in terms of the healing process, the time of healing is not easy to predict and the period of observation can be too long, and during this healing period uncontrolled events may occur.

Despite these difficulties, a positive effect of dietary interventions on pressure ulcer healing cannot be ruled out. Ideally, individual randomization and double-blind nutrient versus placebo trials should be implemented, either in prevention or pressure ulcer healing. Theoretically, it should be possible to attribute the decrease in incidence or the decreased area of a pressure ulcer to the difference in nutrients actually ingested. However, in long-term studies, patients are often poorly compliant with nutritional therapy. Furthermore, the possibility that giving nutritional placebo decreases the final amount of ingested food, particularly in anorexic patients, cannot be excluded. Thus, the observation period should be short both in prevention and in pressure ulcer healing studies. The number of subjects needed to reach statistical significance is therefore high. This implies the implementation of multicenter studies and careful quality control of the data.

The efficiency of nursing staff in pressure ulcer prevention and care is of major importance in such trials. However, even when using standardized training of these nursing staff, it seems unlikely that differences would be avoided in nursing care behavior and in available prevention equipment in the different centers. Thus, statistical models taking into account a potential intracenter correlation would have to be used. The benefits of the intervention on the course of pressure ulcers are also likely to be hidden by other patient characteristics. Thus, it would seem important to monitor each patient's characteristics and in particular the baseline nutritional status. Such difficult studies with numerous patients and variables are likely to be costly. Pressure ulcers are a major concern in hospital care, particularly in elderly patients. Research in this area should therefore be encouraged, to allow progress in prevention and treatment and in particular to understand the role of nutritional support.

GROWTH FACTORS AND WOUND HEALING

The wound healing process is thought to be largely influenced by locally acting growth factors. In fact, this process involves a complex interaction between cells, biochemical mediators, extracellular matrix molecules and the cellular microenvironment. The role of each of these factors is continuously studied and investigated by dermatologists and by all who are interested in new therapeutic approaches to wound treatment[10]. The growth factors are biomolecules, usually small polypeptides. Interacting with specific receptors, they influence the wound repair process by way of cell proliferation, movement and bioactivity. When a wound occurs, the expression of growth factors and corresponding receptors is elevated and subsides once the wound has healed. The growth factors may act as paracrine (produced by one cell type to act on another in the local area) or autocrine (produced by a cell acting on itself) factors.

All growth factors have the following properties:

- Multifunctional properties: they can either inhibit or promote cell growth and differentiation;
- Relationship to oncogenesis: the neoplastic cells produce and respond to the growth factors that they produce;

- Tyrosine kinase activity: the receptors of several growth factors are protein kinase autophosphorylant;
- Competence and progression factors: growth factors can act in synergy with one another.

The growth factors are members of the cytokine family, which includes interleukins and colony-stimulating factors. They may be named according to their function, cell origin or the target cell toward which their action is directed.

The main growth factors involved in the wound repair process are:

- Epidermal growth factor (EGF): a 6 kDa protein made up of a single chain of 53 amino acids. It is produced and released mainly by keratinocytes and platelets. *In vitro* it induces epidermal cellular proliferation. It stimulates epithelial regeneration after partial thickness injuries.
- Platelet-derived growth factor (PDGF): protein made up of two disulfide-linked subunits. It responds to specific receptors (PDGF-r) localized in fibroblasts, glial cells and the smooth muscle of vessels. It is produced by platelets, macrophages and keratinocytes. It has several biological effects: it is a potent vasoconstrictor, induces phospholipase, induces metabolism of prostaglandin, it is a chemotactic molecule and a competence factor; it is a potent mitogen for most mesenchymally derived connective tissue cells. It stimulates angiogenesis and inhibits any EGF occupying its receptor (EGF-r). PDGF stimulates cellular proliferation of connective tissue next to the wound area, facilitating its closure.
- IGFs (insulin growth factors): the IGFs include IGF-1 and IGF-2. They are both able to promote the inclusion of sulfate in

the cartilage; they have insulin activity and a potent mitogenic effect on fibroblasts. They are produced mainly by the liver and also by fibroblasts. The responding receptors for IGFs are detectable in most cells.

- FGFs (fibroblast growth factors): a large family encompassing eight different types. The factors most studied are FGFb (basic) and FGFa (acid). FGFb is a 17 kDa polypeptide. It is produced *in vitro* by fibroblasts, endothelial cells and keratinocytes. The FGFs influence the morphology, proliferation and differentiation of meso-ectodermic cells. FGF-7, -1, -2 promote the proliferation and migration of keratinocytes and the expression of FGF-1,-2,-5,-7 is elevated early in wounds.
- KGFs (keratinocyte growth factors): KGF-1 is a potent mitogen on epithelial cells. It can act as a paracrine factor on responding receptors of keratinocytes. It promotes epithelial proliferation and the formation of granulation tissue.
- TGF-β (transforming growth factor-β): peptides of 25 kDa, detectable everywhere in the body; they have three distinct receptors. TGF-β 1 is produced by various inflammatory cells, such as platelets, leukocytes and fibroblasts. It influences cellular proliferation, angiogenesis and the formation of connective tissue; it stimulates the mitosis of fibroblasts and inhibits the growth of cells such as keratinocytes and endothelial cells. It promotes the deposition of collagen in the extracellular matrix and induces keratinocytes to express cytokeratin K6–K16. The TGFs stimulate the formation of myofibroblasts and may be involved in abnormal scar formation. Enhanced expression of this molecule is thought to be a possible mechanism for fibrous disorders; conversely, antagonists have shown to be potential therapeutic agents for hypertrophic scars.
- GM-CSF (granulocyte-macrophage colony stimulating factor): is a 25 kDa glycoprotein, produced by keratinocytes and leukocytes; it is able to influence wound healing. *In vivo* studies have demonstrated that GM-CSF induces the differentiation of myofibroblasts, thereby facilitating wound contraction, causes local recruitment of inflammatory cells and induces keratinocyte proliferation, all essential for normal wound healing. In addition, GM-CSF activates mononuclear phagocytes, promotes migration of epithelial cells and further regulates cytokine production.
- VEGF (vascular-endothelial growth factor): promotes the permeability membrane of endothelial cells, elevating the amount of fluids and plasmatic elements in the wounded area. It therefore facilitates the recruitment of NK lymphocytes in this area.

These findings have stimulated considerable interest in the use of growth factors as promoters of wound healing. Even if the specific molecular mechanisms involved in healing chronic skin wounds have not been entirely elucidated, it is accepted that specific cytokines and growth factors influence the process. Cell types found within wounds synthesize and express growth factor receptors, and local application of growth factors can speed wound closure *in vivo*. A physiologic basis for managing chronic human wounds with an exogenous recombinant human platelet-derived growth factor (rhPDGF-BB) has been identified with the discovery of PDGF receptors in normal skin and granulation tissue. Clinical trials with rPDGF-BB have shown that it may be effective in improving the healing process by increasing wound fibroblasts and neovessel formation. Important studies were performed by Pierce and co-workers[11] to investigate how rPDGF-BB may induce chronic wounds to heal. In this study, biopsies were taken from the ulcers of 20 patients and evaluated blind by light microscopy for (1) fibroblast content, (2) neovessel formation and (3) collagen deposition. This study showed a significant difference between rPDGF-BB-treated ulcers and placebo-treated ulcers; fibroblast content was higher for the rPDGF-BB-treated ulcers. In all healing wounds, the rPDGF-BB therapy increased fibroblast and neovessel content. These results confirm that induction of fibroblast proliferation and differentiation is one mechanism by which rPDGF-BB can accelerate wound healing and that rPDGF-BB has this effect within the majority of chronic pressure ulcers in man.

Another clinical trial on 20 patients with grade III–IV pressure ulcers, performed by Mustoe and co-workers[12], produced interesting results. Topical PDGF was applied onto wounds and compared with a placebo group. The patients treated with topical PDGF had a faster healing time, but this was not statistically significant. Successive studies performed by El Saghir and co-workers[13] on GM-CSF showed that injections of diluted GM-CSF around and into the ulcer bed every 2–3 days for 2 weeks, then weekly for 4 weeks, promoted the accelerated healing of a sacral pressure ulcer. The ulcer showed 85% healing within 2 weeks and 100% by 2 months. Healing started from the periphery and from within the ulcer bed at sites of GM-CSF injections. Currently, the potential role of other growth factors in pressure ulcers is being investigated and discussed in other clinical trials. Encouraging results have been demonstrated using transforming growth factor beta (TGF-β3) in the treatment of pressure ulcers. TGF-β3 is a recombinant form of the TGF human molecule. To date, an interesting and important study has been performed by Hirshberg and co-workers[14] examining the effectiveness of topical applications of TGF-β3 on pressure ulcers in three groups of patients.

Group 1 received $1.0\,\mu g/cm^2$ of TGF-β3, group 2 received $2.5\,\mu g/cm^2$ of TGF-β3, group 3 received a placebo gel. Efficacy was determined by using target ulcer surface area and volume measurements relative to baseline values taken at the start of the trial. A significant decrease in volume was also seen when comparing group 1 and group 3. This study suggests that TGF-β3 may be effective in the treatment of pressure ulcers, but was significant only at high dosages and during the initial weeks of treatment. The role of other growth factors in wound healing remains to be determined in clinical studies. Extensive research is still needed to determine the effects of the other growth factors and their influence on non-healing wounds[15,16]. When specific growth factors are deficient, it is still not known how much is needed, when it is needed, how much should be applied and when the precise physiologic response will occur. The future of growth factor research may require a greater understanding of how these substances interact with each other. Wound dressings of the future may include several growth factors, each with a specific function. Hence, the application of topically active growth factors to chronic ulcers may be the next great innovation in wound healing[17].

ADVANCED DRESSINGS

Research into pressure ulcer treatment is generally conducted on a small scale and there is insufficient evidence to recommend any particular wound dressing. Treatment of pressure ulcers is based on the management of the general condition of the patient, relief and control of pressure and friction forces and local treatment of the wound. The development of new, advanced dressings has provided great support in wound care, facilitating the management by clinicians of the different aspects of wound healing such as debridement, exudate control, infection management, relief of pressure.

Local treatment should maintain a moist environment on the wound bed and the dressing should be selected according to the condition and location of the wound. The dressing should be maintained *in situ* for an adequately long period or may need to be removed daily to assess the progress of healing[18].

Today, a wide selection of advanced dressings is available with different indications, actions and effectiveness – such as hydrocolloids, hydrogels, hydrofibers, alginates, polyurethane films, polyurethane foams, silver or coal or collagen dressing. The type of dressing depends on the wound bed status, risk of infection, environment and stage of the wound and the compliance of the patient. The study by Winter[19] and the works of Hinman and Maibach[20] showed that epidermal migration was twice as fast in a moist environment as compared to a dry environment. Pressure ulcers treated with hydrocolloid dressing heal 50% faster than those treated with moist saline gauze, as found by Xakellis and Chrischilles[21]. Kim reported that occlusive hydrocolloid dressings for the treatment of stage I–II pressure ulcers were less time-consuming and less expensive compared to conventional saline-soaked gauze dressing[22]. In comparison with wounds treated with gauze and polyurethane dressing, wounds treated with hydrocolloid were consistently found to have lower bacterial burdens and improved healing thanks to the bacterial barrier properties of hydrocolloid dressings[23]. Hydrocolloid dressings provide a moist wound healing with prevention of tissue dehydration and cell death, angiogenesis acceleration, increased removal of fibrin and necrotic tissue, pain reduction and potentiation of growth factors[24]. Clinical studies have shown that hydrocolloid dressings are effective in managing exuding wounds and are commonly used in the management of pressure ulcers[25,26]. Mulder[27] studied the efficacy of three different types of dressings providing moist wound healing such as hydrogel, hydrocolloid and saline solution-moistened dressing on the management of pressure ulcers and found no statistical difference in the healing outcomes. A study comparing a hydrocellular dressing to a hydrocolloid dressing in the management of pressure ulcers showed no significant difference between the two dressing groups in terms of ulcer characteristics, such as changes in appearance, reduction in area, mean ulcer odor and pain. The hydrocellular dressing was found, however, to be significantly easier to remove and quicker to change than the hydrocolloid dressing[28]. There are significant differences according to Bale and Hagelstein[29] in the number of healed wounds observed in patients with pressure ulcers treated with a hydrocellular dressing compared to a hydrocolloid dressing. The external application of hydrocellular dressings is also able to reduce any local effect of pressure due to their hydrocellular structure[30]. Motta and co-workers[31] evaluated the clinical performance and cost of use of a new synthetic polymer hydrogel dressing compared to the leading market hydrocolloid dressing in stage II–III pressure ulcers and found a similar overall healing rate for the two groups. However, the new polymer hydrogel dressing showed more effective support of autolytic debridement, better clinical performance and a more favorable cost of use. Hydrocolloid dressings have been also compared with polyurethane foam dressings in stage II–III pressure sore management, showing a similar wear time but a lower absorbency and ease of removal[32].

An economic evaluation of the treatment of pressure ulcers comparing hydroactive wound dressing in combination with enzymatic ointment against gauze dressing showed a significant reduction in cost of use and duration of treatment in the hydroactive dressing group despite the higher material cost[33]. An evaluation of the efficacy and cost-effectiveness of two treatments of grade IV pressure sores on the heel with a collagenase ointment and a hydrocolloid dressing showed the collagenase treatment to be more cost-effective with a shorter time needed for wound healing[34]. Thomas observed no differences in complete healing of stage I–IV pressure ulcers between an amorphous hydrogel derived from aloe vera and a moist saline gauze dressing[35]. Alginate dressings are now widely used in the management of pressure ulcers. They are most indicated for debridement or in exudative wounds. Healing properties of calcium alginate dressing were compared to those of an established local treatment with dextranomer paste in full thickness pressure ulcers. In this prospective, controlled and randomized trial the alginate wound dressing showed a higher healing rate[36]. A new approach in stage III and IV pressure ulcer treatment is the application of radiant heat through a semi-occlusive dressing. Wounds treated with a radiant heat dressing heal significantly faster than wounds that receive only standard care and furthermore have no adverse effects[37]. Hydrofiber dressings have been shown to be effective in moderate to heavily exuding pressure sores. They can lock exudate away, protecting the surrounding skin and producing a moist environment for optimum wound healing[38]. Hydropolymer dressings have shown no statistically significant differences compared with hydrocolloid dressings in the management of pressure sores[39]. Copolymer membranes are easy to use, promote the healing process and are of particular value in the local treatment of grade II, III and IV pressure ulcers[40].

TOPICAL NEGATIVE PRESSURE

The treatment of pressure ulcers is variable and costly. A device that may improve the healing rate, decreasing the length of hospital stay and health-care cost has recently been introduced. Wound management with negative pressure represents a non-invasive mechanical wound care treatment, using negative pressure to facilitate wound healing. VAC® (vacuum-assisted closure) therapy is used to reduce wound fluid, stimulate granulation tissue formation and reduce bacterial colonization[41]. Negative pressure wound therapy acts by localized and controlled negative pressure applied in continuous or intermittent cycles. The equal distribution of negative pressure to every surface of the wound is ensured by a polyurethane open-cell foam dressing. This foam is trimmed to fit the entire surface of the lesion, placed in the wound bed and sealed with an adhesive drape. Negative pressure is applied via an evacuation tube by a computerized and programmable pump. The target pressure for wound therapy varies from 50 mmHg to 200 mmHg, based on the characteristics of the individual wound. In pressure ulcers, a negative pressure of 125 mmHg is used in a continuous cycle of 48 h. Negative pressure therapy provides a moist wound healing environment, assists in uniformly drawing the wound border, enhances epithelial migration, reduces bacterial colonization and reduces localized edema by increasing local blood perfusion and accelerating the rate of granulation tissue formation[42].

The role of topical negative pressure therapy has been investigated in the management of difficult grade III pressure ulcers. A continuous cycle (75–125 mmHg) for the first 48 h followed by intermittent suction (2 min on, 5 min off) was useful in the achievement of complete healing of the wound, obliteration of the wound cavity to allow surface dressings or closure of the wound by suture or skin graft. During therapy, a more rapid healing was observed in acute wounds with a reduction in the number of bacterial colonies[43]. Stage IV pressure ulcers that were refractory to standard medical and surgical therapy for 10 months have been successfully treated with intermittent cycles of negative pressure therapy[44]. Despite the successful treatment of different wound types, some limitations may occur when attempting to treat certain areas of the body with irregular surfaces surrounding the wounds, such as at the perineum[45].

VAC therapy is indicated in acute and traumatic wounds, dehisced incisions, neuropathic ulcers, stage 3 and 4 pressure ulcers, vascular wounds and chronic debilitating wounds. Split-thickness mesh skin grafts also benefit from VAC therapy. Contraindications for negative pressure treatment include cutaneous malignant lesions, untreated osteomyelitis, necrotic tissue within the wound bed and fistula directly communicating with organs and cavities. Caution should be used when there is active bleeding, unstable local hemostasis, use of anticoagulants or distal diabetic foot lesions. The nutritional status of the patient should be stable (albumin level >3 mg/dl), the patient should be continuously monitored by nurses and should be positioned on a support surface so as to redistribute his/her weight over a large area and reduce pressure. An adequate amount of intact periwound skin for adherent dressing should be available and the ulcer should be free of necrotic tissue or osteomyelitis. The dressing is changed every 48 h or every 12 h if infection is present. The wound bed is cleansed per routine, the sponge is placed in the wound and the evacuating tube is laid on the top of the foam linked to a collection chamber located on the pump. An adhesive clear dressing is placed over the foam and the tube. Duration of therapy varies from 4 weeks to 6 weeks with continuous or intermittent cycles of treatment. Continuous therapy facilitates removal of wound fluids and reduction of edema while intermittent therapy acts as a mechanical stretch and results in the repeated release of biochemical messengers. Wound measurement, tissue and fluid characterization, odor and surrounding skin should be monitored at each dressing change. Negative pressure therapy should be used in pressure ulcers to achieve complete healing or to prepare the wound bed for surgical closure, especially in chronic non-healing wounds of considerable depth, rather than the traditional saline wet-to-moist dressings. Vacuum-assisted closure increases the formation of granulation tissue and the healing rate in chronic, non-healing complicated wounds[46,47].

LARVAE

Recently, there has been intense media interest in the use of sterile fly larvae for the treatment of pressure ulcers. The benefit of an accidental infestation of maggots on wounds sustained in battle has been recognized for centuries. In 1829, Baron Dominic Larrey, Napoleon's Surgeon-in-Chief, reported that many soldiers with infected larvae cutaneous wounds did not develop gangrene[48]. The first well-documented account of a deliberate use of maggots was provided by Zacharias, a medical officer during the American Civil War. The wound-cleansing properties of maggots were also noted during the First World War by Baer, an orthopedic surgeon[49,50]. Following the introduction of sulfonamides and penicillin, which had a big impact upon the prevention and treatment of wound infections, the use of maggots rapidly declined until it disappeared. In the late 1980s, the use of maggots was resumed when in the University of California Sherman once again began to use maggot therapy for treating pressure ulcers and other chronic wounds[51,52]. While maggots of many fly species cause human myiasis, *Lucilia sericata*, a member of the Calliphoridae, is the only maggot currently used medically. The enzymes produced by this species only dissolve dead tissue in human wounds and the maggots are therefore unable to burrow or to damage the healthy tissue. The contents of a fly's egg are sterile, although the outer surface is heavily contaminated with bacteria. Sterilizing the outer surface of eggs and allowing these to hatch in a sterile environment produces sterile maggots. Under favorable conditions, the sterile larvae, initially about 1–2 mm long, will grow rapidly over 3–5 days until they reach about 8 mm. After about 7–10 days, the larvae begin the next stage: the formation of a pupae, a protective capsule in which the maggot changes into an adult fly. As this entire process takes a minimum of 2 weeks from the time the maggots are first applied to the wound, there is no possibility that they could turn into flies between dressing changes. Maggots move over the surface of the wound secreting proteolytic enzymes; these break down dead tissue, liquefying it and then they ingest it as a source of nutrient. Maggots also kill or prevent the growth of microorganisms in the wound during feeding[53]. Maggot secretions increase the pH of the wound to about 8–8.5 due to the production of ammonia, which has an inhibitory effect upon the growth of some bacteria[54]. Maggots secrete chemicals with inherent antimicrobial activity and these may also help to combat infection[55]. It has been shown both in laboratory and clinical studies that maggots are able to combat wound infections caused by methicillin-resistant *Staphylococcus aureus* (MRSA). Therefore maggot therapy can be used in the treatment of pressure ulcers[56,57] and many other types of wounds. The technique used involves the removal of previous dressings, especially if hydrogels were used and application of a hydrocolloid dressing in which a hole is cut to the size of the wound. This dressing protects the surrounding skin, stops the unpleasant sensation caused by the larvae moving and forms the base for a second dressing. The number of larvae suggested is about 10 per cm^2 and they are covered by a thin net stuck to the back of the hydrocolloid. It is important to put a moistened swab on the net to prevent the larvae from drying out.

Then an absorbent dressing is applied that permits the larvae to respire and the exudate to be removed. It is not necessary to place an occlusive dressing, because this could limit the oxygen to the larvae. The advantages of maggot therapy are a more rapid debridement and less pain for patients. The disadvantages are principally in relation to compliance of patients. The contraindications to maggot therapy are bleeding, due to the erosion of the walls of the veins by the maggot enzymes; also, they cannot be applied to fistulae or wounds that might connect with vital organs.

HYDROTHERAPY

Hydrotherapy is frequently used in many countries, principally in patients with leg ulcers. The patient is immersed in special hydrotherapy pools which provide cleansing, pressure-irrigation and hydromassage with the use of water. The hydrotherapy sessions are twice-weekly and each application lasts about 30 min. The cleansing is a useful procedure either to remove secretions and bacteria or to soften wound necrotic material[58]. This procedure is generally performed with saline solution only, with antiseptic solution or other types of detergent solutions used according to wound conditions and dressing compatibility. The pressure-irrigation uses the water pressure to remove the necrotic material from the wound surface. The problem is that, if the pressure used to deliver the irrigation solution is too low, below 4 psi, the lavage will not clean effectively, so pressure irrigation has to be in a range from 4 to 15 psi. A simpler method uses a 35 ml syringe with a 19-gauge needle producing an 8 psi pressure action, which is able to clean a wound without causing damage to new granulation tissue. Another method makes use of hydromassage, i.e. water pressure jets generated in a whirlpool. In this case, the tissue becomes soft in the whirlpool and is removed by the pressure of the jets[59]. Therefore the massage produces an edema reduction on the skin, less inflammation and facilitates improved circulation in ischemic legs. A further refinement of this technique consists of immersing the patient for 20–30 min after a 30-s treatment at maximum pressure. The sessions are twice-weekly. This method is indicated in very exudative wounds, necrotic wounds and eschars, but is contraindicated in clean and granulation wounds. Moreover, there are special new devices that can direct a high-pressure water jet onto lesions and then, with suction, remove the devitalized tissue before it dissolves. Among such instruments, one that deserves particular attention is a device developed by a small Swiss factory, based on high-pressure microjet technology. This device consists of a liquid pump driven by compressed air, which generates high hydraulic pressure liquid directed through a nozzle installed in a hand-piece. The diameter of the nozzle is 0.05–0.12 mm and works with a pressure of 200–800 bars. The major advantage of this debridement technique is the reduction of the duration of treatment. The aim was to provoke a decisive healing impulse in a stagnant wound. Through the nozzle, Ringer solution, NaCl or *aqua ad injectabilia* is injected onto the surface of the wound in the form of a very fine jet with exactly controlled pressure. The duration of each intervention depends on the importance and degree of necrosis of the wound and varies from 10 to 30 min, usually at weekly intervals. Advanced dressings sustain the treatment. The three major results of the application are: shortening of the wound healing process, reduction of the scar tissue and low stress effects for the patients because the treatment is relatively painless. These treatments are contraindicated in patients suffering from anticoagulation, contaminated wounds, tumors and unprotected or open blood vessels.

ELECTRICAL STIMULATION AND ELECTROMAGNETIC TREATMENT

Several studies are evaluating the effectiveness of adjuvant therapy in the treatment of pressure ulcers. The aim of these therapies is to assure healing and reduce healing time in managing chronic pressure ulcers. Electrical stimulation and electromagnetic fields as adjuvant therapy to treat pressure ulcers have been in use for many years[60]. The human body has in fact an endogenous bioelectric system that enhances the healing of wounds. This system is able to attract different types of cells involved in autolysis, granulation tissue formation and anti-inflammatory activity. These cells, including neutrophils, macrophages, fibroblasts and epidermal cells, carry either a positive or negative charge and may be influenced by therapeutic levels of electrical current delivered to the wound tissue from an external source. Electrical stimulation may promote galvanotaxic attraction of these elements into the wound tissue, accelerating the healing process[61]. The effects of alternating and direct current stimulation have been studied on experimental pressure ulcers. When compared to controls, both the alternating and direct current techniques revealed a reduction of healing time and an increased tissue perfusion in the early phases of the healing process. The application of electrical stimulation seems therefore to promote new collagen formation[62]. The Agency for Health Care Policy and Research[18] asserted that electrical stimulation may be considered an adjuvant therapy for stage II–IV pressure ulcers.

The four electrical stimulation modalities usually used are low-voltage alternating current (LVAC), low-voltage direct current (LVDC), high-voltage pulsed direct current (PDC) and pulsed electromagnetic energy (PEM)[63,64]. A study by Kloth[65] on stage IV pressure ulcers treated with high-voltage, monophasic pulsed current showed a mean healing rate of 44.8% with 100% healing over a mean period of 8 weeks, compared to an increase in ulcer size of 29% over a period of 7.4 weeks, which occurred in the sham treatment group. Griffin[66] found that stage II–IV pressure ulcers treated for 1 h/day for 20 consecutive days with high-voltage pulsed current showed a significant decrease in wound area compared with a placebo-treated wound group. Low-voltage pulsed microamperage current was investigated in treating the pressure ulcers of six geriatric patients and resulted in five patients healing within 1 month of treatment, which was performed three times per week for 1 h[67]. Gentzkow[68] investigated 40 non-healing stage III–IV pressure ulcers treated with low-voltage pulsed direct current for 4 weeks. At the end of the study period, the treated group showed an average of 49.8% wound-healing area versus 23.4% in the control group. More recently, Wood[69] studied the efficacy of this modality, treating 43 stage II–III pressure ulcers three times per week for 8 weeks; 25 patients were healed by the end of the 8 weeks. In 1995, Salzberg[70] investigated the efficacy of a pulsed electromagnetic energy in healing stage II–III pressure ulcers and found that the treatment significantly reduced complete healing time with statistically and medically significant advantages for the group treated with PEM. Baker[71] studied the effect of four stimulation protocols on a total of 185 pressure ulcers in patients with spinal cord injury, who received 30 min of daily stimulation with one of the four treatments: asymmetric biphasic waveform, symmetric biphasic waveform, microcurrent stimulation or a sham treatment. The study showed significantly better healing rates in the asymmetric biphasic waveform group, whereas the symmetric one did not differ from the other groups. There are encouraging data on the effectiveness of these adjuvant therapies in relation to wound healing but all the studies suggest that different healing rates are produced with various electrotherapy modalities; therefore further controlled clinical trials are necessary to establish the optimal parameters for electrical stimulation based on specific population, body location, stage and etiology of pressure ulcers, in order to obtain approval by the Food and Drug Administration.

CONCLUSIONS

Important advances have taken place in the world of pressure ulcer treatment during the past decade. These advances are reflected in the high rate of cures being obtained. This, together with the implementation of prevention guidelines, the excellent cost-effectiveness relationship of the techniques described and other factors, means that the field of pressure ulcer management is no more an isolated and self-administered issue in medical practice. The areas discussed above are those in which there will be linear or, in some cases, exponential growth in the decades to come.

References

1. European Pressure Ulcer Advisory Panel (EPUAP). Pressure Ulcer Treatment Guidelines, 1989
2. Thomas DR. Improving outcome of pressure ulcers with nutritional interventions: a review of evidence. *Nutrition* 2001;17:121–5
3. Demling RH. Involuntary weight loss, protein-energy malnutrition, and impairment of cutaneous wound healing. *Wounds* 2001;13 (Suppl D):3D–21D
4. Anthony D, Reynolds T, Russell L. An investigation into the use of serum albumin in

pressure sore prediction. *J Adv Nurs* 2000;32: 359–65

5. Henderson CT. Safe and effective tube feeding of bedridden elderly. *Geriatrics* 1991;46:56–61

6. Lewis B. Zinc and vitamin C in the aetiology of pressure sores. *J Wound Care* 1996;5:83–4

7. Thomas DR. The role of nutrition in prevention and healing of pressure ulcers. *Clin Geriatr Med* 1997;13:497–511

8. Himes D. Nutritional supplements in the treatment of pressure ulcers: practical perspectives. *Adv Wound Care* 1997;10:30–1

9. Strauss EA. Margolis DJ. Malnutrition in patients with pressure ulcers: morbidity, mortality, and clinically practical assessments. *Adv Wound Care* 1996;9:37–40

10. Rothe M, Falanga V. Growth factors. *Arch Dermatol* 1989;125:1390–8

11. Pierce GF, Tarpley JE, Allman RM, *et al*. Tissue repair processes in healing chronic pressure ulcers treated with recombinant platelet-derived growth factor BB. *Am J Pathol* 1994; 145:1399–410

12. Mustoe TA,Cutler NR,Allman RM, *et al*. A phase II study to evaluate recombinant platelet derived growth factor-BB in the treatment of stage 3–4 pressure ulcers. *Arch Surg* 1994;129: 213–19

13. El Saghir NS, Bizri AR, Shabb NS, *et al*. Pressure ulcer accelerated healing with local injections of granulocyte macrophage-colony stimulating factor. *J Infect* 1997;35:179–82

14. Hirshberg J., Coleman J., Marchant B. TGF-β3 in the treatment of pressure ulcers: a preliminary report. *Adv Wound Care* 2001;29:68–73

15. Kallianinen LK, Hirshberg J, Marchant B, Rees RS. Role of platelet-derived growth factor as an adjunct to surgery in the management of pressure ulcers. *Plast Reconstr Surg* 2000;106:1243–8

16. Margolis DJ, Lewis VL. A literature of the use of miscellaneous topical agents, growth factors, and skin equivalents for treatment of pressure ulcers. *Dermatol Surg* 1995;21:145–8

17. Kunimoto BT. Growth factors in wound healing: the next great innovation? *Ostomy Wound Manag* 1999;45:56–64

18. Bergstrom N, Bennet MA, Carlson CE, *et al*. Treatment of pressure ulcers. *Clinical Practice Guideline No. 15*, PHS, AHCPR Pub. No. 95-0652, Rockville, MD, 1994

19. Winter GD. Formation of the scab and the rate of epithelialization of superficial wounds in the skin of the young domestic pig. *Nature* 1962; 193:293–4

20. Hinnman CD, Maibach HI. Effect of air exposure and occlusion on experimental human skin wounds. *Nature* 1963;200:377–8

21. Xakellis GC, Chrischilles EA. Hydrocolloid versus saline gauze dressing in treating pressure ulcers: a cost–effectiveness analysis. *Arch Phys Med Rehab* 1992;73:463–9

22. Kim YC, Shin JC, Park CI, Oh SH, Choi SM, Kim YS. Efficacy of hydrocolloid occlusive dressing technique in decubitus ulcer treatment: a comparative study. *Yonsei Med J* 1996; 37:181–5

23. Mulder G, Kissil M, Mahr JJ. Bacterial growth under occlusive and non-occlusive dressings. *Wounds* 1993;5:295–6

24. Field CK, Kerstein MD. Overview of wound healing in a moist environment. *Am J Surg* 1994;167:2S–6S

25. Yarkony GM, Kramer E. Pressure sore management: efficacy of a moisture reactive occlusive dressing. *Arch Phys Med Rehabil* 1994;65: 597–600

26. Gorse GJ, Messner RL. Improved pressure sore healing with hydrocolloid dressing. *Arch Dermatol* 1987;123:766–71

27. Mulder GD, Altman M, Seeley JE, Tintle T. Prospective randomised study of the efficacy of hydrogel, hydrocolloid and saline-solution-moistened dressing on the management of pressure ulcers. *Wound Repair Regen* 1993;1: 213–18

28. Seeley J, Jeffrey LJ, Hutcherson J. A randomised clinical study comparing a hydrocellular dressing to a hydrocolloid dressing in the management of pressure ulcers. *Ostomy Wound Manag* 1999;45:39–47

29. Bale S, Hagelstein S, Banks V, Harding KG. Costs of dressings in the community. *J Wound Care* 1998;7:327–30

30. Torra I, Bou JE, Rueda Lopez J, Ramon Canton C. Experimental study. Reduction of pressure in areas of risk of developing pressure ulcers with a hydrocellular dressing. *Rev Enferm* 2000; 23:211–18

31. Motta G, Dunham L, Dye T, Mentz J, O'Connel-Gifford E, Smith E. Clinical efficacy

and cost-effectiveness of a new synthetic polymer sheet wound dressing. *Ostomy Wound Manag* 1999;45:41,44–6,48–9

32. Bale S, Squires D, Varnon T, Walker A, Benbow M, Harding KG. A comparison of two dressings in pressure sore management. *J Wound Care* 1997;6:463–6

33. Bergemann R, Lauterbach KW, Vanscheidt W, Neander KD, Engst R. Economic evaluation of the treatment of chronic wounds: hydroactive wound dressing in combination with enzymatic ointment versus gauze dressings in patients with pressure ulcers and venous leg ulcer in Germany. *Pharmacoeconomics* 1999;4:367–7

34. Muller E, van Leen MW, Bergemann R. Economic evaluation of collagenase-containing ointment and hydrocolloid dressing in the treatment of pressure ulcers. *Pharmacoeconomics* 2001;19:1209–16

35. Thomas DR, Goode PS, Lamaster K, Tennyson T. Acemannan hydrogel dressing versus saline dressing for pressure ulcers. A randomised, controlled trial. *Adv Wound Care* 1998;11:273–6

36. Sayag J, Meaume S, Bohbot S. Healing properties of calcium alginate dressing. *J Wound Care* 1996;5:357–62

37. Kloth LC, Berman JE, Dumit-Minkel S, Sutton CH, Papanek PE, Wurzel J. Effects of a normothermic dressing on pressure ulcer healing. *Adv Skin Wound Care* 2000;13:69–74

38. Williams C. An investigation of the benefits of Aquacel Hydrofibre wound dressing. *Br J Nurs* 1999;8:676–7, 680

39. Thomas S, Banks V, Bale S, *et al*. A comparison of two dressings in the management of chronic wounds. *J Wound Care* 1997;6:383–6

40. Honde C, Derks C, Tudor D. Local treatment of pressure sores in the elderly: amino acid copolymer membrane versus hydrocolloid dressing. *J Am Geriatr Soc* 1994;42:1180–3

41. Argenta LC, Morykwas MJ. Vacuum-assisted closure: a new method for wound control and treatment: clinical experience. *Ann Plast Surg* 1997;38:563–76

42. Morykwas MJ, Argenta LC, Shelton-Brown EI, McGuirt W. Vacuum-assisted closure: a new method for wound control and treatment: animal studies and basic foundation. *Ann Plast Surg* 1997;38:553–62

43. Deva AK, Buckland GH, Fisher E, *et al*. Topical negative pressure in wound management. *Med J Aust* 2000;173:128–31

44. Baynham SA, Kohlman P, Katner HP. Treating stage IV pressure ulcers with negative pressure therapy: a case report. *Ostomy Wound Manag* 1999;45:28–32,34–5

45. Greer SE, Duthie E, Cartolano B, Koehler KM, Maydick–Youngberg D, Longaker MT. Techniques for applying subatmospheric pressure to wounds in difficult regions of anatomy. *J Wound Ost Contin Nurs* 1999;26:250–3

46. Evans D, Land L. Topical negative pressure for treating chronic wounds: a systematic review. *Br J Plast Surg* 2001;54:238–42

47. Joseph E, Hamori CA, Bergman S, Roaf E, Swann NF, Anastasi GW. A prospective randomized trial of vacuum-assisted closure versus standard therapy of chronic non healing wounds. *Wounds* 2000;12:60–7

48. Larrey DJ. Observations on wounds and their complications by erysipelas, gangrene and tetanus, *Clinique Chir* 1829;51–52: translated from the French by EF Rivinus. Des vers ou larves de la mouche bleue, Chez Gabon, Paris. Philadelphia: Key, Mielke and Biddle, 1832

49. Baer WS. The use of viable antiseptic in the treatment of osteomyelitis. *South Med J* 1929

50. Baer WS. Treatment and cure of the disease known as osteomyelitis. *Hearings before the Committee on World War Veterans' Legislation, House of Representatives, Seventy-first Congress, Second Session,* April 17, 1930, Washington, US Gov't Printing Office, 1930

51. Sherman RS, Pechter EA. Maggot therapy: a review of therapeutic application of fly larvae in human medicine, especially for treating osteomyelitis. *Med Vet Entomol* 1988;2:225–30

52. Sherman RA, Wyle F, Vulpe M, Levsen L, Castillo L. The utility of maggot therapy for treating pressure sore. *J Am Parapleg Soc* 1993;16:269–70

53. Robinson W, Norwood VH. The role of surgical maggots in the disinfection of osteomyelitis and other infected wounds. *J Bone Joint Surg* 1933;15:409–12

54. Messer FC, McClellan RH. Surgical maggots. A study of their functions in wound healing. *J Lab Clin Med* 1935;20:1219

55. Pavillard ER, Wright EA. An antibiotic from maggots. *Nature* 1957;180:916–17

56. Sherman RA, Wyle F, Vulpe M. Maggot therapy for treating pressure ulcers in spinal cord injury patients. *J Spinal Cord Med* 1995;18:71–4

57. Thomas S, Jones M, Shutler S, Andrews A. Wound care. All you need to know about maggots. *Nursing Times* 1996;92:63–6,68,70

58. Ho C, Burke DT, Kim HJ. Healing with hydrotherapy. *Adv Directors Rehabil* 1998;7:45–9

59. Waspe J. Treating leg ulcers with high pressure irrigation devices. *Nursing Stand* 1996;11:53–4

60. Gentzkow GD. Electrical stimulation to heel dermal wounds. *J Dermatol Surg Onc* 1993;19:753–8

61. Kloth LC, McCulloch JM. Promotion of wound healing with electrical stimulation. *Adv Wound Care* 1996;9:42–5

62. Reger SI, Hyodo A, Negami S, Kambic He, Sahgal V. Experimental wound healing with electrical stimulation. *Artif Organs* 1999;23:460–2

63. Vodovnik L, Karba R. Treatment of chronic wounds by means of electric and electromagnetic fields. Part I. Literature review. *Med Biol Eng Comput* 1991;30:257–66

64. Frantz RA. Adjuvant therapy for ulcer care. *Clin Geriatr Med* 1997;13:553–64

65. Kloth L, Feedar J. Acceleration of wound healing with high-voltage, monophasic, pulsed current. *Phys Ther* 1988;68:503–8

66. Griffin JW, Tooms RE, Mendium RA, Clifft Jk, Vander Swaay R, El-Zeky F. Efficacy of high-voltage pulsed current for healing of pressure ulcers in patients with spinal cord injury. *Phys Ther* 1991;71:433–44

67. Barron J, Jacobson W, Tidd G. Treatment of decubitus ulcers: a new approach. *Minn Med* 1985;68:103

68. Gentzkow GD, Pollack SV, Kloth LC, Stubb HA. Improved healing of pressure ulcers using dermapulse, a new electrical stimulation device. *Wounds* 1991;31:158–70

69. Wood JM, Evans PE, Schalbreuter KU, et al. A multicenter study on the use of pulsed low-intensity direct current for healing chronic stage II and III decubitus ulcers. *Arch Dermatol* 1993;129:999–1009

70. Salzberg CA, Cooper-Vastola SA, Perez FJ, Vrehbeck MG, Byrne DW. The effects of non-thermal pulsed electromagnetic energy (Diapulse®) on wound healing of pressure ulcers in spinal cord-injured patients: a randomized, double-blind study. *Wounds* 1995;7:11–16

71. Baker LL, Rubayi S, Villar F, Demuth SK. Effect of electrical stimulation waveform on healing of ulcers in human beings with spinal cord injury. *Wound Repair Regen* 1996;4:21–8

Mucosal inflammation of the gastrointestinal tract and healing

10

V. Mani

INTRODUCTION

The gastrointestinal tract is lined with mucous membrane from the mouth to the rectum. This protective epithelium varies at different levels according to the functional needs of the organ. Injury to the mucosal lining leads to inflammation, its severity being the determining factor in the production of an ulcer. The factors that determine the size and depth of the ulcer are elements from the lumen and wall of the gut. The major etiologic factors are infection, idiopathic inflammation and neoplasms. Neoplastic and malignant ulcers are chronic ulcers and are not considered in this chapter.

THE NORMAL GUT

The healthy normal gut contains an abundance of inflammatory cells. These are lymphocytes in the epithelial cell layer and lymphocytes, plasma cells and macrophages in the lamina propria. These cells colonize the gut layers in response to a variety of antigens in the lumen, ranging from bacteria to drug and dietary toxins. This has been described as the normal gut in a state of 'physiologic inflammation'. An exaggeration of the inflammatory response results in ulcer formation. This chapter describes examples of the different types of ulcers in the various parts of the gastrointestinal tract.

THE BARRIERS OF THE UPPER GASTROINTESTINAL TRACT AND PATHOGENESIS OF INJURY

The primary defect in the acid-related diseases of the upper gastrointestinal tract, namely gastro-esophageal reflux disease (GERD), gastric and duodenal ulcers, is a defect in the mucosal barrier. This can be either primary or acquired. Malfunction of the lower esophageal sphincter (LES) leads to acid reflux into the esophagus, and the resultant degree of inflammation depends on the volume of the refluxate and the length of exposure. The epithelium of the esophagus is stratified squamous and multi-layered, and is enriched with afferent nerves. When the LES is incompetent, acid reflux causes pain and damage to the epithelium. The tight junctions between the epithelial cells have been demonstrated to be leaky which, in GERD, enables acid penetration leading to pain, damage or both. The intensity of pain bears no direct relationship to the volume of acid refluxed. The same tight junctions (leaky) of the epithelial cells of the LES then allow back-diffusion of the acid. When this happens, the esophageal epithelial secretions, such as mucus and bicarbonate, incompletely neutralize the acid–pepsin fluid. This leads to inflammation and ulcer formation. It has been shown that the average net reflux of bicarbonate is about 78 nmol/30 min/1 cm of human esophagus, regulated by muscarinic receptors. The bicarbonate secretion is incapable of neutralizing the refluxed fluid with a pH below 4, and at pH 2 deeper epithelial layers get acidified. As more superficial layers become eroded, pepsin back-diffusion worsens the damage, leading to ulcer formation. The principles of treatment or healing are by improving the epithelial cell response, the structure of the LES and by acid inhibition to render a pH above 4.

GASTRIC AND DUODENAL MUCOSA AND CYTOPROTECTION

The most relevant factor that prevents auto-digestion of the stomach epithelium is the mucus–bicarbonate barrier. Epithelial cells secrete mucus which forms a thin layer over the surface and forms a part of the gastric barrier that prevents acid back-diffusion and consequent epithelial injury. The bicarbonate (HCO_3^-) secretion occurs both actively and passively. The next important cytoprotective agent is prostaglandin E_2, which is biosynthesized in the gastric epithelial cells. A defect in either of the above leads to mucosal attack by the aggressive agents, acid and pepsin, contributing to ulcer formation. The third and major aggressive factor in ulcerogenesis is the microbe *Helicobacter pylori*, found in association with both gastric and duodenal ulcer disease. The pathogenic variety of *H. pylori* colonizes the antrum of the stomach, initiating a series of biopathogenic mechanisms responsible for ulcer formation.

Healing

The process of healing begins following ulcerogenesis with eventual restitution. The surface cells migrate to the erosive area, secrete mucus and this is followed by renewal of epithelial cells. The major factors that influence healing include prostaglandins, nitrous oxide and histamine, as well as increased mucosal vasculature and blood supply.

In the duodenum, the luminal surface is lined by villous epithelium, a monolayer of cells with brush borders. The cells in the deeper aspect of the epithelium are the dynamic crypt cells, which constantly keep migrating to the tip to replace the damaged cells. The duodenal cells also secrete bicarbonate like the gastric cells. It has been clearly shown that duodenal bicarbonate secretion decreases in duodenal ulceration.

Both gastric and duodenal ulcers occur as a result of disruption and/or malfunction of any of the above-mentioned mucosal barriers. The healing depends upon the ability of the epithelial cells to repair the damage. Under normal physiologic circumstances, a fine balance is maintained between cell loss and cell building or replication. In pathologic states, increased cell loss (apoptosis) will result in atrophy and a disproportionately increased cell production causes hypertrophy. Several trophic factors act in the mechanism of cell building and repair over and around the injured mucosa. The main trophic factors are gastrin, epidermal growth factor (EGF), tissue growth factor (TGF), cytokines and trefoil peptides.

Following the formation of an ulcer, the main healing events that occur are as follows:

(1) Rapid phase of epithelial restitution when the viable cells surrounding the ulcer migrate inward to close the wound.

(2) Proliferation and new cell formation in the area of the ulcer.

(3) Finally laying down of the matrix where the inflammatory cells are replaced by non-epithelial cells in the lamina propria.

This repair process is ably supported by concomitant increase in the mucosal vasculature and blood supply with the help of growth factors.

Role of *Helicobacter pylori*

The documented evidence for the presence of microbes in the gastric mucosa dates back to the 19th century. However, it was Robin Warren and Barry Marshall who cultured *H. pylori* in the gastric mucosal biopsies and published their results in *The Lancet* in 1983. Following their discovery and several years of painstaking research it is now well established that *H. pylori* is the causative organism in both gastric and duodenal ulcer diseases in well over 90% of the population. These pathogens colonize the acidic stomach and elaborate an enzyme, urease. The gastric acidity activates urea transport and urease activity in the organism. Eradication of *H. pylori* by acid suppressants (proton pump inhibitors) combined with antibiotics heal a very high proportion of ulcers. Consequently peptic ulcer disease is now on the decline.

THE MUCOSA OF THE SMALL INTESTINE AND COLON

The major factors responsible for the production of mucosal inflammation in the small and large bowels are: (1) Interphase between luminal contents (antigens) and (2) the permeability of the epithelium to the antigens. An increase in the mucosal permeability for whatever reason will allow entry of the luminal fluid with increased antigenic concentration. This sets off an inflammatory reaction, the severity depending upon antigenic concentration in the permeated fluid as well as the permeability of the epithelium. The pathogenesis of this inflammatory process has two components, cellular and humoral. This has been extensively studied in Crohn's disease, which is a chronic inflammatory condition of the gastrointestinal tract, mostly involving the small intestine and the colon. Cell-mediated changes that occur have been shown to be the major events. The plasma cells, T-cell macrophages and polymorphonuclear (PMN) cells increase in number in the mucous membrane. All these cells release pro-inflammatory molecules which surround the area of inflammation, leading to damage and ulceration. The concentration of these pro-inflammatory molecules determines the severity of the damage. An increase in B-cells (which release immunoglobulins IgG and IgM) has also been noted in the area of inflammation, suggesting their pro-inflammatory effect.

Macrophages

The number of macrophages both in the general circulation and at the site of insult increases as a part of the acute inflammatory process. In Crohn's disease, activated macrophages are found grouped together to form granulomas which are pathognomonic of Crohn's ulcers. Similar lesions have also been identified in the blood vessels around the lesions, causing vasculitis, a predominant lesion in the disease process.

Polymorphonuclear cells

As with any acute inflammatory process, PMN cell population increases in gut injury. Adhesion molecules on the vascular endothelium become up-regulated, attracting PMN cells which then transmigrate through the vascular epithelium to the interstitial space. Several chemo-attractants like bacterial peptides and inflammatory mediators enhance this process.

The populations of eosinophils and mast cells also increase, releasing inflammatory mediators such as platelet-activating factor (PAF).

ROLE OF EICOSANOIDS

Eicosanoids are specific mediators and are the products of arachidonic acid metabolism. These leukotrienes, notably LTB$_4$ and other activated products, become involved in a range of inflammatory activities such as increasing vascular permeability and gut motility, as well as affecting cytokines and other cells. These pro-inflammatory activators also cause some suppression of synthesis and circulation of anti-inflammatory substances, like prostaglandins, thus enhancing inflammation at the site of injury. Other notable specific mediators include activated oxygen radicals, proteolytic enzymes and complement.

CYTOKINES

Cytokines are synthesized and secreted by T-lymphocytes, monocytes, granulocytes, intestinal macrophages, fibroblasts, epithelial and endothelial cells. They are secreted in response to antigenic stimulation and play a key role in the inflammatory cascade. Several of them induce, exaggerate and help the process of inflammation. Many of them, however, act antagonistically and help the healing process. In a normal healthy state, a balance exists between the inflammatory and healer cytokines and a tip in their balance determines the nature and severity of inflammation. The two groups of the various important cytokines are as listed in Table 1.

Table 1 The two groups of the cytokines important in wound repair

Pro-inflammatory cytokines
IL-1; IL-6; IL-8; IL-12; TNF-α
Anti-inflammatory cytokines
IL-1ra; IL-4; IL-10; IL-11; TGF-β

REPAIR

The general principles of the repair process have been well alluded to in the description of Crohn's disease. The major components involved in intestinal mucosal healing are restitution and regeneration of the epithelium, followed by fibrosis, which results in thickening of the submucosal layer(s). The cytokines that are involved act as growth factors by enhancing cell proliferation, neovascularization and deposition of new matrix. The important growth factors in the process are transforming growth factor β (TGF-β), keratinocyte growth factor (KGF) and epithelial growth factors such as trefoil peptides and TGF-α.

CLASSIFICATION

The gastrointestinal ulcers are best classified according to their etiology as: infective, inflammatory, neoplastic and iatrogenic ulcers.

Infective ulcers

The infective agents, as with any infection, are viral, bacterial, fungal and others. Infestations with parasites are also included under this heading. Viral infections are always acute but, rarely, recurrent infections can occur in immunosuppressed patients. Infection with herpes virus is the most common and can occur in any part of the gastrointestinal tract. Healing occurs quickly with early diagnosis and specific antiviral agents. Bacterial infections can be either acute or chronic. *Salmonella* and *Shigella* infections are frequent. Food poisoning salmonellae are the most common and severe infection can cause ulceration of the colon. Typhoid fever is due to *Salmonella* infection where there is small intestinal ulceration. Early diagnosis and specific antibiotic therapy are essential, as delay may lead to complications like hemorrhage and perforation of the ulcers and carry a high mortality rate. The chronic ulcers due to bacterial infections of the gastrointestinal tract are peptic ulcer disease and intestinal tuberculosis. The organism *Helicobacter pylori* as described above has been proven to be the major factor in the causation of both duodenal and gastric ulcers. Once the diagnosis is made, a cure can be offered by what is commonly known as 'triple therapy' with two antibiotics and an acid suppressant, i.e. a proton pump inhibitor for 1 week. The other chronic infective ulcer is due to infection with *Mycobacterium tuberculosis*, which most commonly affects the terminal ileum but can also affect the colon, stomach and esophagus. Diagnosis can sometimes be difficult and delay in diagnosis leads to complications and death in an untreated patient. Triple or quadruple therapy for a prolonged period results in complete healing of the ulcer. Parasitic infestations of the gastrointestinal tract can also result in acute or chronic ulcers. The notable example of this is infestation with *Entamoeba histolytica*, acquired by the oral route. The large bowel is most commonly affected resulting in severe bloody diarrhea and severe morbidity. Stool microscopy identifies the organism. Eradication and complete cure occur following therapy.

Inflammatory ulcers

Most of the ulcers in this category are chronic recurrent ulcers where the etiology is unknown. The gastrointestinal tract is often affected in autoimmune disorders. These are seen in systemic lupus, Behçet's disease and various other conditions. Treatment with corticosteroids and immunosuppressive agents helps to heal the ulcers does not prevent recurrence. Inflammatory bowel disease, which includes Crohn's disease and ulcerative colitis, causes ulceration of the entire gastrointestinal tract. Ulcerative colitis causes ulceration of the colon, which very often starts as acute ulcers which generally heal with appropriate therapy. The condition characteristically waxes and wanes despite therapy, leading to chronicity. Crohn's disease, on the other hand, can affect any part of the digestive tract. Pathologically the ulcers in ulcerative colitis are superficial involving the mucous membrane only, whereas the Crohn's ulcers involve the entire thickness of the bowel wall. The healing process in both conditions leads to fibrosis in due course, causing narrowing of the bowel lumen and resulting in strictures, necessitating surgery. In both diseases, surgery may result in bowel exteriorization and stoma formation. Therapy for inflammatory bowel disease has advanced in the last decade to include immune modulation therapy, besides corticosteroids and immunosuppressive agents. Total healing of the ulcers and fistulae complicating the disease occurs following immune modulatory therapy with anti-TNF-α antibodies in Crohn's disease.

Neoplastic ulcers of the digestive tract

These carcinomas and lymphomas are chronic and malignant. Prognosis depends on the etiology, but is generally poor.

Iatrogenic ulcers

Several of the orally administered drugs cause gastrointestinal ulceration. The most common and well-studied drugs are non-steroidal anti-inflammatory drugs (NSAIDs). These drugs cause peptic ulceration and account for most of the ulcer incidence in the absence of the organism, *H. pylori*. The drugs cause ulceration by inhibiting prostaglandin synthesis in the gastric and duodenal mucosa. Complete healing occurs following withdrawal of the causative drug and treatment with an anti-ulcer agent. Other notable drugs that cause gastrointestinal ulceration are potassium supplement in the form of slow-K tablets, especially affecting the ileum. Anti-malarial tablets, as well as many of the cytotoxic agents given orally, occasionally cause ulcers. Healing of these ulcers occurs when the drugs are withdrawn.

Following bowel resection for inflammatory bowel disease, the small bowel or the colon is exteriorized at the anterior abdominal wall. Great care needs to be involved in the management of stoma. Crohn's ulcer can develop on the stomal surface and management is similar to that of the disease elsewhere. In addition, surgical re-fashioning and re-siting on the abdominal wall may be required if stomal stenosis develops. Mucocutaneous fistulae are known associated lesions of Crohn's disease and ulcerative colitis. These wounds should be managed just as the intestinal disease and occasionally surgical intervention may be required.

CONCLUSION

The introduction of fiberoptic endoscopy over 25 years ago has revolutionized the understanding of the pathogenesis and the healing process of gastrointestinal ulcers. Since the early 1970s, endoscopic healing has been accepted as the clinical end-point in all placebo-controlled clinical trials in peptic ulcer disease. It has been possible to take biopsies at various stages of healing and study the healing process histologically. Discovery of the organism *H. pylori* and further studies of this microbe in the causation of peptic ulcer, followed by eradication therapy, have helped to cure a chronic disease which has plagued mankind for several centuries. Colonoscopy has contributed enormously in studying the behavior pattern and response to therapy of various mucosal wounds and has helped to classify them. This has led to proper classification of the various ulcers. Advances and improved understanding of the various immunologic mechanisms involved in the healing of mucosal wounds have led to the development of immune modulatory drugs which have been shown to be effective in healing the resistant Crohn's ulcer. Currently, a considerable amount of research is being directed at attempting to identify the luminal antigens in the gut which are accepted as being, at least in part, responsible for the causation of the mucosal wounds in chronic idiopathic inflammatory diseases. This is a particularly hopeful prospect.

Bibliography

Modlin IM, Sachs G. *Acid Related Diseases, Biology and Treatment*. Konstanz: Schnetztor-Verlag, 1998

Allan RN, Keighley MRB, eds. Crohn's disease. *Baillière's Clin Gastroenterol* 1998;12:1

From the wound healing laboratory: any evidence for change?

11

R. Mani

INTRODUCTION

Laboratory tests are mainly used to ascertain diagnostic data, though, where relevant, such tests may also be used to assess the efficacy of therapeutic interventions. In wound management, tests to determine changes in the structure and function of the vascular system have gained acceptance and are used widely[1]. For example, the ankle brachial pressure index (ABPI) is used widely to screen patients for peripheral vascular disease and lower extremity wounds. Duplex ultrasound is commonly used to assess deep venous function. However, this caters for only part of the problem, as chronic leg wounds are often slow to heal and recur frequently. Edema, infection and pain are common complications of leg ulcers. Can laboratory tests help in understanding and therefore managing these complications? Do objective tests help with the management of burns? As this book is focused on the evidence for change, this chapter addresses advances in measurement technologies, as well as clinical data, using laboratory tests that could influence wound management. Biochemistry laboratory tests are excluded from this chapter except with reference to wound fluid measurements that are under development.

In seeking to provide common denominators for all chronic wounds, this chapter is presented from the viewpoints of vascular measurements, measurements in the wound milieu and measurements of complications.

ADVANCES IN MEASUREMENT TECHNOLOGIES

At the time of writing, the use of laser Doppler imaging for measuring perfusion in burn wounds[2], the potential of laser imaging to measure oxygen saturation[3] and surface pH measurements[4] all appear to be outstanding. Transcutaneous measurements of tissue oxygen are reliable and recommended to predict tissue viability in diabetic patients with peripheral arterial disease[5].

Optical imaging

Optical imaging to measure dermal perfusion using a laser Doppler scanning system (LDI) offers immense benefits to manage burns that need surgical debridement. This is also discussed in Chapter 7 which is devoted exclusively to burn wound management. LDI is a development of the laser Doppler flowmeter that measures changes in blood flow in dermal vascular bed. The principle of laser Doppler imaging, shown in Figure 11.1, is simple. A low-powered helium–neon laser is used to generate a low-powered beam that is guided by high-resolution plastic or glass fibers and focused using a lens on a spherical mirror. The mirror is rotated through its optical axis using a stepper motor system, permitting the wound bed to be scanned in raster fashion. The back-scattered radiation is detected by semiconductor devices and processed electronically to generate maps of tissue perfusion, as illustrated in Figure 11.2, which shows tissue perfusion over an ankle burn. It is a non-contact technique, a major advantage. As the method uses infrared transducers, LDI may be used on wards in ambient light conditions.

Pape[2] compared LDI estimates of burn depth with clinical assessment and histology. In 43 patients with burns, LDI imaging showed predominantly high perfusion (41/43, 95%) of those healed with no complications. By comparison, clinical assessment over-estimated burn depth damage in (13/43, 30%). In another group, 25 burns showed low perfusion on LDI imaging, consistent with deep damage. Histology of the wounds was 100% correlated with LDI but less so with clinical assessment (21/25, 84%). This evidence is impressive in recommending the use of LDI for objective assessment of burn depth.

Necrotic or infected tissue will impede the transmission of laser light, as will edema, since black, green/yellow colors act as optical filters; this limits the value of the technique. There is a degree of operator skill to be acquired in order to derive good data.

Oxygen saturation

An optical method of estimating oxygen saturation (OS) has been used with some success in animal studies of burn wounds[3]. This system works on the principle that absorption and scattering of light in tissues are wavelength dependent, 633 nm and 805 nm being critical ones. At these wavelengths, the radiation reflected/backscattered is dependent on both the color and the volume of tissue, or the volume alone. The absorption/reflection of light is characterized by Beer's law of exponential decay,

$$I_t = I_o\, e^{-\mu x}$$

where I_t and I_o are the intensities of the transmitted and incident light beams, μ the coefficient of absorption/reflection and x the distance travelled by the beam or the thickness of the sample of tissue irradiated. This model, elegant in its simplicity, is applicable when the slab of tissue under test (ear lobe, finger, or toe) is interposed between the transmitter and detector. In principle, such devices emit beams of either white light or green and near infrared and detect the reflected or backscattered radiation from which the OS of a sample volume of tissue may be computed using the above equation. Devices attempting to measure OS in reflected radiation are disadvantaged compared to those detecting transmitted fractions because the latter work on small volumes to which Beer's law is applicable. However, unless transformed, Beer's law is inapplicable because of multiple scattering. A limitation of devices that work on detecting reflected light is that the multiple scattering which an optical beam undergoes makes Beer's law inapplicable in a simple form. Calculations of OS are complicated and take into account the distances between emitters (source) and detectors[6].

The application of oximetry to study wound healing is recent. In a pig model, Sowa used laser optical imaging to study wound pathology in incision wounds and showed some changes in the images at different stages of wound healing. The method needs development and validation, but has immense potential. Increasing the intensity of incident radiation, best achieved using high-powered laser light, would help to radiate deep dermal tissues. Like LDI, these probes could not interrogate eschar or necrotic wound tissue.

Assessment in diabetic patients

Peripheral arterial disease (PAD) is a manifestation of atherosclerosis with an estimated prevalence of 16.9% in men and 20.5% in women over 55 years of age[7]. PAD is a significant risk factor for diabetic foot disease that leads to critical limb ischemia, limb loss and lower limb ulceration in a significant number of patients[8]. Impaired circulation or excess plantar pressures leading to callus may cause diabetic foot ulcers. In some, ischemia and neuropathy may be present concomitantly. In all patients, it is important to investigate the macro- and the microcirculation.

Macrovascular disease is easily identified by Duplex ultrasound using imaging and spectral frequency analysis, and arteriography. Magnetic resonance imaging is most useful, though its availability is limited to certain centers. In order to manage diabetic foot disease, accurate microvascular assessments are essential, the objective being to determine tissue viability. Most attempts to assess viability are based on transducing skin perfusion, with the exception of video microscopy in which the capillaries are visualized. A summary of these methods is presented in Table 1.

MICROVASCULAR MEASUREMENTS

Direct visualization is an elegant way of studying capillaries, a technique that was frequently described through the 1980s. Tooke[12] measured capillary flow velocity and used the technique to study diabetic foot disease. The technique is not widely used despite its initial promise, possibly because tissue viability is dependent on having patent functional capillaries. In conditions where tissue is ischemic because of peripheral vascular disease or systemic sclerosis, capillaries become resorbed. Microscopy techniques are therefore of limited value. Epidermal thickness and hyperpigmentation also limit this application.

Radioisotope imaging may be used to assess tissue viability; this requires relevant technical skills and nuclear medicine laboratory facilities. The repeatability of such tests is dependent on the radio-isotope having a reasonably short half-life; iodine-125 (using 4-iodo-antipyrine) is a good example. The latter isotope has additional advantages: it clings less to fat molecules and clears in a way that may be accurately modeled using a mono-exponential curve. For these and other reasons, including its ease of use and non-invasiveness, the transcutaneous oxygen sensor is well recommended for measuring tissue viability in diabetics.

The $TcPO_2$ sensor (Figure 11.3) was developed as a non-invasive measure of arterial oxygen in neonates, in whom it correlated well with independent measurements of arterial oxygen from in-dwelling catheters. The sensor is an electrochemical cell with the difference that the cathode is negatively biased with respect to the anode. The electrolyte is an aqueous solution of potassium hydroxide. A gold cathode is used in some models. The sensor has a heater ring that is concentric to the electrode assembly. Oxygen atoms diffusing through skin react with water molecules to generate hydrogen peroxide and free electrons in a continuous process. In correct conditions of biasing, the partial pressure of oxygen diffusing out of skin is linearly proportional to the current generated. $TcPO_2$ machines produce readouts in units of pressure mmHg or kPa. The system is calibrated in air.

Table 1 Various methods useful for measuring tissue viability in patients with ischemia and ulceration of the limbs

Measurement parameter	Method of transduction of signals	Comments
Toe systolic pressure	Strain gauge plethysmography or Doppler ultrasound and narrow cuffs	Directly dependent on blood flow. Operator must be experienced and skilled
Ankle brachial pressure index (ABPI) ratio of systolic pressures	Doppler ultrasound and sphygmomanometer cuff	Well-defined ranges, widely used. Falsely high values are possible in diabetics on account of medial calcification. Difficult to use on patients with large painful legs[9]
Skin blood flow	Clearance of 4-iodo-antipyrine by cutaneous blood flow. Radioactivity detected by small purpose built counters or gamma cameras	Difficult technique though excellent results obtained for amputation level assessments in one center[10]
Vasodilatory status	Transcutaneous measurement of oxygen	Reliable measures of tissue viability in diabetics with peripheral arterial disease at risk of limb loss and foot ulcers[11]
Capillary density and morphology	Capillary microscopy	A visual method limited to studying nail beds. Skin thickness and pigmentation limit use[12]
Skin perfusion imaging	Laser Doppler imaging	Necrotic material on wound surfaces will limit use[13]
Oxygen saturation	Optical assessment of backscattered light using lightguides	Relatively unused in patients with peripheral arterial disease. In a study (41 patients and 12 controls) hemoglobin oxygenation was derived and compared with skin blood flow. Sensitivity and selectivity of 1.0 were derived from data[14]

PROTOCOL FOR MEASURING TISSUE OXYGEN USING SKIN SENSORS

$TcPO_2$ is best measured with patients lying supine in a room free from noise and draughts where the ambient temperature is maintained between 21 and 24°C. Posture regulates flow in the peripheral circulation; in a dependent limb the veno-arteriolar response will reduce blood flow by increasing pre-capillary sphincter resistance. It is advisable to use the antecubital fossa as a control site, though the fifth intercostal space in the mid-clavicular line is ideal. The sensor should be heated ideally between 41 and 44°C using the concentric heater ring. The probe should not be left *in situ* for longer than 2 h to avoid local burns. Skin sites should be prepared carefully; degrease using alcohol swabs and shave, if needed. Patients should desist from tobacco use and avoid stimulants such as coffee or tea for at least 2 h prior to tests. Patients should be well hydrated and rested for at least 10 min prior to the start. All concomitant medication including diuretics should be recorded (Figure 11.4).

Rieber[15] found TcPO$_2$ less than 20 mmHg was associated with risk of amputation, the relative risk being 7.5. Kram[16] examined the accuracy of TcPO$_2$ to predict amputation levels after measuring on anterior and posterior aspects below knees, expressing the values with respect to control measurements derived on forearms distal to the crease of the elbow. The effect of setting the ratio of site to control value at 0.2 on successful amputation yielded 98% accuracy with a positive predictive value of 97% and a negative predictive value of 100%. Kram recommends this method to determine viability of skin flaps prior to below-knee amputation. Olerud and colleagues[17] reported using TcPO$_2$ and other measurements to study differences in wounds in elderly controls and patients with peripheral vascular disease or diabetes mellitus.

Chomard[18] measured TcPO$_2$ on the leg skin of patients with peripheral vascular disease with different degrees of ischemia. He studied the interaction between demographic variables as well as positional changes in skin TcPO$_2$. This group studied 116 patients with Leriche and Fontaine stage III or IV obliterative arterial disease, mean ages 71.9 years and 81.6 years for male and female patients, respectively. Lesion sites studied included aorto-iliac, femoro-popliteal, and multiple sites. The interventions studied were medical, surgical, i.e. revascularization, partial amputation and total amputation. Patients were followed up for a year. TcPO$_2$ was measured at 44°C at the base of the toes on the skin over the second metatarsal space. Control values were measured 5 cm inferior to the right clavicle. Patients were studied resting horizontally and with the affected limb hanging vertically. The effects of 100% oxygen inhalation at 1 and 4 min were measured, though it is unclear which limb position was used during this challenge.

The results of the study support the concept that a TcPO$_2$ ratio of 0.2 (site to chest control) is the limit below which healing cannot occur. The study results also show that dangling the leg vertically leads to significant increases in absolute values as well as in TcPO$_2$ ratio, except when the distal foot is non-viable. The authors have modeled the effects of age, sex and TcPO$_2$ values and propose this equation to derive a viability index. The relevant and important effects of diabetes, as well as smoking, need to be determined in developing a precise model of this measurement that may be used to predict the effects of targeted intervention in ischemic wound disease.

What is TcPO$_2$?

TcPO$_2$ reflects skin nutrition and is dependent on the vasodilatory capacity of skin. Skin thickness as well as edema affect TcPO$_2$; edema impedes oxygen diffusion[19]. As capillaries become resorbed into ischemic tissues, making the diffusion distances longer, oxygen available for healing will decrease.

IS VENOUS INSUFFICIENCY A RISK FACTOR FOR DIABETIC FOOT DISEASE?

Sumpio[8] included venous hypertension as a risk factor for diabetic foot ulcers, though no other details were available. In a recent study in the author's laboratory, venous refilling time (VRT) was determined as a measure of venous hemodynamic function in a study of diabetic foot ulcers[20]. Patients with neuropathic foot ulcers (n = 30, males = 23, females = 7, median age 59.5 years; range 37–77 years) were randomly assigned to two different treatments. Ulcer contour was traced at regular weekly dressing changes and the area enclosed determined by planimetry. VRT was measured using a laser Doppler flowmeter (MBF3 Moor Instruments, UK) placed 10 cm proximal to the medial malleolus following the protocol used in the author's laboratory. Median VRTs were 9.6 and 10.5 s for the ulcerated and control limbs, respectively. These VRT times are short compared with a threshold of much greater than 20 s and usually consistent with the presence of hemodynamic dysfunction in the legs. We considered but excluded impaired mobility of the ulcerated limb as a likely cause, since both legs were similarly affected. No differences were obtained when the ulcers healed. Analysis of covariates yielded an association between longer VRT and better healing, a finding that could have implications for symptomatic management of the diabetic foot.

Other measurements in the milieu

The tests done on skin surface and blood have been discussed so far. These are also mostly widely available. A reason for non-healing wounds frequently discussed in recent literature is the wound surface itself. Wound surfaces carry bacteria, slough and exudate. A commonly espoused view about leg ulcers used to be that, as low-grade infection was common, it was worthless to probe further to understand more the role of microbes in delaying healing. Exudates provoked more frequent dressing changes. Robson[21] proposed that 10^5 counts/g of tissue is a threshold of infection beyond which the wound infection must be actively treated. This necessitates regular wound biopsies.

In order to determine whether concerted action involving microbiologic measurements was indicated, in our center, we chose to begin by examining the feasibility of measuring wound pH as a first step.

Wound surface pH can be measured using a surface electrode[22]. A glass electrode (designed for use on gels) is used after calibration in buff-ers at pH 7 and pH 9, respectively. A drop of deionized water is used to bridge (contact) the wound surface with the electrode and measurements are noted after 30 s. The machine measures surface temperature using a thermistor and adjusts surface pH readings to 37°C. The technique compared well with blood gas analyzer data ($r = 0.83$)[22] and had an accuracy of plus or minus 0.2 pH units. The pH electrode kit used in the author's laboratory is shown in Figure 11.5.

Ulcer surface pH is usually alkaline and a reduction associated with healing has been reported in different studies[23]. In a study of venous ulcers treated using sustained four-layer compression, surface pH reduced in responders. The difference between wound pH and controls was statistically significant ($p = 0.02$)[24]. The absolute values of wound pH were not statistically significant, possibly indicating the relative inaccuracy of the technique or insufficient sample size. In the same study, tissue oxygen tension and surface pH were negatively correlated in responders ($n = 16/20$, $r = -0.544$, $p = 0.02$). In a similar study no statistical differences between wound surface pH in diabetic foot ulcers that responded well to treatment were noted. The technique is simple, safe and reproducible. The effect of tissue bio-burden is unknown; this must be studied before the potential of the technique is explored.

WOUND EXUDATE

Wounds exude fluids. In chronic wounds, the level of exudate can be so high as to soak dressings, necessitating more frequent dressing changes. Soaked dressings are uncomfortable to patients, the leak through making them more conscious of their wound. It is likely that exudates also offer tracks for the ingress of bacteria; this applies equally to all chronic wounds. In practice, patients have different levels of exudate which varies with the state of the ulcer. As wounds heal, the amount of exudate diminishes. There have been several reports describing the constituents of wound fluid[25–27] which suggest differences discovered from chronic venous wounds in comparison with acute controls.

Why study wound fluids? Chronic wounds regardless of etiology are a long-term inflammatory condition. For wounds to heal, there need to be favorable changes in metabolic and tissue repair processes. Exudate studies presuppose that examination of the contents associated with tissue remodeling would lead to the understanding of healing.

There are two hurdles to overcome first; to optimize sampling techniques and to determine significant constituents that are to be measured. Wound fluids have been sampled by lavage, absorption using sponge or filter paper, aspiration and suction using the Vacuum-Assisted Closure (VAC) technique described by Argenta[28]. This technique is referred to elsewhere in this book (in Chapters 7 and 13). Rasmussen[29], using a hydrocolloid dressing fitted with a tap, studied lavage fluid from venous ulcers and measured pre-collagen peptides (PINP and PIIICP) in an attempt to study collagen synthesis. The technique was innovative; the results may have been affected by the dressing used since hydrocolloids are interactive and known to generate exudate. Lavage fluid may therefore represent the effect of the dressing used. However, Rasmussen's work suggested the potential value of wound exudate measurements.

Both sponge and filter paper have been used to absorb wound exudate by Wysocki[25] and Tarlton[26], respectively. A sponge used to absorb exudate is squeezed and the fluid collected while a wound fluid/exudate is eluted from filter paper. The fluid is stored at −20°C for specific examinations to follow. Trentgrove[27] used a different collection technique to the absorption methods.

In their laboratory, Trentgrove and colleagues fast patients overnight. On the morning of the test, patients are seated with legs dependent and asked to drink a liter of water. This process takes 1 h. The leg ulcer is covered by OpSite® (Smith & Nephew, UK) at this time. The fluid collected underneath the dressing is aspirated after the hour. Trentgrove, after measuring a wide range of biochemical constituents, argued that wound fluid obtained this way is different from serous fluid, is an exudate and that wound fluids from chronic venous ulcers are different in composition. In a recent personal communication, Trentgrove stated that fasting was no longer used as part of their protocol.

What to measure in wound fluid?

Several workers have shown significant reduction in matrix metalloproteinase (MMP) activity, notably MMP2 and MMP9, in both venous ulcers and pressure ulcers[25,26]. Tissue-inhibiting metalloproteinase (TIMP) measurements have mirrored results of MMP measurements, lending weight to the argument that extracellular matrix activity and therefore collagen remodeling is likely to be impaired in some chronic wounds. Most studies have used fluids from acute wounds as controls.

Wound fluid studies permit such inflammatory markers as IL-1, IL-6, IL-10 and TNF-α to be studied, which is essential to unlock some of the mysteries of tissue repair. However, the differences in results between laboratories of certain constituents, for example lactate, suggest there could be systematic errors that need identifying and rectifying. There is a need for a standardized protocol before seeking predictive markers in wound exudate.

HOW TO STUDY COMPLICATIONS

As chronic wounds carry a level of bacteria, being open surfaces, routine swabbing of wound surfaces is usually considered without value, as antibiotic therapy, topical or oral, is not initiated except when certain colonizing species are evident. Punch biopsies (3, 4 or 6 mm) are helpful to establish the level of bacterial burden and, using the threshold advocated by Robsen, it is possible to use antimicrobial therapy to treat wounds specifically.

Some wounds are malodorous. Research in conducting polymer technology led to the development of 'electronic noses'[30], an objective method of assessing wound smell. Electronic noses have been used by both the wine-making and perfume industries. The smell from gaseous emissions causes electronic activity in the polymer analogous to transistor technology.

Edema impedes ulcer healing. It has been suggested after ultrasound imaging that, in venous ulcers, edema is usually located in the papillary dermis where it would impede diffusion of nutrients, especially oxygen. Recent work from our laboratory has shown that edema may also impede perfusion[31,32]. While edema may be located ultrasonically, estimating its volume is easily achieved using a tape to measure calf circumference. Barnes[33] demonstrated that this simple method used carefully could show reduction in tissue fluid volume during leg elevation. This simple method should be used routinely.

Leg elevation and compression are used to manage edema. Intermittent pneumatic compression may be of enormous benefit to patients[34] and carers alike. A systematic review of the randomized controlled trials suggested the need for more studies of this simple technique. In recent years, the VAC method[28] is gaining usage as a useful device to speed wound healing in certain difficult circumstances including burns, as discussed in Chapter 7 in this book. The VAC technique ingeniously employs suction (negative pressure) through a sponge applied to the wound. An electric pump sucks at the sponge, drawing fluid from the wound, thereby reducing edema and exudates and thus promoting healing. The method has been well described by the inventor though its mechanism of action is ill understood. It is useful to reduce edema from chronic wounds on the body.

RECOMMENDATIONS

In addition to the well-described techniques to assess the circulation, wound contour should be traced routinely with every dressing change. The area enclosed may be determined graphically by counting squares or using computer software that is easily available. It has been suggested that an area change of less than 15% of the initial area in 4 weeks is not good healing; when wound closure is slower, the treatment plan should be reviewed[35]. This is merely a guideline; complications such as infection, edema and the patient's condition must be assessed regularly. In neurotrophic lesions, depth assessment is essential; in cavity wounds a simple reliable assessment of depth is fundamental to good management[35]. Wound biopsies are recommended in order to treat infection vigorously. Diabetic foot wounds must be managed with a view to preventing and promoting better healing, preferably without amputation. To this end, the specialist team should assess foot tissue viability in patients at risk.

References

1. Mani R. Laboratory evaluation of non-healing wounds. In: Lalanga V, ed. *Wound Healing and the Skin*. London: Martin Dunitz, 2001: 187–201

2. Pape SA, Skouras CA, Byrne PO. An audit of the use of laser Doppler imaging (LDI) in the assessment of burns of intermediate depth. *Burns* 2001;27:233–9

3. Sowa MG, Leonardi L, Payette JR, Fish JS, Mantsch HH. Near infrared spectroscopy of hemodynamic changes in the early post-burn period. *Burns* 2001;27:241–9

4. Romanelli R. In: Mani R, Falanga V, Shearman CP, Sandeman D, *Chronic Wound Healing: Clinical Measurement and Basic Science*. London: Harcourt Brace, 1999:68–80

5. Kram HB, Paul L, Appel MPA. Multisensor transcutaneous oximetric mapping to protect below knee amputation wound healing; use of a critical pO_2. *J Vasc Surg* 1989;9:796–800

6. Turnbull FW. PhD Thesis, University of Strathclyde, 1997

7. Ouriel K. Peripheral arterial disease. *Lancet* 2001;358:1257–64

8. Sumpio BE. Foot ulcers. *N Engl J Med* 2000; 343: 787–93

9. Barnes RW, Shanik GD, Slaymaker EE. An index of healing in below knee amputation – leg blood pressure by Doppler ultrasound. *Surgery* 1976;79:13

10. McCollum PT, Spence BA, Walker WF. Circumferential skin blood flow measurements in the ischaemic limb. *Br J Surg* 1985;72:310–12

11. Hanna GP, Fujise K, Kjellgren O, *et al.* Infrapopliteal transcatheter interventions for limb salvage in diabetic patients: importance of aggressive interventional approach and the role of transcutaneous oximetry. *J Am Coll Cardiol* 1997;30:664–9

12. Tooke J, Oostergren JE, Fagrell B. Synchronous assessment of skin micro-circulation by laser Doppler flowmetry and dynamic capillaroscopy. *Int J Microcirc Clin Exp* 1983;2:277–84

13. Ubbink DT, Spincemaille GHJJ, Renman RS, Jacobs MHJM. Prediction of imminent amputation in patients with non reconstructible leg ischemia by means of microcirculatory investigations. *J Vasc Surg* 1999;30:114–21

14. Harrison DK, McCollum PT, Newton DJ, Hickman P, Jain AS. Amputation level assessment using lightguide spectrophotometry. *Prosthet Orthot Int* 1995;19:139–47

15. Reiber GE, Pecoraro RE, Koepsal TD. Risk factors for amputation in patients with diabetes mellitus. *Ann Intern Med* 1992;117:97–105

16. Kram HB, Paul I, Appel MPA, *et al.* Multisensor transcutaneous oximetric mapping to protect below knee amputation wound healing: use of a critical pO_2. *J Vasc Surg* 1989;9:796–800

17. Olerud JE, Odland GF, Burgess EM, Wyss CR. A model for the study of wounds in normal and elderly adults and patients with peripheral vascular disease or diabetes mellitus. *J Surg Res* 1995;59:349–60

18. Chomard C, Habault P, Eveno D, LeLamer S, Ledemeny M, Haon C. Criteria predictive of limb viability at 1 year in patients with chronic severe ischemia – TcPO2 and demographic parameters. *Angiology* 2000;51:765–76

19. Mani R. Transcutaneous measurements of oxygen tension in venous ulcer disease. *Vasc Med Rev* 1995;6:121–31

20. Roberts GH, Hammad LF, Baker N, *et al.* IIydrocellular against non-adherent dressings to treat diabetic foot ulcers – a randomised controlled study. *Wound Repair Regen* 2001;9: 402

21. Robson MC. Lessons gleaned from the sport of wound watching. *Wound Repair Regen* 1999;7: 2–6

22. Glibbery A, Mani R. pH in leg ulcers. *Int J Microcirc Clin Exp* 1992;11:Suppl 109

23. Romanelli M, Schiapani E, Piagessi A, *et al.* Evaluation of surface pH in venous leg ulcers under Allevyn dressings. In: Suggett A, Cherry GW, *et al.* eds. *Evidence-Based Wound Care*. London: RSM

24. Roberts GH, Hammad L, Collins C, Shearman C, Mani R. Some effects of sustained compression on ulcerated tissues. *Angiology* 2002;53: 451–6

25. Wysocki A, Kusakabe A, Chang S, Tuan T. Temporal expression of urokinase activator, plasminogen activator inhibitor and gelatinase-B in chronic wound fluid switches from a chronic to acute wound profile with progres-

sion to healing. *Wound Repair Regen* 1999;7: 154–65

26. Tarlton JF, Bailey AJ, Crawford E, Jones D, Moore K, Harding K. Prognostic value of markers of collagen remodelling in venous ulcers. *Wound Repair Regen* 1999;7:347–55

27. Trentgrove NJ, Langton SR, *et al.* Biochemical analysis of wound fluids from non-healing and chronic leg ulcers. *Wound Repair Regen* 1996;4: 234–9

28. Argenta LC, Morykwas MJ. Vacuum-assisted closure: a new method for wound control and treatment: clinical experience. *Ann Plastic Surg* 1997;38;563–76

29. Rasmussen L, Jensen L, Avnstorp C, *et al.* Collagen types I and III propeptides as markers of healing in chronic leg ulcers. *Ann Surg* 1992; 216:684–91

30. Armani MEH, Payne P, Persaud KC. Multi-frequency measurements of organic conduct-ing polymers for sensing of gases and vapours. *Sensors Actuators B* 1996;SBBO33 (1–3):137–41

31. Mani R. Science of measurements in wound healing. *Wound Repair Regen* 1999;6:330–4

32. Hammad L. A study of the mechanical and microcirculatory properties in skin subject to venous ulceration. PhD Thesis, University of Southampton, 2000

33. Barnes M, Mani R, Barrett DF, White JE. Changes in skin microcirculation during leg elevation in patients with chronic venous insufficiency. Proceedings of Second Joint British/Swedish Angiology meeting. *Vasc Med Rev* 1991;3:21

34. Mani R, Vowdern K, Nelson EA. Intermittent pneumatic compression for leg ulcer manage-ment. Cochrane Library Software, 2001:4

35. Falanga V. www.woundheal.org

Models for healing

12

F. Gottrup

INTRODUCTION

Models in wound healing aim to improve understanding of the healing process[1,2]. Studies of wound healing in the human organism should be decisive. Legal and ethical reasons, as well as problems of complexity of human wounds, render the need for other models. Models must be accurately representative, not idealized. Presently, there are no models suitable for many of the different types of wounds, leading to the use of acute wounds to represent all healing situations. Clearly, this is incorrect and mistakes have resulted from this policy, especially in relation to the treatment of chronic wounds such as pressure ulcers, leg ulcers, etc. In order to develop a good usable model, there is a need to understand the nature and pathophysiology of the different types of wounds, to define the end aim of the exercise and the applicability of the chosen model. The aim of this chapter is to examine the problem of modeling chronic wounds, the shortfalls in the models described, as well as useful types of models.

MODELS FOR CHRONIC WOUNDS – AN UNREMITTING CHALLENGE

Acute wounds modeled in animals often parallel surgical procedures or other traumatic lesions; it is infinitely difficult to develop chronic wound models using animals. This is a great challenge faced by wound researchers.

The majority of chronic wounds manifest on skin; nonetheless, these are diverse in their etiology. Therapeutic techniques used to treat such wounds are also varied. The majority of chronic wounds are leg and foot ulcers, as frequently described elsewhere in this book. Leg ulcers develop as a result of circulatory dysfunction; either venous or arterial systems may be impaired. Foot ulcers result from excess pressures or ischemia and are common in diabetic patients.

Models of venous ulcers must simulate venous hypertension. In man, chronic venous hypertension leads to changes in the skin microcirculation, as well as in subcutaneous tissues around the ankle. Man alone, of the vertebrate species, is susceptible to postural venous hypertension since humans stand upright and walk. Animal modeling of these changes is fraught with difficulties. Some efforts were made to study the effects of surgically induced venous hypertension in a canine model, which suggested associated changes in capillary permeability and density[3]. This study led to the suggestion of the fibrin cuff hypothesis as the cause of venous ulceration[4]. This theory, however, has been difficult to substantiate in the human pathophysiology of ulcers. Other attempts to replicate the chronic nature of venous ulcers have been made on guinea-pigs using chemical injuries (tetradecyl sulfates) in skin of the flank[5]. This creates a sloughy wound, which, however, healed within 2 weeks, similar to an acute type of wound healing. Furthermore, this model contains no venous hypertension in the pathogenesis of the wound. There are no reports of any replication of this model. For reasons similar to the above, modeling diabetic lesions is very difficult. Diabetes may be induced in animals and acute lesions created in these. How closely do such lesions represent diabetic foot ulcers that are often triggered by ill-fitting shoes, sharp foreign bodies such as nails in shoes, lack of physical activity and restrictive clothing?

Differences in anatomic construction augment the problems in using animal models. Human wounds are most often a combination of impaired circulation, poor nutrition, chronologic age, restricted physical activity and physiologic imbalance. It may be impossible to develop models of this complexity. For these reasons, investigators have focused on isolated segments of the problem to reproduce cost-effective methods, in order to demonstrate that healing is impaired. Such models that seek to simplify human wounds are used to study the efficacy of therapeutic agents or interventions. Such models should be described as 'impaired' wound models; the tendency to term these 'chronic' models is erroneous and misleading.

Impaired healing models may be used to study systemic impairment, biologic local healing impairment and so on. Systemic impairment can be caused by immune suppression, diabetes, aging, nutrition, zinc deficiency and renal failure, all of which may be induced[6]. A further sub-division can be performed in relation to the type of drugs used, type of induced disease and type of nutritional deficiencies. Biologically impaired models can be achieved by the use of infections; the use of the Brown Recluse spider venom permits tumor necrosis factor alpha (TNF-α) over-expression to be modeled. The use of bacteria also permits modeling of this common wound complication.

Models with local healing impairment are typically those where ischemia is induced either surgically or mechanically by restricting blood flow, applying pressure or local radiation. Restriction of blood flow can be induced in flaps, pedicles or arterial or skin ligation. External pressure to reduce flow has been investigated in a canine model[7,8].

Chemically impaired healing models are produced in dermis by the use of cytotoxic dermonecrosis vesicants, by caustic agents in epidermis and by calcium in cornea and gastric mucosa. In each group different types of chemicals can be used to induce tissue lesions. Models of the future may derive from genetic manipulation of mice and other species, an area that has advanced much in the last decade.

Mathematical models, a theoretic approach to wound healing studies, are used to evaluate quantitative data[9]. Mathematical models may be derived from graphic representation of experimental findings. For example, if the change in wound areas in response to different treatments was plotted and lines of best fit derived, a mathematic relationship could be derived. Such a relationship would permit the change in area to be predicted with some restrictions. Simple mathematical models have been used to analyze wound healing data from different wound healing experiments. A specialized computer package has been developed for simulation, curve fitting, statistic analysis and graphic plotting in mathematic models used in the life sciences. These types of models have been used to study data from different wound healing experiments, such as accumulation of collagen in the wound site, recovery of wound strength during healing, recruitment of inflammatory cells and collagen orientation. Exponential models have been developed and different wound healing parameters like cell numbers, epithelial thickness, glycosaminoglycans (GAG) content, etc., can be evaluated against time. Mathematical models have also been used in the description of the different types of forces involved in the development of pressure ulcers (pressure–distribution factor)[8]. As with animal modeling, theoretic or mathematical models are based on compartmental description of a problem; as such, these are restrictive in their perspective.

As mentioned by Hunt and co-workers[10], clinical wound healing research has been delayed for many years by the old statement 'to make a difference, there must be a difference'. Most clinicians have used this as proof for the only way to study wound healing clinically is to actually use wound complications as the end-point of the study. This would mean, however, that each improvement in management of human wound healing would require the recruitment of large numbers of patients and still the specific problem may not be solved because of the complexity of the end-points. There is a need, therefore, for experimental models to relate an objective measure of one or more wound healing components to actual clinical events.

Rats have been used as a model, despite the fact that they heal faster with fewer infectious complications than humans[11]. Most human infectious complications take place in the subcutaneous layer, but, of all species used for this type of research, only the pig and perhaps monkeys have a total comparable subcutis to man. Another problem has been that no animal models of chronic wounds such as venous leg ulcers, diabetic ulcers or even pressure ulcers are presently available. For these reasons, the use of human models, in spite of ethical and methodologic problems, is to be preferred in all wound healing research. However, only a few human models or methods are presently available[1,2].

ANIMAL MODELS

The Greek physician and philosopher Galen carried out anatomic studies on apes and pigs in the second century AD. The concept of animal models was introduced in 1865 by French physiologist Claude Bernard for introduction of chemical and physical diseases in experimental situations[12]. The use of animals in research began mainly in Germany and France and rapid advances followed in the understanding of medical physiology. Since then, experiments with animals have developed into an essential part of most biomedical research including wound healing.

It was assumed when studying animals that humans are identical to other animals in body function. This assumption is erroneous. 'Animal' derives from the Latin word anima, meaning soul/spirit, to imply living organisms that are animated[11]. Through history it has been discussed whether humans are part of this group, but it would be a linguistic and scientific mistake to imply that humans should not be part of the animal 'species'.

'Models' are defined as 'a representation of a real or actual object' (Oxford English Dictionary). A model is an object of imitation, something that accurately resembles something else, a person or thing that is a likeness or image of another[13]. The US National Research Committee on Animal Models for Research on Aging attempted to define the term 'laboratory animal model' as 'an animal model in which normative biology or behavior can be studied or in which spontaneous or induced pathologic processes can be investigated and in which the phenomenon in one or more respect resembles the same phenomenon in humans or other species of animals'. This extended definition tries to cover the whole area, but is very long. One of the problems with the term animal model is that it would be more correct to define it as 'a model of humans'[11].

The objective of modeling is to 'simplify a complex problem and to clarify thinking followed by development of a hypothesis'. Models must not substitute creative thought[14] though the use of models is not without limitations. Is it possible to transfer the results to the situation that initiated the use of the model? Are we looking at pharmacologic concentrations versus physiologic? Are there ethical or legal problems with using the model? There may also be a limitation in experimental psychologic conditions and it has to be taken into consideration that the researcher is part of the model used.

The ideal animal model should reflect the etiology and pathogenesis of the wound chosen and it should illustrate the clinical situation. Unfortunately, no existing model fulfills all these criteria.

Types of animal models

The literature often describes four main groups of animal models. These are induced, spontaneous, negative and orphan models[11]. Induced models are images in which the condition under investigation is experimentally induced e.g. a disease like diabetes mellitus. This type of model allows the researcher a free choice of species. It must to borne in mind that a close phylogenetic relation to man does not guarantee validity of extrapolation. One example is the unsuccessful chimpanzee model in AIDS research[15]. A specific type of induced disease image is the transgenic animal model. These animals carry artificially inserted, foreign DNA in their genomes. Mice are the preferred animal species in this group. Spontaneous models of human diseases utilize naturally occurring genetic variants. A well-known example is the nude mouse, which has been used in cancer research. Negative models, unlike the spontaneous and induced types, are unable to develop particular diseases. Their main application is in the study of the mechanism of resistance to pathophysiologic conditions. In orphan models, a disease not yet described in humans occurs naturally in a non-human species. The disease can then be

'adopted' when a similar disease is described later in humans, e.g. bovine spongiform encephalopathy or 'mad cow disease'.

Rules for choosing models may be generalized as: (1) is the problem worth investigating/resolving; (2) if so, has someone else already solved the problem?; (3) could a human model be developed and; (4) if not, is an animal model appropriate and if so is the chosen species appropriate? Further thinking must determine whether genetic and environmental variations can be assessed/controlled, whether the health status of animals can be controlled during the project and is the choice of animal model sound? The use of or attempts at using models for personal convenience, inadequacy of local facilities, financial, ethical or legal restraints, lack of availability of species, lack of inter- or intra-departmental cooperation and laboratory traditions and convenience should be avoided. Finally, it should be questioned whether rates and routes of metabolism of a substance to be tested are comparable in the model.

Extrapolation

Human response is difficult if not impossible to predict with accuracy and consistency. This adds to the problems of modeling, especially using animals. For example, the drug Thalidomide® produced no birth defects in rats or many other species[16] but had tragic effects on humans, crippling the children of mothers who took the drug when pregnant. In other words, the animal model to be studied should have been primates, though it is easier to be wise in hindsight. This incongruity, i.e. interspecies reactivity, was a serendipitous finding. In spite of numerous anatomic and physiologic differences, many of the animals that are inadequate, predictive models nevertheless continue to be used extensively.

In considering extrapolation from animal models to humans, it is important to remember the striking cultural, dietary and environmental differences among and between our societies. For example, walking without shoes is culturally acceptable in some societies such as in South Asia. In Europe, this would be unacceptable and unbearable in the prevailing climate. This is relevant to the modeling of foot ulcers. Dietary habits are very varied and therefore extremely difficult to account for in modeling effects on metabolism. Environmental differences are relevant in modeling reactions on skin and its microcirculation. This can have special significance in the area of wound healing, where the patient population varies considerably.

These considerations are the background for numerous scientific and political debates and public views are especially sensitive to poor quality research. For this reason, it is of special importance that mistakes be avoided. This can to a certain degree be obtained by focusing on some vital requirements before the final study plan is accepted: (1) take a pluri-species approach, if needed use two species, as in most toxicology screening; (2) metabolic patterns and rate must match between species, primarily for drug and toxicity studies; (3) confounding variables of metabolism must be controlled. Differences due to age, sex, diet, season, daily temperature, distress and so on must be accounted for; (4) experimental design and the life situation of the target species must correspond.

In wound healing research, it has become obvious that there are often problems when extrapolating results from animal studies to clinical work. In animals models, growth factors have been shown to have beneficial effects on the healing process, but these effects have until now been of doubtful clinical importance. Different experimental conditions, e.g. acute wounds in young healthy animals compared to non-healing chronic wounds in old patients with many complicating diseases,

may account for lack of clinical significance observed in humans.

Differences in biology between the different species have to be taken into account. Most human infectious complications take place in the subcutaneous layer, but, of all species used for this type of research, only the monkey and pig have a comparable subcutis to man. For these reasons, the use of human models, in spite of ethical and methodologic problems, is to be preferred in all wound healing research.

It can be concluded that general rules for the extrapolation of results achieved in one species to another are difficult to provide. Each experiment has to be individually evaluated and often the result can be found after the first studies of the target species. An overview of this area, especially related to toxicologic research, has been performed by Calabrese[17].

Some advantages of animal models

Human skin is unique and variable according to age, sex, race and region of the body[18,19]. Despite differences between humans and animals, they share simple basic structures and patterns of cell proliferation and differentiation[20]. Animal models allow similar wound environments and morphologic conditions to be studied. The pig is used extensively to model for epithelialization on account of similarities with human skin. The dermis of pigs is relatively poorly vascularized and contains only apocrine glands. Pigs are therefore unable to sweat like humans, but the similarities in respect of size and other functions of skin are sufficient to allow useful comparisons[21]. In the case of collagen repair, most mammalian species are similar to humans, although differences exist. Rats have been extensively used for this type of wound healing study, but, in spite of a higher collagen production in wounds compared to humans[22], this species does not produce keloid or hypertrophic scars and the collagen production comes from the subcutaneous panniculus carnosus muscles[23]. Production of collagen also requires ascorbic acid (vitamin C) in humans, while some mammals are capable of synthesizing this cofactor.

CHOOSING A MODEL

When a model is needed for an experiment, the first question is: 'Which model to use?'

From a general point of view, the choice of models in wound healing research is dependent on several factors such as: 'type of investigation' (tissue repair physiology or pathophysiology, biologic agent efficacy, dressing efficacy, safety evaluation, pharmacokinetics, etc.); 'type of method' (*in vitro/in vivo*, acute/impaired/fetal, animal/human, etc.); 'animal or human studies' (animal type, anatomy, biology, extrapolation, ethical aspects, etc.); 'variability' (intra/inter-organism variation, variability of involved measurements, etc.); 'outcome measurements' (wound size [area/volume], wound strength, granulation tissue/collagen, blood supply, resurfacing, visual assessment, etc.); 'recruitment criteria' (age, sex, species, strain, statistic consideration, etc.)[14,24].

The ideal 'experimental animal model' is a living organism with an inherited, naturally acquired or induced pathologic process that, in one or more respects, closely resembles the same phenomenon in man[11]. It may vary from a one-cell protozoan to a chimpanzee, depending on the purpose of the study. To find a good and appropriate model, some criteria have to be fulfilled[1,25]: (1) accurately reproduce the lesion; (2) possibility for multiple investigations; (3) exportability; (4) allow multiple biopsy samples; (5) fit into animal facilities; (6) be easy to handle; (7) be available in more than one species and; (8) be usable for a long enough time.

The models available can be divided into *in vitro* and *in vivo*. The choice depends on the problem itself but also on some important practical factors such as: (1) the space and physical facilities required for animal studies; (2) laboratory facilities; (3) technical expertise; (4) financial resources; (5) time; and (6) ethical and legal factors. *In vitro* models can generally be used as cell cultures or organ cultures. The cells most studied in wound healing research are fibroblasts, keratinocytes, macrophages, epidermal or endothelial cells. *In vivo* models relate to healing of tissue and organs and can involve both animal and human models.

As in other types of research using animal models, wound healing research uses *in vitro* and *in vivo* models. The decision on the type of model should be based on the type of parameters relevant to describe the problem under consideration. The advantage of *in vitro* models in wound healing research is the direct examination of the effect of an environmental change or substance on the tissue, without influencing the other tissue components. The major disadvantage is the difficulty in extrapolation of results to the wounded tissue in an otherwise normal organism.

The advantages of an *in vivo* model in wound healing research are that wounded tissue is similar to wounds found in clinical practice and, in the case of skin wounds, can be made in human subjects. The disadvantages are that direct examination of single tissue components is difficult and, in the case of human skin wounds, only small, clean wounds can be produced and even this may be an ethical problem.

In order to investigate the efficacy of a therapeutic compound, different parameters can be used. *In vivo*: biomechanic and biochemical studies of the healing tissue, observation of healing macroscopically, measurements of different wound healing markers, cellular response and immunologic responses. *In vitro*: cultures of cells (fibroblasts, keratinocytes, macrophages, epidermal or endothelial cells etc.) and observation of activity in these

Table 1 Models in wound healing research (modified from ref. 1)

In vitro models	
Single cell systems	Monolayers, 3-D
Multicellular systems	Co-cultures, 3-D
Organ cultures	Intact skin
In vivo animal models	
Artificial models	Subcutaneous chamber/sponges, subcutaneous tubes, others
Tissue models	Excisional wounds, incisional wounds, superficial wounds, burn wounds, others

* 'Impaired healing models' are established by altering the healing response by: local factors: ischemia, infection etc.; systemic factors: age, diseases, infection etc.; outside factors: radiation, agents, etc.

cultures by monitoring differences in collagen metabolites, amino acids, glycosaminoglycans, etc., or following the modulation of cultures by cloning of cells or adding types of wound fluid or tissue factors. Organ cultures of the skin can also be used. Migration of the epidermis can provide information on the first phase of wound healing and the system is easily used for studying the influence of intrinsic as well as extrinsic factors.

Before the final decision on which model to use, two factors are important: (1) the problem itself and (2) the degree of simplification which will be acceptable. In investigation of the efficacy of a topical component, the model used depends on the stage of the component in the clinical development and which purpose the test should fulfill. Is it a preclinical pharmacologic and/or toxicologic investigation? – an animal (*in vitro* or *in vivo*) model probably will be used. Is it a product efficacy study? – in phases I–III a human model will be used.

TYPES OF MODELS AVAILABLE

In this section, the different types of models available will be described (Table 1). In order to obtain more detailed knowledge of each model, specialized articles and chapters should also be consulted[1,6,10,14,24–26].

In vitro models

In vitro systems are generally rapid to set up, simple, less costly and involve less ethical considerations compared with *in vivo* wound models. *In vitro* models also permit several pharmacologic agents at different concentrations to be investigated simultaneously free from extraneous influences. Furthermore, *in vitro* models are appropriate to study the mechanism of action of a compound, which is complicated *in vivo*. However, the ultimate test of a wound healing agent is in a complete animal.

This section describes the increasing complexity of the *in vitro* test systems, i.e. more and more *in vivo*-like, beginning from single-cell systems, then multicellular systems in artificial three-dimensional (3-D) matrices and on to organ cultures[1]. To mimic the wound environment, especially the effect of the inflammatory response, the medium can be supplemented and/or replaced with wound fluid from various wound types at different stages. Wound fluid contains the major mediators released during the inflammatory response, such as

151

cytokines, growth factors, proteases and intact and degraded matrix molecules.

Single-cell systems

Monolayers

Cells in monolayer are usually grown directly on the plastic surface of culture dishes, although it is possible to use other substrates such as collagen, fibrin, fibronectin, vitronectin or laminin in static systems. The cyclic mechanical stress that cells are subjected to *in vivo* can be mimicked *in vitro* using an ingenious instrument that applies vacuum in cycles to the bottom of plastic dishes with cultured cells.

Commonly, wound closure is simulated *in vitro* by simply creating defects in cell monolayers. The cell-free area is then re-populated by adjacent cells through the combined action of migration and proliferation. To eliminate the role of proliferation on the closure of the defects, cells can be pre-treated with a DNA synthesis inhibitor. The progression of re-population of cells in the different systems is examined by microscopy and analyzed using image analysis systems.

Three-dimensional

Cells commonly composed of collagen type I or fibrin alter their phenotype drastically when cultured in 3-D matrices. Dramatic phenotypic changes of contraction-generating fibroblasts cultured in 3-D matrices are found depending on the mechanical tension in the systems. Presumably, 3-D systems are more representative of normal wound physiology than two-dimensional systems. It is well known that collagen production is decreased, whereas collagenase is increased, by fibroblasts incorporated in relaxed collagen type I gels compared with 2-D systems. These effects are presumably mediated by integrins. The increased number of apoptotic fibroblasts seen in maturing granulation tissue *in vivo* has also been reproduced in fibroblasts cultured in collagen gels. The composition of the gel can be modified by, for example, incorporating different types of collagen, fibronectin or glycosaminoglycans to mimic more closely the early granulation tissue deposited during wound repair.

Multicellular systems

Co-cultures

The importance of cell–cell interactions can be investigated in different systems. Convenient prefabricated two-well Transwell systems are available.

Three-dimensional

Apart from Transwell systems, 3-D gels with incorporated fibroblasts and with keratinocytes cultured on the apical side of the gel are common. These systems are laborious and require experience. There are also commercially available skin equivalents (Apligraf ™, Novartis), although they are costly. Wounds of varying depths can be made in the equivalents using a punch biopsy.

Organ cultures

Usually, intact human skin is utilized in wound healing studies. In contrast to skin equivalents described above, all the cellular, including skin appendages and matrix, elements are included in skin explants. One disadvantage is that skin explants cannot be modified in respect of cellular or matrix composition. It is recommended that skin from the same donor is used in an experimental series. Skin explants are cultured at the air–liquid interface or submerged in the culture medium. Studies have also been performed where healing is followed from explants placed directly onto plastic dishes. In most cases, epithelialization is the primary variable (end-point), although the development of tensile strength of full-thickness skin incisions occurs and can be monitored *in vitro*. Standardized burn wounds can also be inflicted in skin explants and epithelialization can be assessed by histomorphometry. It is also possible to carry out morphologic studies of the connective tissue. It should be emphasized that skin explants should be cultured in physiologic concentrations of calcium and for not more than 2 weeks, to prevent detachment of epidermis and degradation of the connective tissue, respectively.

In vivo models

No consensus has been achieved in the classification of *in vivo* models. One way could be to differentiate models in sub-groups related to which parts of the healing process is being investigated[1]. This can be epithelialization, neovascularization, dermal reconstitution, production of granulation tissue, contraction, etc. From a more practical point of view, animal and human models can be subdivided into models of foreign materials (artificial models) and of living tissue (tissue models)[1]. All the mentioned models can be used in animals while only selected models can be used in humans.

Artificial models

These models are primarily usable in the evaluation of the effect of systemic or local application of different substances on the wound healing process (e.g. growth factors, growth hormone, pharmacologic agents, etc.). Most often, the subcutaneous tissue has been investigated.

Subcutaneous implanted chambers and sponges

A variety of models in this group have been used. The original materials used were subcutaneous implanted sponges of polyvinyl, polyurethane and cellulose sponges, polyvinyl alcohol (PVA) sponges and stainless steel wire mesh chambers.

THE WIRE MESH CHAMBER MODEL. This was deployed by filling subcutaneously with wound fluid and connective tissue matrix. Fluid and tissue inside the cylinders can be measured by histologic, histochemical and biochemical analysis.

The advantages of these chambers are frequent sampling and they harvest large quantities of wound fluid and granulation tissue. The disadvantages are size and the time required to obtain granulation tissue. The use of this model is restricted to animal studies.

THE POLYVINYL ALCOHOL (PVA) SPONGES MODEL. This model can be placed percutaneously in animals as well as humans. It comprises three small preweighed PVA sponges placed inside a perforated silicone tubing. The model can be used for investigating granulation tissue histologically and biochemically. In humans the yield of collagen, however, is lower and the variability of the results higher than observed with the use of the expanded polytetrafluoroethylene (ePTFE) model. The advantages of this model are that histology can be evaluated, that it is easy to insert and remove and early phases of healing can be studied. The disadvantages are low collagen growth and relative high variability.

Subcutaneous implanted tubes

These devices are usable in man. The miniature porous ePTFE (Gore-Tex®) model is inserted subcutaneously and allows the in-growths of connective tissue, which can be evaluated by histology and measurement of collagen. More recently, a less expensive material of ePTFE (formerly Impra®) with a higher in-growth has been used.

THE EXPANDED POLYTETRAFLUOROETHYLENE (ePTFE) TUBING MODEL. This porous material allows diffusion of gas and fluid through the device. Like chambers, the ePTFE tubes most often are inserted in the anesthetized animal in the dorsal region. In man, the ePTFE tube is most often inserted in the lateral part of the upper arm under local anesthesia or in general anesthesia during surgery. The tubes are removed after 7–14 days.

This model has been widely used and specifically by our group for investigation of the influence of growth factors, major trauma and surgery, collagenase and smoking. The ePTFE model is well suited for controlled studies, because the patient may serve as his own control by the implantation of another ePTFE in the contralateral arm for administration of a placebo drug. In animal studies, it has been shown that the amount of hydroxyproline accumulated in the ePTFE model correlates with the tensile strength of incisional wounds.

The advantages of this model are high collagen yield, and the potential for DNA assessment and histology. The disadvantages are relatively few and based on a moderate variability. The method is less suitable for the study of early wound healing and a certain degree of encapsulation of the tube occurs, producing adhesions to the surrounding tissue.

VISCOSE CELLULOSE SPONGE INSIDE A SILICONE MATERIAL (CELLSTICK®). The model can be used in animals as well as in humans. The device is inserted as a drain. In this model, wound fluid is analyzed during the first 2–3 days after wounding. A cell-rich exudate is trapped in the sponge matrix. The contents of the sponges have been analyzed using histology, enzyme histochemistry, biochemistry, cytology or electron microscopy. This model is suitable for studies on wound fluid components in the early inflammatory phase of wound healing.

The major advantage of this model is the possibility of studying the early inflammatory response of the healing process and investigat-ing wound fluid. The disadvantage is that interpretation of the results is complicated. Only a few centers have experience using this methodology.

Tissue models

In these models, the normal tissue of the animal or human is an integral part. Measurements of outcome most often are made discontinuously.

Excisional wound models

This type of wound fulfills many of the aforementioned criteria of a good animal model as it can be accurately reproduced. These models are also available for multiple investigations.

The wound(s) can be made anywhere on the body surface and the shape of the wound depends on the purpose of the study. The effect of different types of dressings, dermal substitutes and local agents can be investigated by this model, where the outcome measurements will be an evaluation of wound size by measuring primarily changes in area as well as histology.

These models have primarily been used as wounds in skin and ears of experimental animals. Biopsies are used in humans.

Skin wound models

An excision of a full thickness piece of skin is made and the open defect will heal by re-epithelialization, dermal reconstitution and contraction. The following processes can be detected: epithelialization, contraction, dermal reconstitution, inflammation, chemotaxis, angiogenesis, matrix production/organization and cosmetic and functional outcome.

The skin can be removed using a pair of scissors, a knife or a dermatome. This model is mainly used in animals, while in humans a punch biopsy instrument or a trephine can be used for biopsies.

The advantage of this model is that it is a wound often found in clinical life. The model is economic when using small experimental animals or many wounds in larger animals.

The disadvantages of this model are that the defect heals from the edges by epithelialization as well as by contraction. The chronic leg ulcer is known to heal with minimal contraction and almost entirely by re-epithelialization and granulation tissue formation. In these cases, the ear wound model may be more suitable because it heals without contraction and has an avascular cartilage wound bed.

Ear wound models: the hairless mouse ear model

This model has been used in burn studies, reperfusion injuries and flap necrosis. The model consists of full thickness dermal wounds created on the dorsal aspect of the ears. In order to visualize wound epithelialization and neovascularization, the anesthetized animal is placed with the ear wound transilluminated in a trinocular compound microscope.

The advantages of this model are that virtually all healing observed is attributed to epithelialization and subsequent granulation accompanying the neovascularization. The healing is without contraction. The effect of different topical agents on epithelialization and vascularization can be evaluated in a clinically relevant way. The architecture of the hairless mouse skin, however, in many ways is different from human skin. This model has also been used to study impaired healing during pathologic processes (diabetes, immunosuppression and ischemia).

The rabbit ear model. This model is an analog to the hairless mouse ear wound model and has been used as an ischemic model as well as for investigating hypergranulation. In this model, several wounds on each ear can serve as treated group or controls. Tissue explants of the new tissue can be labeled in culture for new collagen, protein, glycosaminoglycans or DNA synthesis. The rabbit ear has the additional advantage of a very constant anatomy of the three major vascular pedicles. When two of these are divided, the ear is rendered reproducibly ischemic but yet it survives. This allows an examination of different agents during ischemic conditions with impaired healing.

Incisional wound models

Like the excisional wounds, this type also fulfills many of the mentioned criteria of a good animal model because it can be accurately reproduced and be available for multiple investigations. The wound(s) can be made anywhere on the body surface as well as in most other organs. The shape of the wound depends on the purpose of the study. This model can be used to investigate the wound healing process and the influence of different systemic and local compounds as well as dressings. During the last century, it has been extensively used in skin and all organs available for surgery (retina, tendons, fascia, inside the body cavities, etc.) and the outcome measurements have primarily been wound strength, collagen content and histology. Breaking strength parameters or bursting pressure measurements can evaluate incision wounds and anastomoses in hollow organs.

Superficial wound models

This type of model is mainly used in experiments related to skin. Different techniques are used to separate the layers of the dermis (dermatome, sucking, tape stripping, etc.) in order to make a wound which does not involve the layers beneath the dermis. Using this procedure, it is possible to evaluate epidermal regeneration and matrix production. The influence of different compounds and drugs can be investigated. This model can be used both in animals and in humans as it only produces minor trauma in the tissue, leaving no scar but in some cases a hyperpigmented area. Assessments of these models are provided by histology and barrier integrity.

The blister wound model. This can be used both in animals and in humans for evaluation of epidermal regeneration and the influence of different compounds and drugs. Suction procedures in the same anatomic area or different locations on the body can produce one or more blisters. A scalpel blade can then remove blister roofs. This procedure creates identical superficial wounds of similar diameter and uniform depth.

Absorption of drugs or compounds in different solution or molecular weight and transepidermal water loss (TEWL) can be measured daily and used as a measure for the effect of the barrier function of epidermis. The advantages of this wound model are that all wounds are created at the same time under identical conditions; the wounds are of identical surface area and depth and they can be compared side by side in the same field on the same body area. The disadvantages are that these superficial wounds may be of no relevance to deeper dermal wounds.

The tape stripping skin model. In this model successive stripping of the epidermis using adhesive tape disintegrates the skin barrier. The disintegration of the barrier can be estimated by evaporimeter measuring TEWL. Twenty successive stripping procedures using adhesive tape will normally produce a humid skin surface. However, this method is more damaging for the epidermis than the blister model, leading to changes in physiologic processes like TEWL, which is increased compared to the blister wound.

Partial thickness excisional skin wound model. This type of wound is produced by a hand-held or electrical dermatome. The depth of the wound can be adjusted to the desired type of wound. This model can be used for evaluation of local environmental factors and topical agents. The advantage is that there is small or no wound contraction, the model can be used in animal as well as man, the surface area can be calculated exactly and the wound is stable and easy to handle. The main disadvantage is that it is a surface wound with no possibility of measuring matrix and collagen development. Donor sites are widely used as one of these models in humans.

CONCLUSIONS

The focus of this chapter is on models useful in the study of acute and chronic wounds. Chronic wounds such as venous leg ulcers and diabetic foot ulcers are complex and extremely difficult to model uniquely. To a certain extent, some modeling has occurred, leading to better understanding of the wound problem as well as the science of modeling. In reality, chronic wounds are incredibly difficult to represent in experiments, be these in animals or in other conditions. This chapter has examined the principles of modeling and the role of animal models as well as the potential of other means of modeling.

When choosing the correct model in wound healing, many different factors have to be taken into consideration. Is there a human model available? Especially, the choice of models for different sequences in the wound healing process and for wounds in the clinical life have been problematic. The background for choosing a model has been discussed and the models normally used in adult soft tissue wound healing research described and advantages and disadvantages mentioned.

It is useful to emphasize that wounds are heterogeneous, and wound healing is a multi-factorial process. This renders the interpretation of clinical trials difficult. In commenting on the slow progress in clinical wound healing research, it has been said: 'to make a difference, there must be a difference'. Most clinicians have used this as a guide that makes legitimate their attempts at using wound complications as an end-point in healing studies. For this approach to be universally successful, large numbers of patients would need to be enrolled in studies and yet the specific problem may not be solved owing to the complexity of the end-points. There is a need, therefore, for experimental models to relate an objective measure of one or more wound healing components to actual clinical events – this is the model that we seek.

References

1. Gottrup F, Ågren MS, Karlsmark T. Models for use in wound healing research: a survey focusing on *in vitro* and *in vivo* adult soft tissue. *Wound Repair Regen* 2000;8:83–96

2. Gottrup F. Experimental wound healing research. The use of models. *EWMA Journal* 2001;1:5–8

3. Burnand KG, Clemenson G, Whimster I, Gaunt J, Browse NL. The effect of sustained venous hypertension on the skin capillaries of the canine hind model. *Br J Surg* 1982;69:41–4

4. Browse NL, Burnand KG. The cause of venous ulceration. *Lancet* 1982;2:243–5

5. Manna V, Bern J, Marks R. An animal model for chronic ulceration. *Br J Dermatol* 1982;106:169–91

6. Davidson JM. Animal models for wound repair. *Arch Dermatol Res* 1998;290 (Suppl):S1–11

7. Reswick JB, Rogers JE. Experience at Los Amogos Hospital with devices and techniques to prevent pressure sores. In: Kendi RM, Cowden JM, eds. *Bed Sore Biomechanics*. London: Macmillan, 1976;301–10

8. Staarink HAM. *Sitting Posture, Comfort and Pressure*. Delft: Delft University Press, 1995

9. Bardsley WG, Sattar A, Armstrong JR, Shah M, Brosnan P, Ferguson MWJ. Quantitative analysis of wound healing. *Wound Repair Regen* 1995;3:426–41

10. Hunt TK, Goodson WHI, Scheuenstuhl H. A strategy for human studies: thoughts on models. In: Janssen H, Rooman R, Robertson JIS, eds. *Wound Healing*. Petersfield: Wrightson Biomedical Publishing, 1991:177–87

11. Salén JCW. Animal models – principles and problems. In: Svendsen P, Hau J, eds. *Handbook of Laboratory Animal Science, Vol II: Animal Models*. Boca Raton: CRC Press, 1994:1–6

12. Bernard C. *An Introduction to the Study of Experimental Medicine (1865)*. Translated by Green HC. New York: Dover, 1957

13. *The Compact Edition of the Oxford English Dictionary*. Oxford: Oxford University Press, 1971

14. Gottrup F. Physiology and pathophysiology of wound healing. In: Jeppsson B, ed. *Animal Modelling in Surgical Research*. London: Harwood Academic Press, 1997:29–35

15. King NW. Simian models of acquired immunodeficiency syndrome (AIDS): a review. *Vet Pathol* 1986;23:345–53

16. Lewis P. Animal tests for teratogenicity, their relevance to clinical practice. In: Hawkins DF, ed. *Drug and Pregnancy: Human Teratogenesis and Related Problems*. Edinburgh: Churchill Livingstone, 1983:17–21

17. Calabrese EJ. *Principles of Animal Extrapolation*. Chelsea, MI: Lewis, 1991

18. Johnson S, Kile R, Fliegelman M, Fix JC. Differences in skin surfaces according to age in age groups by subjective methods. *J Toilet Goods Assoc* 1951;16:35–8

19. Montagna W. Cutaneous comparative biology. *Arch Dermatol* 1971;104:577–91

20. Landsdown ABG. The mammalian skin: structural variations and responses to injury. *Biologist* 1986;33:253–60

21. Mount LE, Ingram DL. *The Pig as a Laboratory Animal*. Academic Press: London, 1971

22. Jorgensen LN, Kallehave F, Karlsmark T, Vejlsgaard GL, Gottrup F. Evaluation of the wound healing potential in human beings from the subcutaneous insertion of expanded polytetrafluoroethylene tubes. A methodologic study. *Wound Repair Regen* 1994;2:20–30

23. Cohen IK, Moore CD, Diegelmann RF. Onset and localization of collagen synthesis during

wound healing in open rat skin wounds. *Proc Soc Exp Biol Med* 1979;160:458–62

24. Svendsen P, Gottrup F. Comparative biology of animals and man in surgical research. In: Jeppsson B, ed. *Animal Modelling in Surgical Research*. Philadelphia: Harwood Academic Press, 1998:1–15

25. Gottrup F. Experimental tissue trauma and healing. In: Jensen SL, Gregersen H, Shokouh-Amiri MH, Moody FG, eds. *Essentials of Experimental Surgery: Gastroenterology*. Chapter 34. Amsterdam: Harwood Academic Press, 1996: 1–11

26. Gottrup F, Ågren M, Karlsmark T. Wound healing. In: Gabard P, Elsner P, Surber C, Treffel, eds. *Dermatopharmacology of Topical Preparations*. Berlin: Springer–Verlag, 1999: 417–41

The role of surgical intervention in chronic wounds

13

C. P. Shearman

This chapter will examine the potential ways in which surgical intervention may aid healing either by direct action on the wound itself or by correcting the underlying pathology that has led to the problem. There have been many enthusiastic reports of benefits of intervention, but generally there is lack of robust evidence to draw firm conclusions about efficacy and, in particular, cost-effectiveness. Currently, the decision to intervene has to be based on the merits of the individual case.

GENERAL PRINCIPLES

Many of these lesions will occur in elderly frail patients with significant co-morbidity. Before considering intervention, other conditions such as anemia or heart failure should be optimized, both to improve the chances of healing as well as to reduce the risk of surgery. Ulcers associated with acute inflammatory conditions such as rheumatoid arthritis rarely heal unless the primary condition is brought under control medically. Drugs such as steroids or antimitotic agents may impair healing and it is important to determine whether it is possible to stop them or reduce the dose in the individual patient. Poor social conditions, including nutrition, contribute to the prognosis of ulcer healing and the chance of recurrence and so, if possible, should be improved[1]. This is sometimes not possible but needs to be taken into account if contemplating intervention, as it

will significantly affect the prognosis for long-term success. Similarly, limited mobility, especially if the patient is chair-bound, increases lower limb edema and carries a poor outlook for successful healing[2].

Rehabilitation of patients back into the community can be very time-consuming and they may occupy acute hospital beds for a long period. During a prolonged hospital stay, many patients will lose their network of social support, making return even more difficult. If hospitalization is required, a clear management plan needs to be agreed with targets to be achieved so that the appropriate time to discharge can be clearly identified.

A confident diagnosis of the underlying etiology is essential if intervention is going to be of any benefit. This can be very difficult in ulcers of mixed etiology. For example, in leg ulcers of mixed venous and arterial etiology, the relative contribution of each component must be carefully assessed to avoid unnecessary revascularization procedures or inappropriate compression therapy. In some conditions, predictors of poor outcome such as deep venous insufficiency associated with venous ulcers should be taken into account[3]. In an unfit patient with a poor chance of success, intervention should be avoided and conservative treatment pursued.

Anesthetic techniques need to be carefully selected by an experienced anesthetist depending on the planned procedure and the health of the patient. Regional techniques such as spinal, epidural or local blockade are often the most suitable for lower limb surgery. Although the surgery itself will often be relatively minor, great care needs to taken to balance the perceived benefit to be gained against the risk to the patient and use of resources. Unless there is a significant chance of benefit, surgery is often best avoided.

Investigation and selection of patients for intervention requires a focused team effort and protocols. If it is policy to offer surgery to patients with venous ulcers and superficial venous disease, all patients will require a venous duplex ultrasound scan to identify those likely to benefit. This needs planning and resources, but units which have developed multidisciplinary teams and clear protocols regarding intervention achieve better results. The Gloucestershire Vascular Group, UK, increased the 12-week venous ulcer healing rates from 12% to 47% and reduced the 12-month recurrence rate from 50% to 17%[4].

LOCAL WOUND CARE

The removal of dead or infected material from the wound is a basic surgical principle. This may need to be done urgently in a patient at risk of developing sepsis, but, when minor, can often be achieved by carefully separating the dead tissue with sharp dissection in the clinic or by the use of topical desloughing agents. Maggots are especially useful for this purpose in chronic wounds of the lower extremity and can be used in the community or hospital[5]. They separate necrotic tissue from living tissue without causing damage to the living tissue, allowing healing to continue at the same time. This may be particularly useful in patients with wounds infected or colonized with antibiotic-resistant bacteria. Chronic wounds sometimes develop a fibrous chronic edge and surgical

excision of this area may accelerate healing. Whether this is due to the build-up of chronic scar tissue that prevents healing or perhaps stimulates the release of growth factors is unclear, but has been recognized to be beneficial for many years[6]. Some groups favor complete excision (shaving) of the ulcer in venous disease with split skin grafting. While this is quite a major undertaking for the patient, it does seem, in non-controlled series, to have long-term benefit[7].

Skin grafting of ulcers will reduce the time to healing and often reduces pain. For small wounds, pinch grafting can be very useful. In the clinic, small discs of skin are harvested under local anesthetic and placed on the chronic wound. Larger areas can be covered by meshed split skin grafts (Figure 13.1). The chronic wound must be clean and free from infection, especially *Streptococcus* and *Pseudomonas*. Early results are often encouraging, but, unless the underlying pathology has been corrected, the ulcer recurrence rate generally will be high[8]. This is particularly true in venous ulcers. Bioengineered skin substitutes have been reported to accelerate wound healing in long-standing ulcers[9]. However, large-size randomized controlled studies are needed to assess the potential role of skin grafting in general compared to standard compression therapy[10].

Topical negative pressure may improve the rate of wound healing. Vacuum-assisted closure (VAC) devices exert a constant suction under an impermeable dressing. This removes excess tissue fluid, reduces the size of the wound by sucking it together and may help to remove necrotic tissue. VAC pumps have been used to aid healing of toe amputation wounds in diabetics left to heal by secondary intention[11] but may have a much wider application to chronic wounds. However, to date there have been no studies of sufficient quality to assess the real effect of these devices[12].

VENOUS ULCERS

These are the commonest cause of leg ulcers in the Western world. The exact pathophysiology of the ulcers remains unclear but is associated with failure of the calf venous pump and subsequent failure of the ambulatory venous pressure to fall. This is commonly caused by valvular incompetence in the deep venous system, calf perforating veins or superficial veins resulting in reflux. Less commonly, it is associated with chronic venous obstruction. Either way, this results in venous hypertension that has adverse effects on the microcirculation leading to ulceration. Surgery has focused on methods to correct venous incompetence that should promote ulcer healing and prevent recurrence. There have been no large randomized studies of surgery compared to compression, but generally results have been disappointing. This may be due to incomplete understanding of the pathology of the condition and the importance of the microcirculation or failure to correctly identify or correct the venous abnormalities.

Some patients with ulcers will have saphenous incompetence alone. The number varies from series to series and depends on how the patients are investigated, but probably includes 20–40% of all venous ulcer patients[13]. Saphenofemoral ligation (with or without stripping of the long saphenous vein) or saphenopopliteal ligation may lead to healing and prevent recurrence in over 90% of these patients[14]. In a recent large community-based study, patients who had surgical correction of superficial venous reflux did not have improved healing rates compared to those on conservative treatment, but did have significant reductions in recurrence rates from 28, 30 and 44% at 1, 2 and 3 years in non-operated patients, respectively, to 14, 20 and 26% in those who had surgery[15]. The morbidity and mortality for this procedure are very low and it can be readily performed under local anesthesia[16] (Figure 13.2).

Perforator incompetence alone is relatively uncommon – occurring in 0–8% of patients with ulcers – and the role of surgery is controversial and unproven. Despite this, there has been considerable recent interest in the treatment of these with subfascial endoscopic perforator surgery (SEPS), as the technique can be carried out utilizing small incisions remote from the ulcerated area which heal without the problems of direct perforator surgery. Initial uncontrolled reports suggest that SEPS may aid ulcer healing either alone or in combination with saphenous vein surgery[17], but no controlled studies have evaluated either the role of perforator surgery or SEPS in particular.

Patients with deep venous incompetence and superficial venous incompetence have been shown to benefit from treatment of the superficial component of their problem. However, as only around 40% of ulcers may heal with such treatment[4], it is important to try to select those patients likely to benefit. At present, this is difficult to do but those who have evidence from either the history or imaging of postphlebitic damage to the vein seem to fare badly. Attempts to repair or reconstruct deep venous valves alone or in combination with ligation of perforating veins seems to improve venous valve function, but it is unclear to what extent this may benefit patients with ulceration[18].

Venous reconstruction for patients with occluded deep veins is only occasionally undertaken. Methods using the contralateral long saphenous vein to bypass an occluded iliac vein (the DePalma operation) can improve the venous drainage, but results, especially long-term, are variable and should only be undertaken in patients with intractable symptoms not controlled with conservative measures[19]. Radiologic techniques such as venous dilation and stent placement have been shown to work in some situations, offering a less invasive alternative if it is felt necessary to recanalize an occluded vein[20].

ARTERIAL (ISCHEMIC) ULCERS

Chronic ischemia is a common contributing factor to failure of wound healing. Peripheral arterial disease (PAD) is very prevalent in the Western world and the commonest cause of ischemia of the lower limbs. In a community-based study of males and females over 55 years of age, 4.5% had symptomatic PAD and a further 24.6% were found to have evidence of atheromatous disease[21]. Wounds can occur directly due to the lack of tissue perfusion but often they follow minor trauma, such as chafing from footwear, in an ischemic, but previously asymptomatic limb.

Identification of ischemia is based on general principles such as history, examination and basic tests such as ankle blood pressure. Other more sophisticated tests have been used such as transcutaneous oxygen tension $(TcPO_2)$[22] and laser Doppler[23]. The most common problem encountered, though, is not the identification of underlying ischemia but whether it is severe enough to prevent wound healing. Disappointingly, there are no objective tests which can be widely applied to wounds which will predict healing, especially in those where there is borderline ischemia. Clinical judgement is often the best tool and careful observation of a wound can identify signs of healing.

The role of surgery is to optimize the wound environment by removing dead and infected tissue and draining abscesses. This must sometimes be undertaken urgently to control spreading soft tissue infection and sepsis. If, on the criteria outlined above, it is felt necessary to revascularize the limb, several options are available. Conventional angioplasty is appealing but, for lesions below the inguinal ligament, the long-term patency is disappointing. The development of subintimal angioplasty, largely by the group in Leicester, UK, has allowed endovascular treatment to be offered to patients with more extensive disease, particularly of the calf vessels[24]. In this technique, the guide wire is deliberately passed into the artery wall above the diseased segment with X-ray screening. The wire is then advanced, passing through the media, effectively creating a dissection or false lumen. When beyond the diseased segment, the wire is manipulated back into the true lumen (Figure 13.3). This technique can be difficult to master but excellent results have been obtained. Other groups have been unable to achieve long-term patency rates as good as this and considerable debate surrounds the value of subintimal angioplasty[25]. What does seem apparent is that angioplasty is a much less invasive technique than bypass surgery and possibly more appropriate for elderly frail patients. Even if the angioplasty site reoccludes, it will often stay open long enough to allow tissue healing and remove the immediate risk of limb loss[26].

Bypass surgery has been the mainstay of treatment. Procedures can be divided into those that increase blood flow into the femoral artery (inflow procedures) and those that bypass diseased arterial segments below the groin. Increased experience with iliac angioplasty has reduced the numbers of surgical inflow procedures being undertaken. For iliac artery disease treated by angioplasty, patency rates at 1 year of 75–94%[27] can be expected for stenoses and 64% for an occlusion[28]. Most surgical inflow procedures are undertaken using prosthetic bypass material and, in limbs with chronic wounds, this increases the risk of infection considerably. Vascular graft infection is a life-threatening complication and endovascular techniques such as angioplasty can avoid this complication, so should be used preferentially whenever possible in patients with open lower limb wounds. The use of antibiotic impregnated grafts has disappointingly failed to reduce rates of infection[29].

Inflow procedures are either anatomic, e.g. aortobifemoral or iliofemoral, or extra-anatomic, e.g. axillofemoral or cross-femoral bypasses. Extra-anatomic bypasses tend to be less invasive and more suitable for frail patients but may have less good long-term patency.

To bypass arterial disease below the groin, superior patency rates are obtained using the patient's own vein, either by reversing it or by cutting the valves and ligating the branches (*in situ*)[30]. Even for short bypasses, above the knee vein is superior to prosthetic material over the longer term. If the long saphenous vein is not available, vein harvested from the arm or short saphenous vein may be used[31]. Vein also has the advantage that it is more resistant to infection and therefore more suited to patients with chronic wounds. The exception to this are patients infected with methicillin-resistant *Staphylococcus aureus* (MRSA). The mortality and morbidity of vascular graft infections with MRSA are very high and vein seems to be vulnerable. In patients with active MRSA infection, it is best to avoid surgical bypass if at all possible and, if there is no alternative, to try to eradicate infection first and to cover the procedure with appropriate antibiotics[32].

In patients with critical limb ischemia, disease often extends distally into the calf vessels necessitating bypass to that level (Figure 13.4). Using autologous vein, good results can be obtained, with limb salvage rates of 70–75%. Some patients, particularly diabetics, will have gangrene of the foot with occluded calf vessels and a patent popliteal artery. They may benefit from popliteal to pedal bypass. The vein can be harvested from above the knee so that only a small incision at the ankle or foot needs to be made.

In patients requiring bypass to the calf vessels, prosthetic grafts give very poor results. There is some evidence to suggest that using an adjunctive hood or patch made of autologous vein at the distal anastomoses can improve patency results[33]. This remains controversial and currently there is no randomized controlled evidence to show that this is a cost-effective method of managing critical limb ischemia.

In some patients in whom vein is not available, the distal run-off vessels are poor or the extent of tissue loss on the foot is extensive, primary amputation is the only option available. It should always be borne in mind that the worst result for the patient functionally and the most expensive for the health economy is a failed bypass that comes to amputation.

Amputation of dead tissue is often delayed after bypass unless overtly infected. In our unit, we have tended to carry out any adjunctive amputation of a digit or dead tissue at the time of bypass. This prevents further returns to the operating theater and delays in rehabilitation. The only exception is when ischemia is borderline and it is not clear whether the tissue will survive with the improved blood supply. In this situation, delayed excision may result in less tissue loss.

COMBINED ARTERIAL AND VENOUS ULCERS

Some patients are found to have venous ulcers with a moderate degree of arterial disease with ankle brachial pressure indices (ABPI) of 0.6–0.8. With care, these can be managed with modified compression. Those with more marked arterial disease (ABPI < 0.6) usually need revascularization, preferably angioplasty, but occasionally bypass surgery. This seems to have an impact with over 50% of ulcers healing, but postphlebitic ulcers seem to respond least well[34].

THE DIABETIC FOOT

Seven to ten percent of patients with diabetes mellitus will develop a foot ulcer and in many this will ultimately result in a major lower limb amputation[35]. Patients with diabetes have an increased risk of arterial disease and neuropathy and these are often compounded by infection of the soft tissues and bone. In many patients, all three components are apparent and the patient presents as an emergency (Figure 13.5). Initial treatment includes intravenous antibiotics and fluids, removal of dead and infected material and drainage of any collection of pus. The clinical signs can be deceptive due in part to the neuropathy and impaired immunologic response, and it is often found that the extent of tissue damage and infection is far greater than expected and a plain X-ray of the foot may reveal extensive bone destruction and gas in the tissues (Figure 13.6). Surgical exploration of the foot should be carried out as soon as possible, irrespective of the underlying pathology, as rapid deterioration can occur.

Once the situation is stabilized, assessment can be undertaken to ascertain the principal cause of the problem. Approximately 50% will be neuropathic, 10% ischemic and 30–40% will be neuroischemic. Neuropathic ulcers usually require pressure-relieving measures such as initial bed rest, walking casts or specifially designed footwear. The limb may need revascularization with angioplasty or surgery. The same principles apply to chronic ulcers except that magnetic resonance scanning can be helpful in determining the extent of underlying tissue damage and infection. Neuropathic ulcers are often surrounded by a thick ring of keratin (Figure 13.7) which needs removal to allow healing.

When the condition is reversed, the foot can be reconstructed (Figure 13.8). It is vitally important that the patient receives advice about risk management for vascular disease and foot care to try to reduce recurrence[36].

SUMMARY

Surgical intervention has a lot to offer in the management of many chronic wounds. The key lies in correct diagnosis of the underlying pathology and selecting patients who are most likely to benefit from the intervention. Above all else, there is a need for well-conducted, randomized controlled studies to evaluate the effectiveness of the intervention.

References

1. Callum MJ, Harper DR, Dale JJ, Ruckley CV. Chronic leg ulceration: socio-economic aspects. *Scot Med J* 1988;33:358–60
2. Ryan TJ. Common denominators for the low-cost management of leg conditions. *Lower Extremity Wounds* 2002;1:62–7
3. McDaniel HB, Marston WA, Farber MA, *et al.* Recurrence of chronic venous ulcers on the basis of clinical, etiological, anatomic, and plethysmographic criteria and air plethysmography. *J Vasc Surg* 2002;35:723–8
4. Ghauri ASK, Taylor MC, Whyman MR, Earnshaw JJ, Heather BP, Poskitt KR. Influence of a specialised leg ulcer service on management and outcome. *Br J Surg* 2000;87:1048–56
5. Mumcuoglu KY. Clinical applications for maggots in wound care. *Am J Clin Dermatol* 2001;2:219–27
6. Browse NL, Burnand K, Irvine AT, Wilson NM. *Diseases of the Veins*. London: Arnold, 1999:581
7. Scmeller W, Gaber Y. Surgical removal of ulcer and lipodermatosclerosis followed by split-skin grafting (shave therapy) yields good long term results for 'non-healing' venous leg ulcers. *Acta Derm-Venereol* 2000;80:267–71
8. Turczynski R, Tarplia E. Treatment of leg ulcers with split skin grafts: early and late results. *Scand J Plast Reconstr Hand Surg* 1999;33:301–5
9. Brem H, Balledux J, Sukkarieh T, Carson P, Falanga V. Healing of venous ulcers of long duration with a bilayered skin substitute:

results from a general surgery and dermatological department. *Dermatol Surg* 2001;27: 915–19

10. Jones JE, Nelson EA. Skin grafting for venous ulcers (Cochrane Review). In: *The Cochrane Library*, Issue 2, Oxford; Update Software, 2002

11. McCallon SK, Knight CA, Valiulus JP, Cunningham MW, McCullo Farinas LP. Vacuum-assisted closure versus saline-moistened gauze in the healing of postoperative diabetic foot wounds. *Ostomy Wound Manag* 2000;46: 28–32

12. Evans D, Land L. Topical negative pressure for treating chronic wounds. (Cochrane Review). In: *The Cochrane Library*, Issue 2, Oxford: Update Software, 2002

13. Darke SG. Can we tailor surgery to the venous abnormality? In: Ruckley CV, Fowkes FGR, Bradbury AW, eds. *Venous Disease*, London: Springer-Verlag, 1999:139–49

14. Darke SG, Penfold C. Venous ulceration and saphenous ligation. *Eur J Vasc Surg* 1992;6:4–9

15. Barwell JR, Taylor M, Deacon J, *et al.* Surgical correction of isolated superficial venous reflux reduces long-term recurrence rate in chronic venous leg ulcers. *Eur J Vasc Endovasc Surg* 2000;20:363–8

16. Bello M, Scriven M, Hartshone T, Bell PR, Naylor AR, London NJ. Role of superficial venous surgery in the treatment of venous ulceration. *Br J Surg* 1999;86:755–9

17. Lee DW, Chan AC, Lam YH, *et al.* Early clinical outcomes after subfascial endoscopic perforator surgery (SEPS) and saphenous vein surgery in chronic venous insufficiency. *Surg Endosc* 2001;15:737–40

18. Abidia A, Hardy SC. Surgery for deep venous incompetence (Cochrane Review). In: *The Cochrane Library*, Issue 2, Oxford: Update Software, 2002

19. Jost CJ, Gloviczki P, Cherry KJ, *et al.* Surgical reconstruction of ileofemoral veins and the inferior vena cava for non-malignant occlusive disease. *J Vasc Surg* 2001;33:320–8

20. Razavi MK, Hansch EC, Kee ST, Sze DY, Dake MD. Chronically occluded inferior venae cavae: endovascular treatment. *Radiology* 2000:214:133–8

21. Leng GC, Lee AJ, Fowkes FG, *et al.* Incidence, natural history and cardiovascular events in symptomatic and asymptomatic peripheral arterial disease in the general population. *Int J Epidemiol* 1996;25:1172–81

22. Romanelli M, Falanga V. Measurement of transcutaneous oxygen tension in chronic wounds. In: Mani R, Falanga V, Shearman CP, Sandeman D, eds. *Chronic Wound Healing*. London: WB Saunders, 1999:68–80

23. He C, Cherry GW. Measurement of blood flow in patients with leg ulcers. In: Mani R, Falanga V, Shearman CP, Sandeman D, eds. *Chronic Wound Healing*. London: WB Saunders, 1999: 50–67

24. Nydahl S, Hartshorne T, Bell PRF, Bolia A, London NJM. Subintimal angioplasty of infrapopliteal occlusions in critically ischaemic legs. *Eur J Vasc Endovasc Surg* 1997;14:212–16

25. McCarthy RJ, Neary W, Roobottom C, Tottle A, Ashley S. Short-term results of femoropopliteal subintimal angioplasty. *Br J Surg* 2000;87:1361–5

26. Lofberg AM, Lorelius LE, Karacagil S, Westman B, Almgren B, Berqvist D. The use of below-knee percutaneous transluminal angioplasty in arterial occlusive disease causing chronic critical limb ischaemia. *Cardiovasc Intervent Radiol* 1996;19:317–22

27. Rutherford RB, Durham JA, Kumpe DA. Endovascular intervention for lower extremity ischemia. In: Rutherford RB, ed. *Vascular Surgery*, 4th ed. Philadelphia: WB Saunders, 1995: 858–74

28. Leu AJ, Schneider F, Canova CR, Hoffman U. Long term results after recanalisation of chronic iliac artery occlusions by combined catheter therapy without stent placement. *Eur J Vasc Endovasc Surg* 1999;18:499–505

29. Braithwaite BD, Davies B, Heather BP, Earnshaw JJ on behalf of the Joint Vascular Research Group. Early results of a randomised trial of rifampicin-bonded Dacron grafts for extra-anatomic vascular reconstruction. *Br J Surg* 1998;85:1378–81

30. Michaels JA. Choice of material for above-knee femoropopliteal bypass graft. *Br J Surg* 1989;76:7–14

31. Tisi PV, Crow AJ, Shearman CP. Arm vein reconstruction in limb salvage: long term outcome. *Ann R Coll Surg* 1996;78:497–500

32. London NJM, Nasim A. Management of methicillin-resistant *Staphylococcus aureus* infection in vascular patients. In: Earnshaw JJ, Murie JA, eds. *The Evidence for Vascular Surgery*. Shropshire: TFM Publishing 1999:183–8

33. Wijesinghe LD, Beardsmore DM, Scott DJA. Polytetrafluoroethylene (PTFE) femorodistal grafts with a distal vein cuff for critical ischaemia. *Eur J Vasc Endovasc Surg* 1998;15: 449–53

34. Treiman GS, Copland S, McNamara RM, Yellin AE, Schneider PA, Treiman RL. Factors influencing ulcer healing in patients with combined arterial and venous insufficiency. *J Vasc Surg* 2001;33:1158–64

35. NHS Centre for Reviews and Dissemination. Complications of diabetes. *Effect. Health Care* 1999;5:1–12

36. Valk GD, Kriegsman DMW, Assedenlft WJJ. Patient education for preventing diabetic foot ulceration (Cochrane Review). In: *The Cochrane Library*, Issue 2, Oxford: Update Software, 2002

Conclusion

14

C. P. Shearman and R. Mani

The overall aim of this book has been to discuss the current evidence for change in the management of chronic wounds and to speculate on the direction this field will take over the next decade. It is now widely recognized that chronic wounds, such as diabetic foot ulcers and venous leg ulcers, are a major cause of morbidity in society and place an enormous burden on the health economy. The impact on the quality of life of such patients is considerable and comparable with many more high-profile conditions that receive more resources for treatment and research. Disappointingly though, despite recent increases in awareness of the problem, there is little to suggest that the outlook for patients with these wounds has changed dramatically. The failure to achieve the reduction in amputation rate in the diabetic population is a depressing example of this failure. Why is this and how are we to respond to this challenge?

Increased understanding of the biology of wound healing has perhaps not produced the dramatic improvements for which we hoped. The disappointing results with growth factors have illustrated the complexities of the healing process. One of the most neglected areas has been in prevention. Many patients who suffer deep vein thrombosis will subsequently develop leg ulcers and yet are given little advice about methods to reduce this risk. Patients with diabetic neuropathy often present again with further foot ulcers that with better care could have been avoided.

Prevention is obviously the best solution for the patient and usually the most economic. National Service Frameworks (NSFs) in the United Kingdom have been developed for some diseases and determine the standard of care to be expected. Considerable emphasis tends to be placed on prevention and patient education. The NSF in diabetes, which is coming out in stages, directs attention to this area[1]. The challenge is how to facilitate this process and achieve good patient compliance.

Some of the most dramatic results of wound healing have come from units that have formed multidisciplinary teams across the community and hospital settings[2]. It is often unclear whether the apparent improvement is due to better methods of treatment or simply the enthusiasm that tends to be generated for an often-neglected condition. Whatever the reason, it illustrates what has been accepted in many other fields that chronic wound care does require teams with expertise. It is relevant to mention that the understanding, and therefore the management, of mucosal ulcers in the gastrointestinal tract has changed dramatically since the correlation between infection and pathology was accepted. Chronic wound management needs such dramatic developments to occur for the course to change favorably.

There can be no doubt that, against this background of prevention and improved delivery of wound care, further advances in the understanding of wound biology will continue. Interest in the balance between environmental and inherited factors has stimulated new therapeutic options in some areas. The genotype of some individuals makes them susceptible to specific diseases or respond poorly to stimuli such as trauma. The inherited components of wound healing have largely been unexplored and may offer new options for intervention.

We hope this book, if nothing else, has stimulated interest and enthusiasm for the treatment for what is globally an enormous, but sadly neglected, problem.

References

1. Department of Health. *National Service Framework for Diabetes*. London: Department of Health. http://www.doh.gov.uk/nsf/diabetes/index.htm

2. Gottrup F, Holstein P, Jorgensen B, Lohmann M, Karlsmark T. A new concept of a multidisciplinary wound healing centre and a national expert function of wound healing. *Arch Surg* 2001;136:765–71

Chronic wound management illustrated

List of illustrations

Figure 1.1 Remoulding of a wound during healing may result in unacceptable scarring such as keloids

Figure 1.2 Orientation of new capillaries around wounds

Figure 1.3 Mid-twentieth century wound healing studies in a hamster cheek pouch

Figure 1.4 Lymphedema in an immobile patient in the UK

Figure 1.5 Community shoe worker

Figure 1.6 Acupuncture practiced at a Chinese Traditional Medicine Clinic in Beijing

Figure 1.7 Movement rather than a focus on exercise characterizes Asian practice

Figure 1.8 Site of expansion of the upper dermis

Figure 1.9 Ultrasound of the skin showing different colorations indicating relative water content

Figure 1.10 The Koebner phenomenon in a patient with psoriasis

Figure 1.11 Pyoderma gangrenosum is a spontaneous necrosis of the skin, often at the site of minor injury and often associated with inflammatory bowel disease

Figure 1.12 Painless non-inflammatory deepy-pierced skin wounds in some Asian ceremonies

Figure 4.1 Typical brown skin discoloration characteristic of severe, long-standing venous disease and ulceration with associated typical chronic venous ulceration

Figure 4.2 'Atrophie blanche'

Figure 4.3 Inter-relationship of factors thought to be associated with chronic venous hypertension

Figure 4.4 Effect of compression on the venous system

Figure 4.5 Inverted champagne bottle deformity of the limb due to scarring secondary to chronic venous disease

Figure 4.6 Difficult limb shapes affecting bandage application and performance

Figure 4.7 Class 3c elastic bandage (Surepress) incorporating markers to allow the bandager to gauge the correct application tension

Figure 4.8 Applying orthopedic wool as a protective and absorbent layer prior to the application of compression bandages

Figure 4.9 Short stretch bandage applied in a spiral with 50% overlap

Figure 4.10 Class 3a Litepress bandage applied in a figure-of-eight as part of a four-layer bandage system

Figure 4.11 Cohesive class 3b bandage applied in a spiral as part of a four-layer bandage system

Figure 4.12 Completed four-layer bandage

Figure 4.13 Elastic high compression class 3c bandage (Surepress)

Figure 4.14 The relationship between compression, ankle brachial pressure and the risk of tissue damage

Figure 4.15 Management strategy for the use of compression in patients with a reduced ankle brachial pressure index

Figure 4.16 Reported healing rates from a trial of alternative four-layer compression systems

Figure 5.1 Burn wound on the left arm of a child covered with silver sulfadiazine cream and dressed with a plastic glove taped to the skin

Figure 5.2 Abscess cavity packed with gauze soaked in glycerine and ichthammol in a patient with HIV infection and tuberculosis of the cervical lymph nodes

Figure 5.3 Purple oral Kaposi's sarcoma tumor on the hard palate of an HIV-infected man

Figure 5.4 Endemic Kaposi's sarcoma lesions on the foot of a 55-year-old man

Figure 5.5 Dry gangrene of the toes in a 30-year-old man with HIV infection and a history of smoking

Figure 5.6 Wound breakdown after distal amputation in the same patient as in Figure 5.5

Figure 5.7 Bilateral gangrene of the lower limbs in a 22-year-old HIV infected man who refused amputation for 3 months

Figure 5.8 Necrotizing fasciitis in a 27-year-old woman with AIDS

Figure 5.9 Clean, granulating wound in an HIV-infected woman before split skin grafting

Figure 5.10 Split skin graft failure 1 week after operation of the wound shown in Figure 5.9

Figure 5.11 Thyroid abscess after incision and drainage with a corrugated rubber drain

Figure 6.1 Flowchart outlining the current approach in the management of diabetic foot with ulceration/infection

Figure 6.2 A large non-infected chronic ulcer with hypertrophied edges of more than 2 years' duration which had undergone failed skin grafting twice

Figure 6.3 The same patient as in Figure 6.2 was treated with pulsed galvanic stimulation using silver-mesh stocking electrodes

Figure 6.4 The same ulcer as in Figures 6.2 and 6.3 after 4 months

Figure 6.5 Acute thermal injury to the lateral three toes of the right foot

Figure 6.6 Commercially manufactured collagen membrane derived from sheep's intestine

Figure 6.7 Commercially manufactured collagen membrane derived from reconstituted bovine collagen membrane from the Achilles tendon of sheep

Figure 6.8 Commercially manufactured collagen membrane derived from reconstituted human amniotic collagen membrane

Figure 7.1 Rule of nines

Figures 7.2 Blister is present in second-degree burns

Figures 7.3 After 2–3 days, the blister opens and is a source of potential infection

Figure 7.4 Mixed aspect of superficial and deep second-degree burns of the face

Figure 7.5 The aspect is white over the dorsal aspect of an index finger with third-degree burn

Figure 7.6 Schematic diagram of TransCyte™ showing the temporary colonization by fibroblasts and the presence in this product of growth factors secreted by the cells

Figure 7.7 Integra recently applied on a child's neck

Figure 7.8 After 3–4 weeks, the revascularized collagen can be covered using a thin split-thickness graft

Figure 7.9 Keratinocyte culture is presented in a double container on a semisolid hydrogel

Figure 7.10 Histologic aspect of skin reconstruction after keratinocyte culture using Epibase®

Figure 7.11 Fresh second-degree burns of the hands

Figure 7.12 VAC can be applied in order to reduce edema, a factor which improves vascularization and reduces inflammation

Figure 7.13 Postgrafting local infection

Figure 7.14 Keloid will develop preferably in the adolescent

Figure 11.1 Principle of the laser Doppler imager

Figure 11.2 Laser Doppler image of a thermal burn on an ankle

Figure 11.3 TcPO$_2$ sensor

Figure 11.4 TcPO$_2$ sensors on a patient

Figure 11.5 Wound pH meter

Figure 13.1 Meshed split skin graft to chronic venous ulcer

Figure 13.2 Saphenofemoral junction displayed at surgery just prior to ligation

Figure 13.3 Angiogram showing disease of the tibioperoneal trunk in a patient with diabetes and a foot ulcer, and after successful subintimal angioplasty

Figure 13.4 Distal bypass to the peroneal artery in a patient with critical limb ischemia

Figure 13.5 Neuroischemic diabetic foot with extensive infection

Figure 13.6 X-ray of foot of a diabetic with extensive destruction of the 2nd metatarsal

Figure 13.7 Neuropathic ulcer with keratin ring

Figure 13.8 Reconstructed foot in a diabetic following femoroposterior tibial artery bypass

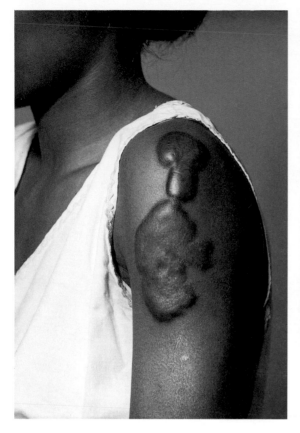

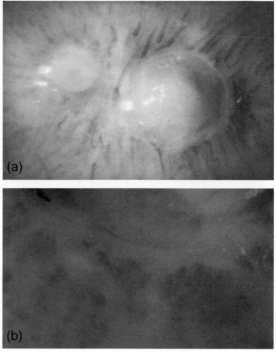

Figure 1.2 (a) Uniform orientation of new capillaries around a healing wound edge; (b) lack of orientation of new capillaries around a non-healing wound

Figure 1.1 Remoulding of a wound during healing may result in unacceptable scarring such as keloids

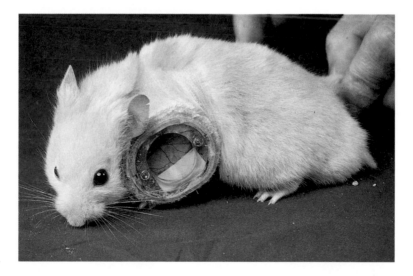

Figure 1.3 Mid-20th century wound healing studies in a hamster cheek pouch, which has now largely been replaced by *in vitro* and human models

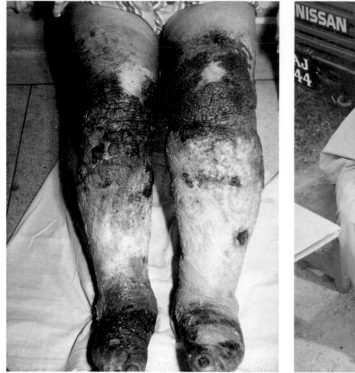

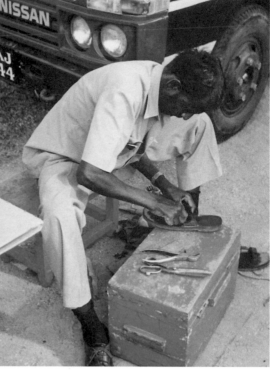

Figure 1.4 Lymphedema in an immobile patient in the UK

Figure 1.5 Community shoe worker at work with his nails! A likely cause of foot ulceration in a patient with leprosy

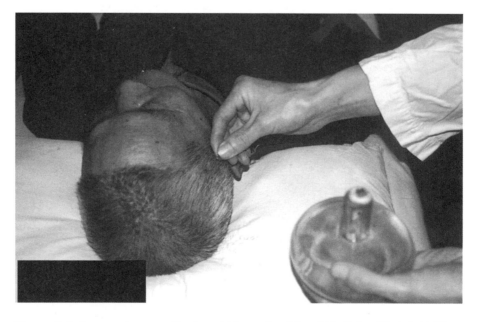

Figure 1.6 Acupuncture practiced at a Chinese Traditional Medicine Clinic in Beijing

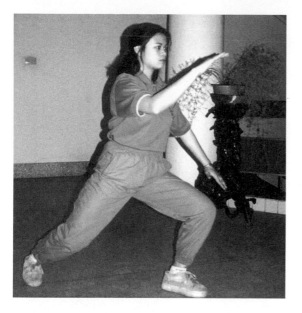

Figure 1.7 Movement rather than a focus on exercise characterizes Asian practice

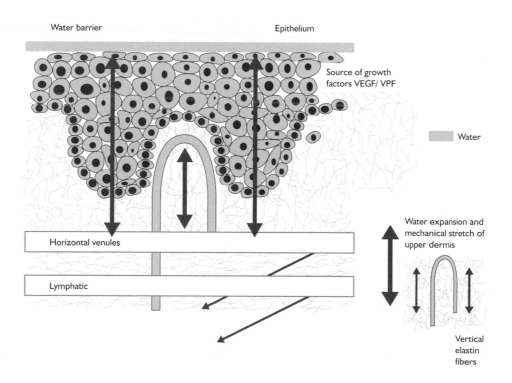

Figure 1.8 Site of expansion of the upper dermis which may be mediated by permeability factors, such as VEGF, that enhance mechanical distortion and lengthening of the upper dermal vasculature

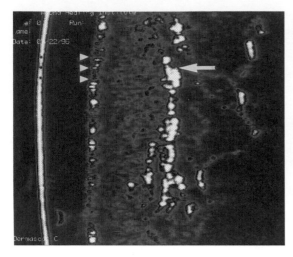

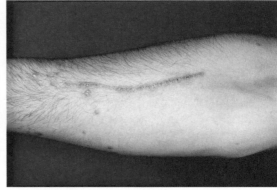

Figure 1.10 The Koebner phenomenon in a patient with psoriasis. A secondary lesion to a recent scratch psoriasis has developed at the site of injury

Figure 1.9 An ultrasound picture of the skin showing different colorations indicating relative water content. It has been shown that the upper dermis contains more water but that it can be easily expanded and, as such, it is usually followed by angiogenesis. Arrowheads, epidermis. Reproduced with permission from reference 20

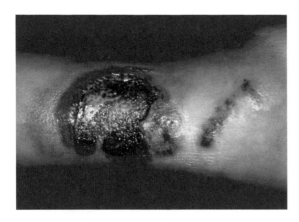

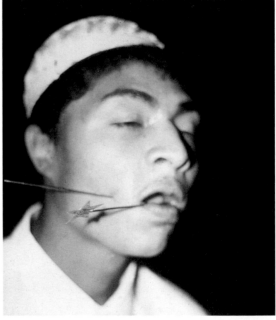

Figure 1.11 Pyoderma gangrenosum is a spontaneous necrosis of the skin, often at the site of minor injury and often associated with inflammatory bowel disease

Figure 1.12 Painless non-inflammatory, deeply-pierced skin wounds in some Asian ceremonies

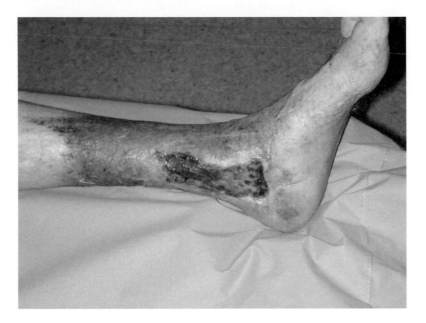

Figure 4.1 Typical brown skin coloration characteristic of severe, long-standing venous disease with associated typical chronic venous ulceration

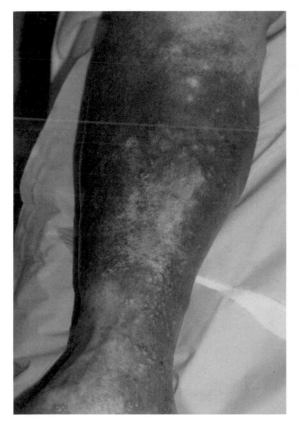

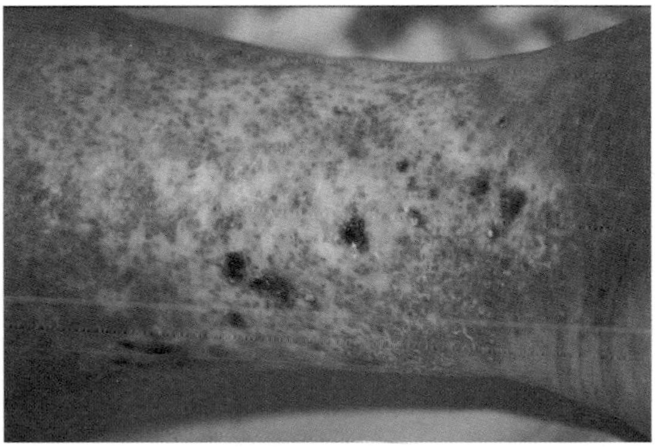

Figure 4.2b 'Atrophie blanche'

Figure 4.2a 'Atrophie blanche'

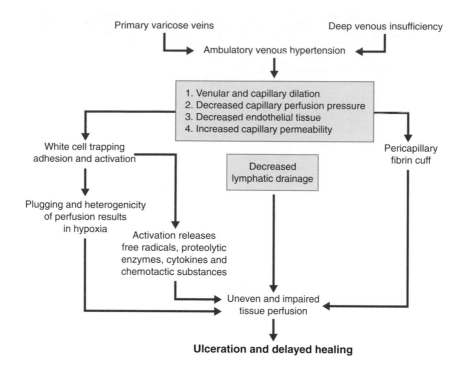

Figure 4.3 Inter-relationship of factors thought to be associated with chronic venous hypertension and venous insufficiency

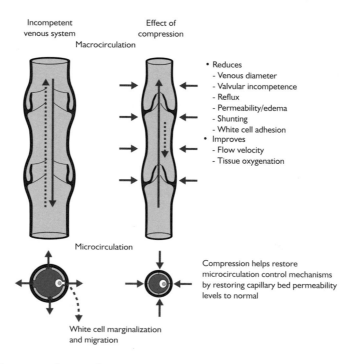

Figure 4.4 Effect of compression on the venous system

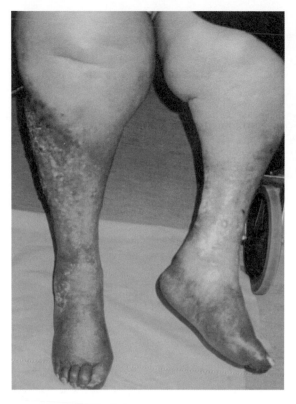

Figure 4.5 Inverted champagne bottle deformity of the limb due to scarring secondary to chronic venous disease

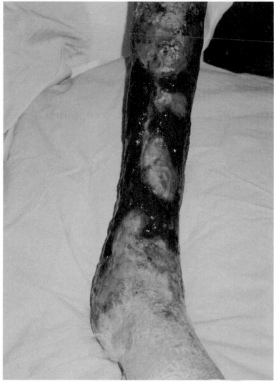

Figure 4.6 Difficult limb shapes affecting bandage application and performance

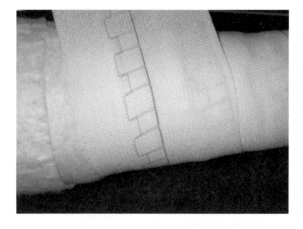

Figure 4.7 Class 3c elastic bandage (Surepress) incorporating markers to allow the bandager to gauge the correct application tension

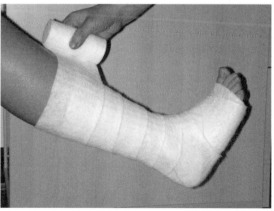

Figure 4.8 Applying orthopedic wool as a protective and absorbent layer prior to the application of compression bandages

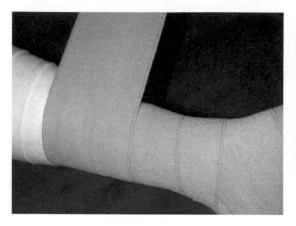

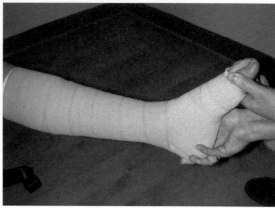

Figure 4.9a Short stretch bandage applied in a spiral with 50% overlap

Figure 4.9b Short stretch bandage applied in a spiral with 50% overlap

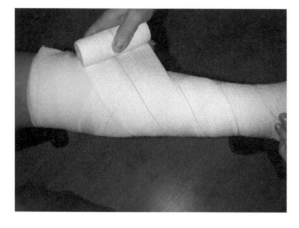

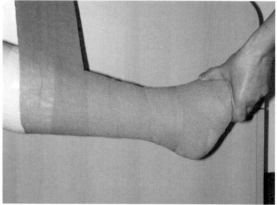

Figure 4.10 Class 3a Litepress bandage applied in a figure-of-eight as part of a four-layer bandage system

Figure 4.11 Cohesive class 3b bandage applied in a spiral as part of a four-layer bandage system

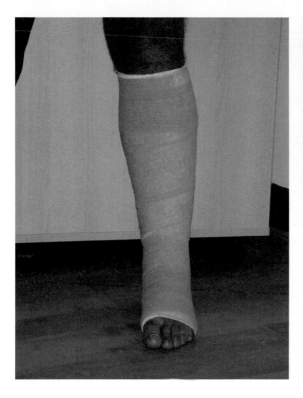

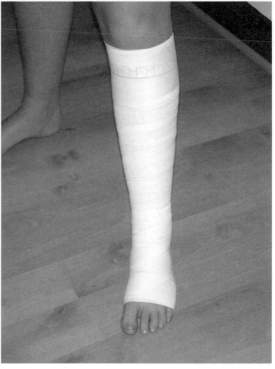

Figure 4.12 Completed four-layer bandage

Figure 4.13 Elastic high compression class 3c bandage (Surepress)

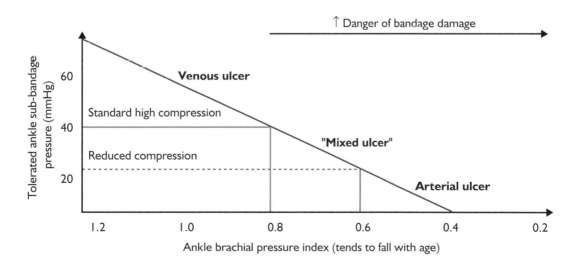

Figure 4.14 The relationship between compression, ankle brachial pressure and the risk of tissue damage

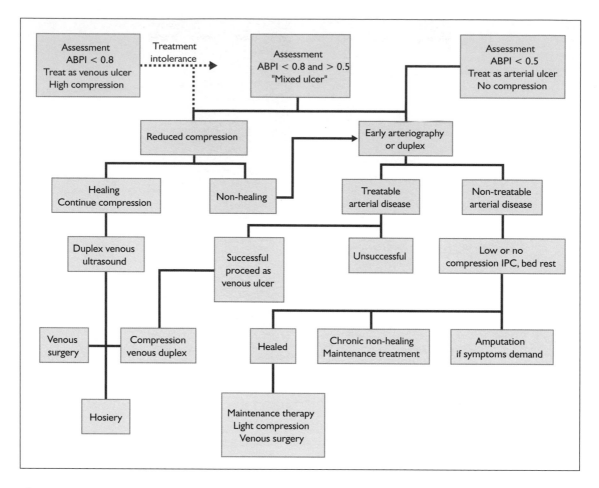

Figure 4.15 Management strategy for the use of compression in patients with a reduced ankle brachial pressure index (ABPI)

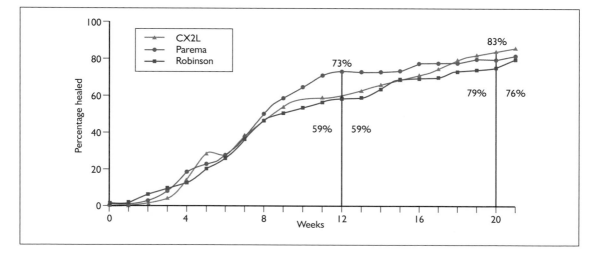

Figure 4.16 Reported healing rates from a trial of alternative four-layer compression systems

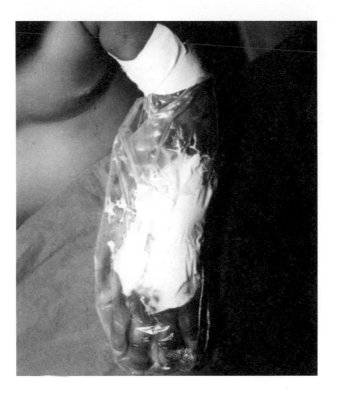

Figure 5.1 Burn wound on the left arm of a child covered with silver sulfadiazine cream and dressed with a plastic glove taped to the skin

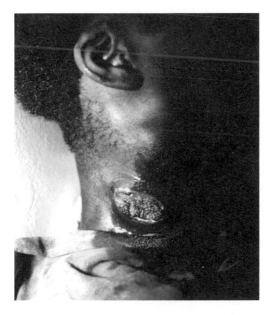

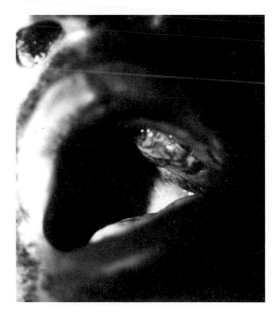

Figure 5.2 Abscess cavity packed with gauze soaked in glycerine and ichthammol. Tuberculosis of the cervical lymph nodes in a patient with HIV infection

Figure 5.3 Purple oral Kaposi's sarcoma tumor on the hard palate of an HIV-infected man

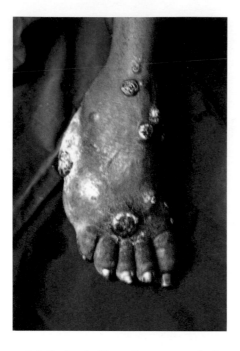

Figure 5.4 Endemic Kaposi's sarcoma lesions on the foot of a 55-year-old man

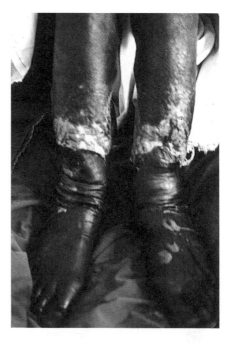

Figure 5.5 Dry gangrene of the toes in a 30-year-old man with HIV infection and a history of smoking

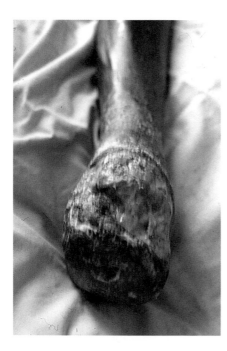

Figure 5.6 Wound breakdown after distal amputation in the patient shown in Figure 5.5

Figure 5.7 Bilateral gangrene of the lower limbs in a 22-year-old HIV-infected man who refused amputation for 3 months. Healed well after bilateral above-knee amputations

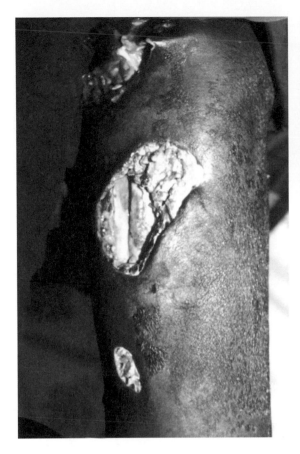

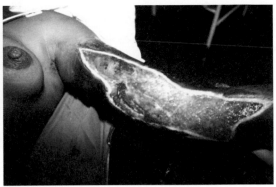

Figure 5.9 Clean, granulating wound in a HIV-infected woman before split skin grafting

Figure 5.8 Necrotizing fasciitis in a 27-year-old woman with AIDS. After multiple limited surgical excisions, she was able to leave the hospital for home-based care

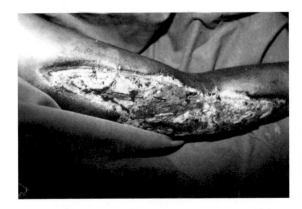

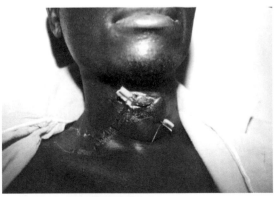

Figure 5.10 Split skin graft failure 1 week after operation of the wound shown in Figure 5.9

Figure 5.11 Corrugated rubber drain positioned through a thyroid abscess after incision and drainage

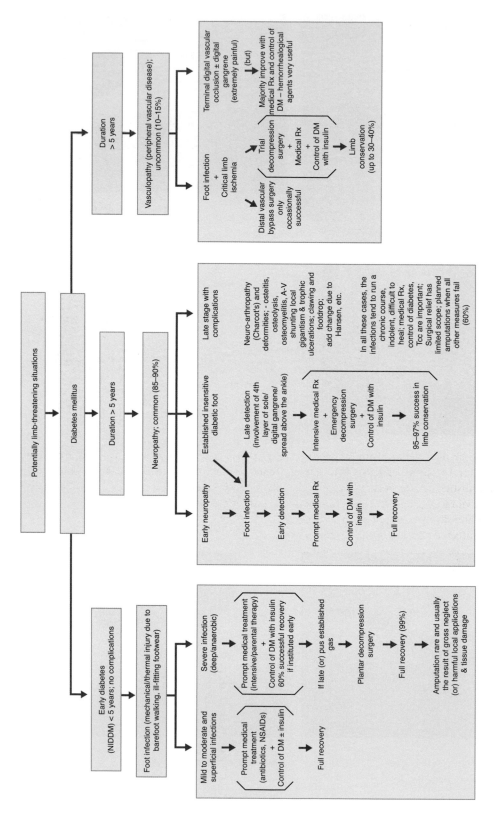

Figure 6.1 Flow chart outlining the current approach in the management of the diabetic foot with ulceration/infection. Reproduced with permission from www.diabetopaedia.com

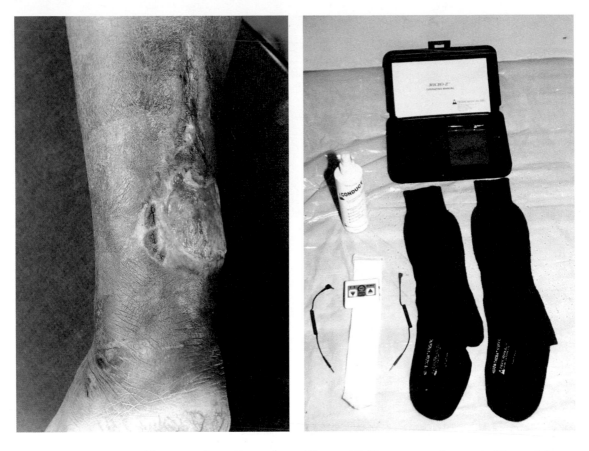

Figure 6.2 A 45-year-old woman from Singapore, a known diabetic for 14 years, NIDDM with polyneuropathy (diminished ankle jerks), preserved sensations of pain, vibration, heat and cold, full foot pulses present bilaterally, presented with a large 6.0×4.5 cm non-infected chronic ulcer and hypertrophied edges of more than 2 years' duration and failed skin grafting twice

Figure 6.3 The same patient as in Figure 6.2 was treated with pulsed galvanic stimulation using silver-mesh stocking electrodes for 4–6 h daily in an outpatient setting

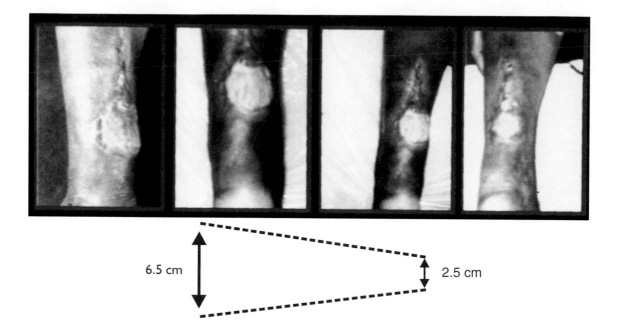

6.5 cm   **2.5 cm**

Figure 6.4 After 4 months, the ulcer in Figures 6.2 and 6.3 reduced in size from 6.5 cm to 2.5 cm

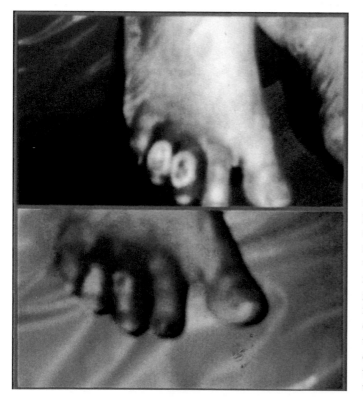

Figure 6.5 A 55-year-old female NIDDM (but presently insulin-requiring) patient had a severe degree of sensorimotor polyneuropathy and classical diabetic foot. She presented with acute thermal injury to the lateral three toes of the right foot (dorsal aspect). After 2 weeks of dressings and medication, skin grafting was considered to accelerate healing. This was unsuitable as she had cardiomyopathy and other problems. She did not want to undergo anesthesia and opted for the alternative modality of therapy. She responded well to daily application of the silver-mesh stocking electrodes with pulsed galvanic stimulation to the affected foot. The bluish coloration of the third digit at presentation improved in color with 1 week's therapy and the entire dorsal ulcers, which had exposed the tendons, epithelialized within 4–6 weeks

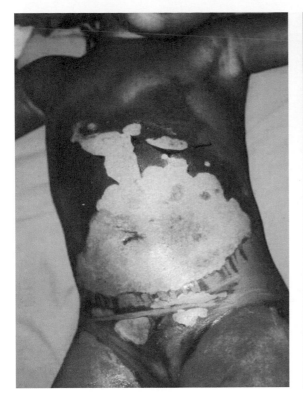

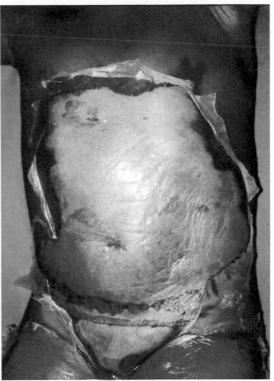

Figure 6.6 Commercially manufactured collagen membrane derived from sheep's intestine is used in superficial partial thickness burns as a biological dressing

Figure 6.7 Commercially manufactured collagen membrane derived from reconstituted bovine collagen membrane from the Achilles tendon of sheep is used in superficial partial thickness burns as a biological dressing

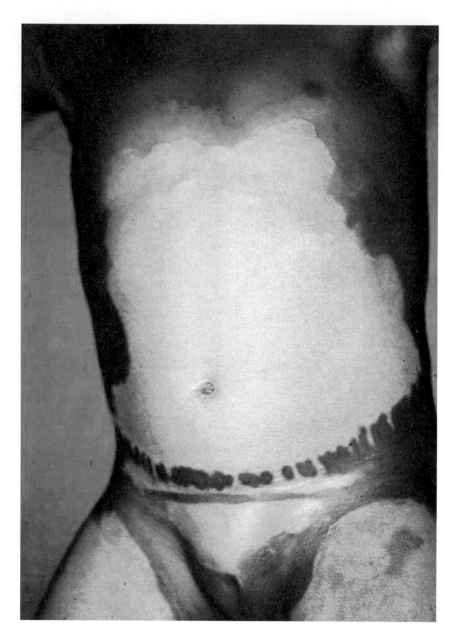

Figure 6.8 Commercially manufactured collagen membrane derived from reconstituted human amniotic collagen membrane is used in superficial partial thickness burns as a biological dressing

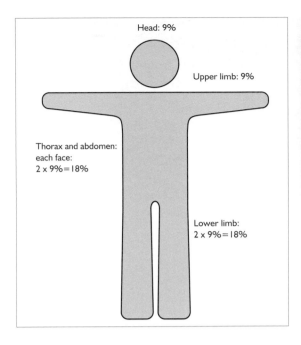

Figure 7.1 Rule of nines. This assessment technique can roughly determine the extent of TBS involved. The palm of the hand roughly corresponds to 1% of TBS

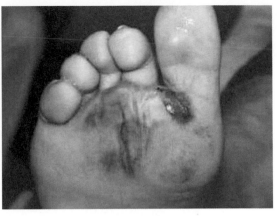

Figures 7.2 Blister is present in second-degree burns. After 2–3 days it opens, a source of potential infection. Removal of the blister is recommended in burns

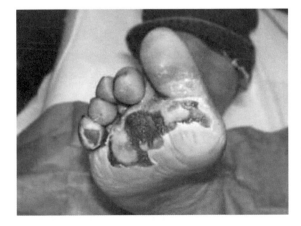

Figure 7.3 Blister is present in second-degree burns. After 2–3 days it opens, a source of potential infection. Removal of the blister is recommended in burns

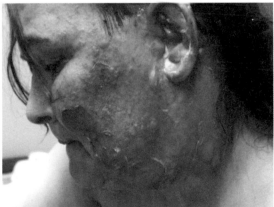

Figure 7.4 Mixed aspect of superficial and deep second-degree burns of the face. Some areas are red and extremely painful, others are more pale (deep second-degree)

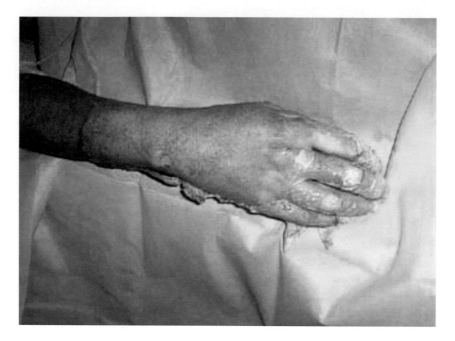

Figure 7.5 In third-degree burns, as here over the dorsal aspect of the index finger, the aspect is white. The skin does not adhere any more and can be easily removed when passing a gauze over the lesion. Pain is absent when touching the lesion

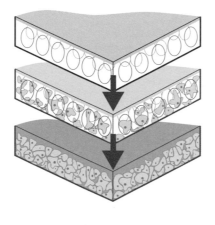

Synthetic epidermis
Knitted nylon scaffold

Fibroblasts proliferate and
form dermal elements

Final product TransCyte™
Dermal components of
importance include:
  1. Structural proteins
  2. Provisional matrix proteins
  3. Glycosaminoglycans
  4. Bound growth factors

Figure 7.6 Schematic diagram of TransCyte™ showing the temporary colonization by fibroblasts and the presence in this product of growth factors secreted by the cells

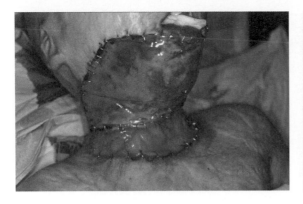

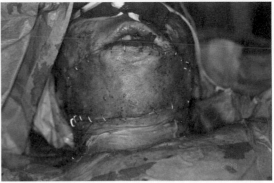

Figure 7.7 Integra recently applied on a child's neck. This is the first stage of this two-step procedure. Note the overlying sheet of silicone covering the collagen

Figure 7.8 After 3–4 weeks, the revascularized collagen can be covered using a thin split-thickness graft

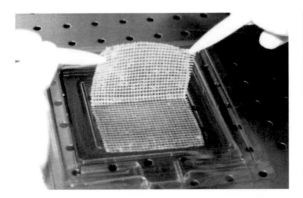

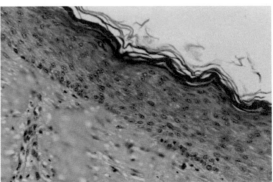

Figure 7.9 Keratinocyte culture, Gerevrier (Epibase®) is presented in a double container on a semisolid hydrogel

Figure 7.10 Histologic aspect of skin reconstruction after keratinocyte culture using Epibase®. Day 14, thoracic area on a 80% total body surface area burn patient

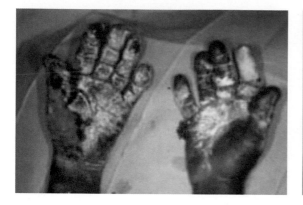

Figure 7.11 Fresh second-degree burns of the hands

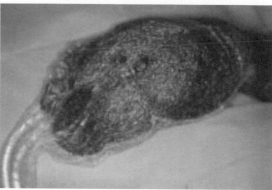

Figure 7.12 VAC can be applied in order to reduce edema, a factor which improves vascularization and reduces inflammation

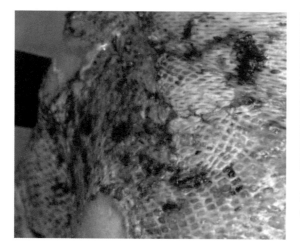

Figure 7.13 Postgrafting local infection. A source of skin loss, often leading to a regrafting procedure after local treatment

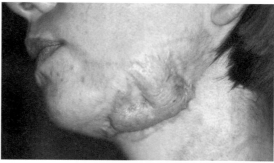

Figure 7.14 Keloid will develop preferably in the adolescent

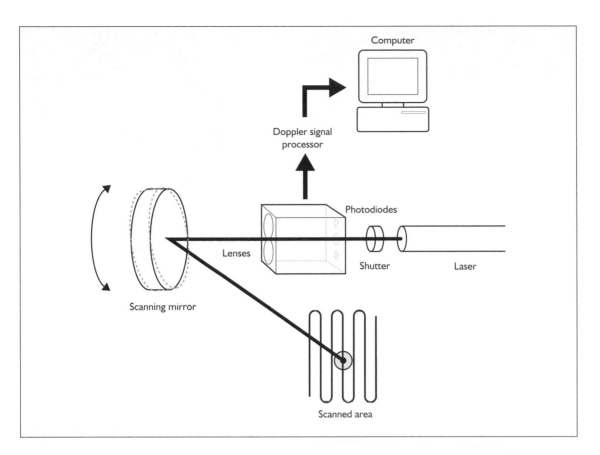

Figure 11.1 Principle of the laser Doppler imager

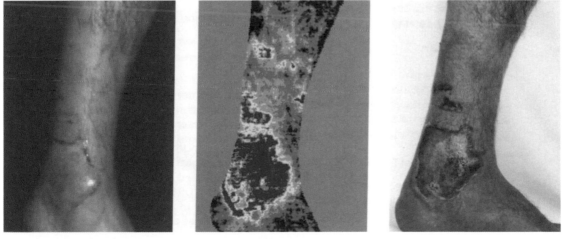

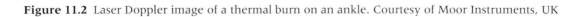

| LDI 'photo' image | LDI flux image | Clinical photograph |

Figure 11.2 Laser Doppler image of a thermal burn on an ankle. Courtesy of Moor Instruments, UK

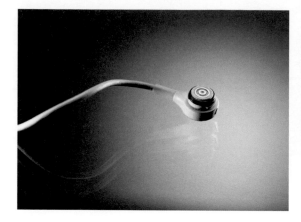

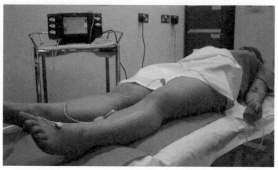

Figure 11.4 TcPO$_2$ sensors on a patient

Figure 11.3 TcPO$_2$ sensor. Courtesy of Radiometer, UK

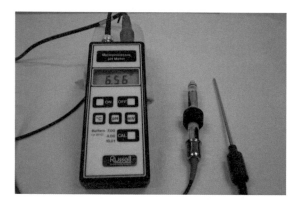

Figure 11.5 Wound pH meter. Courtesy of Russell pH, Fife, UK

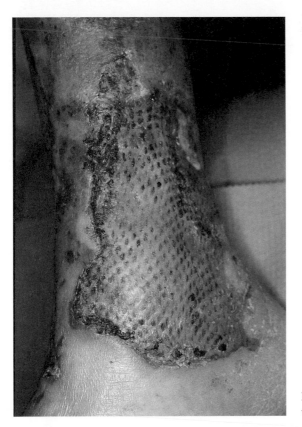

Figure 13.1 Meshed split skin graft to chronic venous ulcer

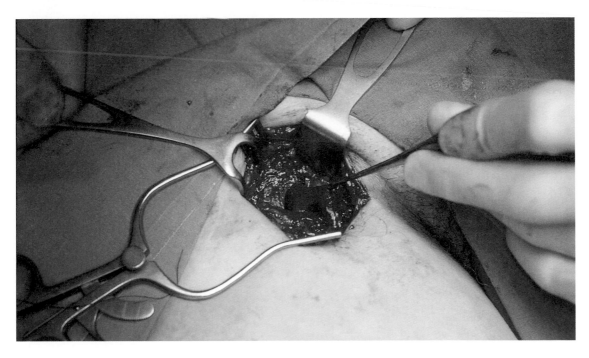

Figure 13.2 Saphenofemoral junction displayed at surgery just prior to ligation

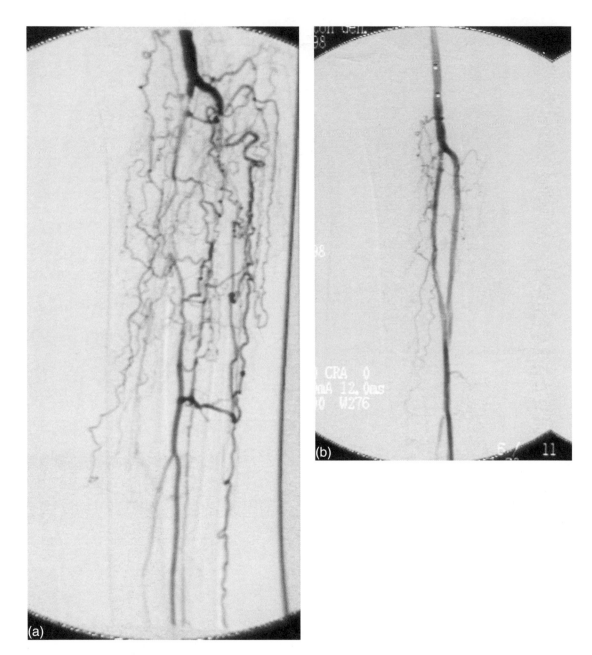

Figure 13.3 (a) Angiogram showing disease of the tibioperoneal trunk in a patient with diabetes and a foot ulcer; (b) angiogram of the same patient after successful subintimal angioplasty. Reproduced with permission from Odurny A. Treatment of the critically ischemic limb. *Int J Lower Extrem Wounds* 2002;1:33–42

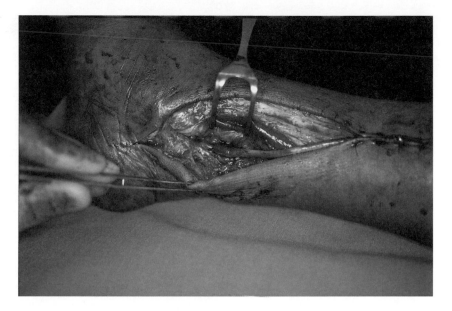

Figure 13.4 Distal bypass to the peroneal artery in a patient with critical limb ischemia. The long saphenous vein has been used *in situ* and anastomosed to the peroneal artery via the medial approach

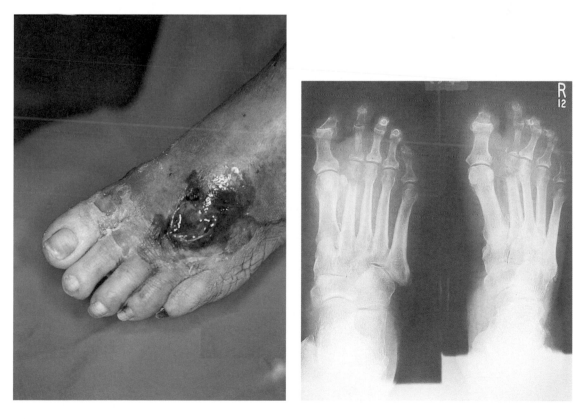

Figure 13.5 Neuroischemic diabetic foot with extensive infection

Figure 13.6 X-ray of foot of a diabetic with extensive destruction of the 2nd metatarsal

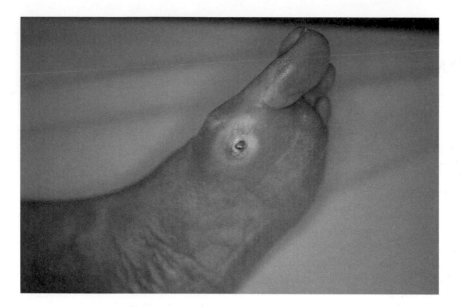

Figure 13.7 Neuropathic ulcer with keratin ring

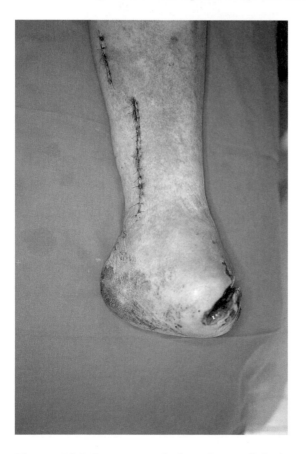

Figure 13.8 Reconstructed foot in a diabetic following femoroposterior tibial artery bypass

Index

abdominal surgery, HIV infection 61–2
accident prevention 3–4
Acticoat 86
advanced dressings, pressure ulcers 118–19
aesculin 77
AIDS *see* HIV infection and AIDS
Aircast boot 100
alginic acid 77
Alloderm, skin substitute 84
allogenic skin 84
aluminum hydroxide 26
amniotic membrane 76
anal lesions 60–1
anatomy and pathophysiology, lower limb veins
    38–9
anemia 114
angiography, Duplex examination 103
angioplasty 103
animal models 147–56
  advantages 149–50
  choice 150–1
  extrapolation to man 148–9
  types 146, 151–6
    in vitro 151–3
    in vivo 153–6
ankle brachial pressure index (ABPI)
  and compression therapy 43–4
  hand-held Doppler 97, 138
  mixed ulcers 46–7
anorexia 114
anti-platelet agents 99
antibiotics
  cellulitis 105–6
  diabetic foot 103
  leg ulcers 24–5
  neuroischemic ulcer 103
  osteomyelitis 106–7
  wet/dry necrosis 109–10
Apligraf 102
arterial calcification, hand-held Doppler 97
arterial ulcers 162–3
  see also peripheral arterial disease
arterial–venous ulcers 46–7, 163
atrophie blanche 39
autoimmune disorders, GI tract 133

bandages *see* compression therapy
becaplermin 27
biological dressings 76
biosignals, transduction, mechanical forces 6
burn management 81–91
  Acticoat 86–7
  assessment of burn wounds 82–3
  biological dressings 76
  cooling 83
  elderly patients 90
  epidemiology 89
  HIV infection 66–7
  in India 75–6
  laser Doppler imaging 83, 89
  moist exposed burn ointment (MEBO) 87
  pain 83
  problems of skin maturation 88–9
  scar prevention 89
  skin substitutes 28–9, 84–5
  socioeconomic factors 89–90
  surgical excision and grafting 87–8
  topical creams 85–6
  types of burns 81–2
  vacuum-assisted closure (VAC) 87
bypass, ischemic ulcers 162–3

calf muscle pump 38–9
  perforator vein incompetence 161
callus, debriding agents 101
caring, multicultural aspects 8
case-control study 14–15
cellulitis 104–7
cerium silver sulfadiazine 86
champagne-bottle limb deformity 40
Charcot (diabetic) foot 98–100
chronicity, defined 1
collagen
  Apligraf 102
  artificial dermis 84–5
  Promogran 102
  reconstituted amniotic membrane 76
colon, mucosal inflammation 131
compression therapy for venous leg ulcers 30,
    35–55
  assessment of patient 43–4

complications 44–6
economic aspects 37, 49–50
expected healing rates 47–8
mixed ulcers 46–7
mode of action 39–40
optimal levels 40–1
patient compliance 48–9
systems 36–7
    application, monitoring pressure 44, 45
    compression hosiery 42
    dynamic/intermittent pneumatic compression
        (IPC) 42–3
    elastic bandages 41
    multi-layer bandages 42, 43
    reduced compression 47
    short-stretch bandages 41–2
    see also venous leg ulcers 42-3
Crohn's disease 131, 132–4
cytokines 132

debridement
    for callus 101
    for necrosis 108
debriding agents 20
    NICE Report 19–21
dehydration 114
dental surgery, HIV infection 62
DePalma operation 161
Dermagraft 28–9, 101–2
dermis, artificial, collagen-based 84–5
developing world, traditional medicine 5–6
diabetic foot
    classification 95–6
    natural history 96
    presentation/management 30–1, 96–110
        high-risk foot 98–100
        ulcerated foot 100–4
        ulcerated foot with cellulitis 104–7
        ulcerated foot with necrosis 107–10
    risk factors, venous insufficiency 139–40
    surgery 163
DNA repair, and wound healing 76–7
duodenal ulcer 129–34
Duplex ultrasound 137

economic scarcity 4–5
edema 142
    diabetic foot 98
    venous leg ulcers 40
eicosanoids 132
electrical stimulation 123–4
Entamoeba histolytica infection 133
ephedrine, dosage 98
epidermal growth factor, properties 116

ePTFE models 153–4
equivalence trials 14
evidence-based healthcare 11–22
    hierarchy of designs 13–16
        case series 14
        case–control study 14–15
        quasi-experimental study 15
        randomized controlled trial 15–16
    strength of evidence 13
    theorems and proof 12–14

falsifiability 12
fiber orientation, skin 6
fibroblast growth factors, properties 117
fibroblasts, skin substitute 84–5
footwear 98
Fournier's gangrene, HIV infection 63

gangrene see necrosis
gastrointestinal mucosal inflammation 129–34
gold leaf 26
grafts 162
    burns 87–8
        HIV infection 66–7
    bypass 162–3
    Dermagraft 28–9, 101–2
Graftskin 28–9
granulocyte CSF (GCSF) 27–8
granulocyte-macrophage CSF (GMCSF) 117
growth factors 26–8
    properties 116
    types 116–18

Hansen's disease, India 78
Helicobacter pylori 130, 131
heparin 76
herbal preparations 77–8
historical aspects 2–3
    compression therapy for venous leg
        ulcers 35
    evidence, theorems and proof 12–14
HIV infection and AIDS 57–72
    burns 66–7
    epidemiology 60
    resistance to wound infection 64–6
    wounds in adults 61–6
    wounds in children 60
honey 77
hosiery, compression 36–7, 42
Hume, D, on general statements 12
hyaluronic acid, Hyaff 102
hydrocolloid dressings 87, 119
hydrogel dressings 119
hydropolymer dressings 120

hydrotherapy 122–3
hypercholesterolemia 114
hypotheses, theorems and proof 12–14

iatrogenic ulcers 133–4
implanted chamber models 153–4
India
   burn management 75–6
   epidemiology of wounds 74–5
   Hansen's disease 78
   herbal preparations 77–8
   wound definition and natural history 73–4
infective ulcers 133–4
inflammatory ulcers 134
insulin growth factors, properties 116–17
Integra, skin substitute 84
intermittent pneumatic compression (IPC)
      systems, venous leg ulcers 42–3
iron 26
ischemia, detection 97, 162
ischemic ulcers 162–3

Kaposi's sarcoma 59–60
keratinocyte cultures 85
keratinocyte growth factors, properties 117
Koebner phenomenon 7

laboratory tests 135–44
Laplace's law 40, 41
larvae (greenbottle fly) 101
   pressure ulcers 121–2
laser Doppler imaging, burns 83, 89
leg ulcers
   medical therapy 23–33
      antibiotics 24–5
      pentoxifylline 23–4
      nutritional therapy 25–6
   see also arterial ulcers; diabetic foot; pressure
      ulcers; venous leg ulcers
lower limb
   anatomy and pathophysiology, veins 38–9
   arterial disease 43–4
   see also venous leg ulcer
lymphedema, compression bandages 41, 42

macrophages, mucosal inflammation 131
mafenide acetate 86
maggots (greenbottle fly) 99, 121–2
magnesium 26
mechanical forces, transduction of biosignals 6
methicillin-resistant Staph. aureus (MRSA) 122
microcirculation, measurement 137, 138
mixed leg ulcers 46–7, 163
models of healing 145–58

animal models 147–56
impaired healing 145–7
mathematical 146–7
mucosal inflammation, GI tract 129–34
Mycobacterium tuberculosis infection 133
Mycobacterium ulcerans infection 59

necrosis
   HIV infection 62–4
   management 108–10
   presentation 107–8
necrotizing fasciitis, HIV infection 63
negative pressure see vacuum-assisted closure
      (VAC)
neuroischemic and neuropathic foot 95–6
neuropathic foot
   vs neuroischemic foot 95–6
   test 97
   ulceration 100
   see also diabetic foot
NICE (National Institute for Clinical Effectiveness,
      UK) 11
   report on wound care technology 19–21
NSAIDs 29–30, 133
null hypothesis 12
nutrition
   oral supplementation 114–15
   and pressure ulcers 113–16
   vitamin C 25–6

optical imaging 135–6
osteomyelitis 104–7
oxygen (hyperbaric) therapy 30, 107
oxygen saturation (OS) 136–7, 138–9

pain management 7–8, 29–30
   burns 83
   complex regional pain syndrome 7–8
pentoxifylline 23–4
peptic ulcer 129–34
perforator vein incompetence 161
peri-anal lesions 60–1
peripheral arterial disease 109, 137
   ABPI 43–4, 46–7
platelet releasate 26–7
platelet-activating factor 131
platelet-derived growth factor
   PDGF-BB (becaplermin) 27
   properties 116
   Regranex 101
   rhPDGF-BB 117–18
Pneumocystis carinii infection 62
polymorphonuclear cells 131–32
popliteal vein reflux 48

Popper, K, on falsifiability 12
povidone iodine 86
pressure ulcers 113–27
   adjunctive therapies 30
   advanced dressings 118–19
   defined 113
   electrical stimulation and electromagnetic
      treatment 123–4
   growth factors 116–18
   hydrotherapy 122–3
   larvae 121–2
   nutrition and 113–16
   topical negative pressure 120–1
Promogran 102
pulsed electromagnetic treatment 124
PVA models 153
pyrophosphate scintigraphy 83

randomized controlled trials 15–16
   advantages/disadvantages 16–17
   vs non-randomized studies of same therapy 17,
      18
   quality control 18
Regranex 101
resistance to wound infection,
      immunocompromised patients 64–6
rutosides 26

saphenous veins
   anatomy and pathophysiology 38–9
   ligation 161
scar formation 1
scar prevention, burn management 89
scintigraphy 137
   Tc-99m 83, 99
Scotchcast boot 100
shoes 98
Shwartzman phenomenon 7
silver nitrate 86
silver sulfadiazine 86
skin
   fiber orientation 6
   maturation, burn management 88–9
   sensors, oxygen saturation (OS) 136–7, 138–9
   substitutes 28–9, 84–5
skin cleansing agents 25
skin grafting see grafts
small intestine, mucosal inflammation 131
spectroscopy, near infrared 83
subfascial endoscopic perforator ligation 161
surgical intervention 159–66

Tc-99m scintigraphy 83, 99
TcPO$_2$ sensor 137–9
thyroid abscess, HIV infection 63
topical creams, anti-infectious 85–7
topical negative pressure see vacuum-assisted
      closure (VAC)
traditional medicine, developing world 5 6
TransCyte, fibroblast skin substitute 84–5
transepidermal water loss (TEWL) 156
transforming growth factors, properties 117, 118
tuberculosis, and HIV infection 61
typhoid fever 132–3

ulcerative colitis 133–4
ultrasound 83

vacuum-assisted closure (VAC) 87, 102, 120–1,
      141, 160–1
vascular-endothelial growth factor 117
   angiogenic effect 6
venous anatomy and pathophysiology 38–9
venous hypertension 145
venous insufficiency, risk factor 139–40
venous leg ulcers
   compression therapy 30, 35–55
   cost issues 37, 49–50
   epidemiology 37
   expected healing rates 47–8
   laboratory tests 135–44
   mixed ulcers 46–7, 163
   models 145–58
   quality of life 37–8
   recurrence rates 49
   surface pH 140
   surgical intervention 161–2
   variables adversely affecting healing 48
   see also compression therapy
vitamin C 25–6, 114
vulnerability concept 6–7

wound healing, and DNA repair 76–7
wounds
   complications 141–2
   definition and natural history 73–4
   edema 142
   epidemiology 74–5
   exudate 140–1
   pH 140

zinc 26